BEING AN EVALUATOR

Being an EVALUATOR

Your Practical Guide to Evaluation

Donna R. Podems

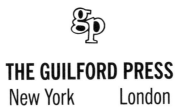

THE GUILFORD PRESS
New York   London

Copyright © 2019 The Guilford Press
A Division of Guilford Publications, Inc.
370 Seventh Avenue, Suite 1200, New York, NY 10001
www.guilford.com

Printed in the United States of America

This book is printed on acid-free paper.

Last digit is print number: 9   8   7   6   5   4   3   2   1

Library of Congress Cataloging-in-Publication Data

Names: Podems, Donna, author.
Title: Being an evaluator : your practical guide to evaluation / Donna R. Podems.
Description: New York : Guilford Press, [2019] | Includes bibliographical references
    and index.
Identifiers: LCCN 2018021202| ISBN 9781462537808 (pbk.) | ISBN 9781462537815
    (hardcover)
Subjects: LCSH: Evaluation research (Social action programs) | Evaluation.
Classification: LCC H62 .P5725 2019 | DDC 001.4—dc23
LC record available at *https://lccn.loc.gov/2018021202*

The comics that appear in Chapters 3 and 6 and the icons were created
by Christopher Lysy. Images on the game pieces are from Dreamstime.com, LLC.

I dedicate this book to four very important people in my life:

*To my mom, Elizabeth Podems, who, since the first time
I could pick up a pencil, always encouraged me to write*

*To my dad, Gary Podems, who gave me the courage
to write what I wanted with that pencil*

*To my children, Gemma and Rhys, who bring amazing joy,
laughter, and fulfillment to my life— and without whom
I would have completed this book 3 years ago!*

A Conversation with My Readers

I have written this book just for you: the practicing evaluator; the emerging evaluator; the "I am thinking about being an evaluator" nonevaluator; the "I do monitoring" evaluator; the "I was unceremoniously dumped into evaluation" evaluator; the "I just got out of grad school, and now I have to practice evaluation" evaluator; the "I do not do evaluations [yet]; I just need to know about evaluative thinking" nonevaluator; the researcher; and the person who needs to know how to work with evaluators.

I take each of you on a journey that demystifies evaluation, explores what it means to be an evaluator, and shares some well-kept trade secrets along the way. This is not an evaluation theory book, nor is it a research book. It is a book about being an evaluator who uses evaluation to explore, describe, explain, and eventually judge (in some way) how, and the extent to which, something does or does not work where, for whom, and why. The chapters offer various ways to engage with evaluation information and knowledge—ways that cement learning and encourage reflection. Structured guidance shows you how to untangle various evaluation situations through facilitation, negotiation, and listening. Some core aims of this book are to encourage you to experiment with different ways of thinking; consider multiple perspectives; and acknowledge and engage with the formidable roles that context, power, politics, culture, language, and values play throughout the *entire* evaluative journey.

HOW THE BOOK IS ORGANIZED

I start at the beginning, as one should when writing a book, and then build each chapter on the previous one, providing scaffolding on which to engage in any evaluative process. However, the book does not need to be read sequentially. I have written the book to support your unique evaluation adventure, which may begin in Chapter 3 or Chapter 14, then jump to the last section of Chapter 5, and then circle back to a paragraph in Chapter 2. The book provides a structure that untangles the messiness of evaluation by informing and guiding the many choices faced, and the various discussions held, in an evaluation journey; at the same time, it allows for a realistic sense of unpredictability and differences found in each one.

The book has two parts. Part I lays the foundation for exploring any evaluative process: It breaks down and takes you through what an evaluator needs to know, whether it is an evaluative process for learning, reflection, improvement, accountability, social justice, or judgment. Part II focuses on working as an evaluator and exploring evaluation: It is aimed at fostering reflection on, and thoughtfulness and awareness of, the many kinds of evaluation that exist; discussing the many evaluative roles that can be filled; and exposing some common challenges and pitfalls often encountered in the field, but rarely described in textbooks. Fused together, Parts I and II demystify evaluation and provide a firm basis for candidly engaging with any monitoring or evaluation process, no matter what role you fulfill.

Throughout the book, I dive into the murky sea of evaluation and guide you through it all. Although I provide strategies and processes, I do not provide a "do this and then do that" model, which may work in some situations, and then not in others. Rather, I offer a way to *think* through any evaluative process so that you can comfortably engage with a peer, colleague, boss, beneficiary, or client in any evaluation situation. The book will support your work in almost any evaluation context—whether you work for a nonprofit, a community-based organization, a donor, a government, a university, an institute, or a foundation, or for some other group that aims to fix, change, influence, or in some way make something better in the social world.

THE LEARNING APPROACH

People learn in different ways and at different speeds. A concept that seems easy to grasp for you may be a stumbling block for others. This is true in most of life. Some people find it harder than others to tell time by using an analog clock, or instantaneously to know their left from their right. Often there is something in our daily lives that we find more challenging to do or understand than the people around us; often we do not talk about this. The same is true in evaluation. With this recognition, I draw on different ways of learning, including facilitated interactive activities, self-learning exercises, areas for reflection, sections for discussion, and practical applications. Furthermore, we all have lives outside of practicing evaluation. Some days I find I have a few minutes where I can quickly watch or listen to something, and some evenings I find an hour or two to read. Once in a blue moon, I find more focused time. Acknowledging that reality, I provide further ways to learn about each chapter's topic that meet your varying needs—carefully balancing how much more you want to learn with how much time you have to learn more.

Remember Aesop's fable about the Tortoise and the Hare? The overconfident, sleek, fancy-looking Hare bragged about how fast he could run. Tired of hearing him boast, the Tortoise challenged him to a race. The race was long and challenging, and the Hare sprinted ahead, while the Tortoise approached the race in a precise and methodical way. All the animals in the forest gathered to watch the race, which was won by the wise Tortoise. In the book, we (you and I) are Tortoises. We do not rush to the end to assess and judge; rather, we thoughtfully engage and delight in each step of the evaluative process.

My Perspective

Making sense of things in the social world is not an easy task for anyone. Being asked to judge something, and in doing so to value that thing, can be daunting. There is no perfect template. An evaluator needs to engage in the academic theory and the practical side of evaluation; it is not an either–or decision. Theory informs practice, and practice informs theory. An evaluator educates when appropriate, to ensure engagement, learning, and meaning in the process and in its results. An evaluator comfortably negotiates where necessary, and acknowledges and engages with culture, language, power, politics, and values that constantly swirl in the evaluation process and influence all decisions, including her own. (See "My Use of Pronouns," below.) Through demystifying the process, an evaluator invites people into it and enables them to join in; he actively takes that responsibility, and in doing so through evaluation makes the world a bit better off, even if just a tiny bit.

Why I Wrote the Book

The reason I am an evaluator is not that I enjoy judging things or being critical. I am an evaluator because I believe that evaluators have the potential to make the world a better place to live in. I have written this book to provide a way of thinking that supports an evaluator—not to intimidate others with knowledge, but to engage and guide them through a transparent process.

All over the world, especially where funds dedicated to social improvement are finite, thoughtful, kind, knowledgeable, and skillful evaluators can offer appropriate evaluative processes that inform decisions that affect people's lives, animals' lives, and the environment. Capable evaluators can fulfill an important societal role, while incompetent ones can be a detriment.

Some Guiding Icons

In an evaluation report, it is very common to have a page that lists all the abbreviations used in the report, along with their full terms; this provides a quick guide that you can refer to when reading the report. In this book, I use eight icons to draw your attention to how various features support you in more easily engaging with the text. The icon list follows.

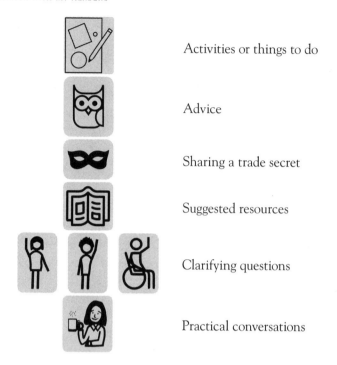

Activities or things to do

Advice

Sharing a trade secret

Suggested resources

Clarifying questions

Practical conversations

THE USE OF PRONOUNS

The use of pronouns is a funny thing. In older books, there is a constant use of *he*. Being a *she* myself, I find that a bit bothersome. On the other hand, when I am reading, it is not always a smooth experience to read *he/she*. For some reason, when I read *he/she*, my brain always reacts with "Wait, so which is it? A he or a she?" This makes me stop reading the sentence, decide if it is a he or she, and then reread the sentence with my chosen pronoun. So I decided to alternate between using *he* and *she* throughout the book. But this then got me thinking: "What about people who do not identify with those pronouns? Perhaps I should use the pronoun *they*?" However, the use of *they* as a singular pronoun is not yet that common, and some early reviewers of the book kept thinking I was incorrectly using the plural *they*. So a note to my readers is that I use *he* and *she* alternately throughout the book, sprinkled with a few uses of *they*, to refer to a person.

Furthermore, I often switch in the book to using the term *we* instead of *you*, when you are technically not part of the *we* conversation just yet. I often find that using the term *you* can be heard as too direct, too confrontational, or too "othering." That is, it can be perceived as an attack that puts people on the defensive or makes them feel isolated. Of course, there are times when only *you* is appropriate, or indeed is the only option. However, using the term *we* underscores that we (you and I) are on the evaluation journey together.

Acknowledgments

If someone asked me to describe how this book came about, it would be a very long story. The story starts with my parents, Elizabeth and Gary Podems, who stood behind me and supported me in whatever I decided—whether it was passing up law school to join the Peace Corps, leaving a paying job to take a volunteer fellowship in South Africa, or living in Bosnia or Somaliland, because, as I explained to them, it just seemed right to me. All those journeys, and many more, informed the kind of evaluator I am. Mom inspired my love of writing by giving me my first journal at the age of 9, and then a new one every year after that.

Michael Quinn Patton entered my life at the beginning of my evaluation journey as my teacher, and has continued in the role of mentor and friend. Throughout my career, he has encouraged me not to conform to evaluation norms when they did not resonate with me (or my clients), to stay true to my principles and values, to march to the beat of my own drum (not his or anyone else's), and to write. He gave me the greatest gift: He believed in me.

I would not even be an evaluator had it not been for Paula Bilinsky, who plucked me out of nowhere and put her trust in a newbie just back from the Peace Corps; she patiently explained the basic ropes of evaluation, and has remained a constant and valued friend in my evaluation journey. Jennifer Greene grounded me in qualitative research and introduced me to feminist and democratic evaluation, all of which heavily influence my practice. She then went on to encourage me to edit my first book, which gave me the courage (and experience) to finish this one. After grad school, I approached C. Deborah Laughton and asked her guidance on how to publish a book; she provided a path that I diligently followed over the next 13 years, which proved to be excellent advice. I thank her for continued support during the making of this book.

Over the years, several of my colleagues and clients provided insights found in this book, as well as much-needed encouragement, for which I am most grateful. The book was a whisper of an idea when Catie Lott encouraged me. As it was taking shape, Kerstin Rausch Waddell provided a calming and insightful voice, which I relied on heavily throughout the journey. Anna Davis never stopped asking me when I was going to write the book, read multiple drafts, and gave me sage advice and thoughtful feedback. I stalled in the middle, and Tessie Catsambas provided a timely nudge. Benita Williams offered courage when I needed it most, along with her quantitative insights and the best-ever pep talks. Susan Tucker provided inspiring weekend and evening conversations that kept me on my toes. A book does not get written overnight (at least this one did not), and during the 5 years of writing, many other people have informed its shape and its content. I thank Leanne Adams, Daleen Botha, Cindy Clap-Wincek, E. Jane Davidson, Svetlana Negroustoueva, Tim Reilly, Gäelle Simon, Liezel de Waal, and Lauren Wildschut.

Robin Miller asked me to fill in for her and teach her evaluation foundation course at Michigan State University when I was a few years into writing the book. Teaching that class provided new insights, and Robin's thoughtful feedback on the second part of the book inspired me to think harder. Aimee N. White was supposed to be a "blind" peer reviewer; however, she knows my writing and stories so well that she guessed it was me. Her funny and sincere support, and meticulous feedback in the final, crucial stretch to the book's completion, were invaluable. I also thank the many peer reviewers who did not recognize me, and whose thoughtful criticism made this a better book: Mary E. Arnold, College of Public Health and Human Sciences, Oregon State University; Penny Burge, School of Education, Virginia Tech; Janice Fournillier, Department of Educational Policy, Georgia State University; John Klemanski, Department of Political Science, Oakland University; and Neil J. Vincent, Department of Social Work, DePaul University. Among the important elements of my book are its icons, comics, and game pieces, and I thank Christopher Lysy for enhancing the book with these fun and "totally me" additions.

Two very important people during the whole process were my children, Gemma and Rhys. I thank them for giving me the peace and quiet time to write (OK, I admit, it was often in exchange for iPad time) and for always asking, "How's the writing going, Mom?" Thank you, my Munchkins.

Contents

Purchasers can access an online supplement at *www.guilford.com/podems-materials*
that contains some of the activities and games described in the book.

PART I

DOING EVALUATION
AND THINKING EVALUATIVELY

An evaluator should understand how to gather data and use that to make a finding, a value judgment, and then develop a recommendation. I think being able to sustain that type of clearly articulated thinking throughout the conceptual pathway is a rare talent. . . .
—DUGAN FRASER, Chairperson of the South African M&E Association (2015)

CHAPTER 1
Speaking the Language

An evaluator is a human being living in a complex world. She (or he or they) engages with other human beings through a process that values something that is important to someone in some way. That process is called the **evaluative process,** and its findings are used to learn, improve, judge, or in some way inform decisions. How an evaluator thinks, who and what shapes her thinking, and how she views evaluation's role in society are all germane to how she defines herself as an evaluator. (For my use and choice of pronouns, please see page x in "A Conversation with My Readers" at the start of the book.)

Consider that the multidisciplinary field of evaluation includes pluralist philosophies that draw on multiple methods, criteria, measures, assessments, perspectives, audiences, and interests, as well as a plethora of traditions that have emerged from different social science disciplines (e.g., anthropology, psychology, sociology). Add to all this the roles of politics, power, culture, language, and values, and you can begin to see the many difficulties of definitively explaining what an evaluation is and how to design and implement one. Nonetheless, definitions and guidance abound, although of course they do not always agree.

Mix into this conversation the many roles that an evaluator can play, and you begin to see the complications of defining who is an evaluator, or drawing a boundary around what an evaluator does. Since the late 1980s, evaluation associations and societies, governments, international aid organizations, foundations, institutes, and other groups and institutions have been exploring ways to define who is an evaluator. However, evaluation differs from the medical, accounting, or legal fields, for example, in that no formal certification process is needed to practice evaluation: Anyone can claim to be an evaluator (McKegg, 2017; Podems & King, 2014).

Defining and clarifying what an evaluator does, how to be an evaluator, and the essence of being one constitute this book's core focus. Being comfortable with discussing the common language of evaluation provides a starting point from which to demystify evaluation and explore how to be an evaluator. If you would like to skip ahead to an in-depth discussion of what it means to be an evaluator, read Chapters 2 and 11. Otherwise, join me at the start of our evaluation journey, with a discussion of evaluation language.

THE POWER OF WORDS

I begin with a memory of an awkward moment.

> "I grew up in a small town in New Jersey, and moved to South Africa in 1998. Back in those early days, I did not know too many people in South Africa. As the December holidays drew near, I received several invitations to holiday parties, and was especially glad to accept an invitation to join my neighbors for Christmas dinner. I was raised never to go to someone's house empty-handed, so I immediately asked what I could bring to the meal. My neighbor asked me to bring some crackers. I was glad for such an easy request. So I showed up on Christmas Day with two boxes of crackers; one salted and one flavored with rosemary. My hostess graciously accepted them. As we sat down to dinner, her husband loudly asked, 'Where are the crackers?' Since they were on the table, I pointed to them, at which point everyone burst out laughing. Apparently crackers are also small, prettily wrapped pieces of round cardboard, each containing a small prize; when you pull one open, it makes a small pop, like a firecracker. Who would have thought? I mean, who stops to ask, 'Tell me, what do you mean by a cracker?'"

Words may have different meanings to different people, in different contexts, and points in time. Sometimes the same word simply has multiple meanings for the same person. How and why people choose the words they use, and how their meanings are interpreted, are all part of everyday life; they are also relevant to any evaluative process. A critical part of being an evaluator is speaking the language. To do this, an evaluator needs to know the difference between evaluation words, terms, and concepts with concrete definitions that an evaluator should confidently know and be able to explain, such as *random sampling* (see Chapter 5), and words with meanings that vary by user and context, where evaluators often need to negotiate or clarify definitions and practical applications, such as the term *impact*. Although throughout the book I provide concrete definitions for evaluation terms and concepts that have them, the present chapter specifically looks at words and concepts with meanings and practical applications that need to be clarified prior to engaging in any evaluative process.

Language is a powerful tool, and a separate, broader conversation (which builds on the one found in this chapter) on how language influences evaluation is provided in Chapter 13. We start the evaluative journey here by exploring words, terms, and concepts that often perplex through their various definitions, interpretations, and applied meanings, and that have the potential to derail any evaluative process if they are not properly considered.

Before delving into examples for the evaluation field, let's start with some from everyday life. What would you think if someone said that the movie they just watched was "bad" or "sick"? Depending on the tone, the expression, the age of the speaker, and the cultural context, it would likely have different meanings, from "The movie was awful" to "It was fabulous." And because words have these nuances, there are always times in our lives where we feel we are the only ones in the room (or the world) who do not understand a term, or completely misunderstand it. Recently a younger colleague of mine asked what I was doing for the weekend. I responded that I was working on this book. She muttered something that sounded like "FOMO." I laughed and she laughed, but I was thinking, "What in the world is FOMO?" For those who do not know, it means Fear Of Missing Out. I now know this, but I didn't know it then.

Consider a time when someone used a word or mentioned a concept that you thought you should know but did not, or you thought everyone else in the room knew and you did not. Most likely you nodded and pretended that you understood, and then did a web search on it later (or perhaps in the moment, if you had a chance to do so surreptitiously). Nearly everyone has been in this situation when it comes to working in the evaluation field. Ironically, it almost always starts with the mere mention of the field's most fundamental concept: evaluation.

The term **evaluation**; its cousin, **monitoring**; and the phrase and acronym that link them together, **monitoring and evaluation (M&E),** are among some of the more problematic terms in the field. While some definitions differ only slightly, others blatantly disregard and sometimes flat-out disagree with each other. These factors alone can create a breeding ground for intimidation (and perhaps insecurity, frustration, exasperation, or confusion, to name a few descriptors mentioned by colleagues and students) in the evaluation field. As one of my peers, Anna Davis, once told me, "In so many situations, I am sure I know what I am talking about with regard to monitoring or evaluation. Then someone comes along who has more power than me, uses a term in a different way, and tells me otherwise. . . . It is bullying by M&E!"

Thus an evaluator, or any person in a position of power, can indeed be a bully (either knowingly or unknowingly) or can be perceived as one when flinging about evaluation concepts or terms. Or the evaluator can choose to engage in a process that leads to a common understanding of a term. This approach lays the foundation for an evaluation process that is likely to be more useful to all involved.

> **BOX 1.1. Evaluative Process**
>
> Throughout Part 1, the term **evaluative process** is used to describe anything in an evaluation, from conceptualizing the intervention through to the judgment of it. Essentially, the evaluative process can be any part of a process where questions can be unearthed or answers can be found to address the "what," "when," "why," "where," "how," and "for whom" questions.

Why Evaluation Terms and Concepts Can Be Perplexing

Stand a little bit closer to me; I am going to share a trade secret. Evaluation terms and concepts abound, and for many, so do their definitions and their applications. More challenging is that sometimes differences in definitions are not always clear; the differences may lie in the nuances or the unspoken interpretation (as demonstrated through its application) of a definition in a specific setting. There are a few commonplace reasons for why this happens.

- Evaluation has emerged from diverse social science disciplines (e.g., anthropology, psychology, sociology), and these disciplines themselves use words and terms differently.
- Groups or individuals in positions of power, such as governments, donors, institutes, and foundations, are emboldened to define evaluation terms and concepts, and do so within their own worldviews. Their power stems from various sources; the two I mention here, money and influence, are tightly connected. Briefly, those who hold the purse strings can often define and apply words in any way they wish. If a program or intervention wants to receive funds, for example, more than likely it is the donor's definition that is used. This is often true even if that definition varies from other, more common understandings and uses.
- The innumerable evaluation textbooks, websites, evaluation guides, and blogs, which offer varying definitions of the same term, do not escape blame.

Why an Evaluator Should Clarify Terminology

Engaging explicitly with others about the meanings of evaluation terms and concepts *before* the start of any evaluative task will lay the foundation needed for a useful evaluation. These conversations help to avert misunderstandings, frustrations, potential conflicts, and possibly grave disappointment at the end. Furthermore, clarifying the terminology at the start of an evaluation process is a neutralizing activity. The start of an evaluative process is often nerve-wracking for those being evaluated, and creating the space to clarify terminology provides a neutral, nonjudgmental place in which to calm nerves and encourage dialogue and transparency.

Never assume that people understand evaluation terms or concepts, what they look like in practice, or how they influence an evaluation. When you are clarifying evaluation terminology, separate the terms into two groupings (Patton, 2012). The first group should contain words and concepts with concrete (though often misunderstood) definitions. Address these first. The first step for each of these terms is to provide a clear definition. The second step, and where the discussion is concentrated, is to describe how that term will be applied and how that application will influence the evaluation. An example of a word with a specific definition that commonly needs a thorough discussion is the term *causality*. The term has a concrete definition; there is no negotiation along the lines of "I think it means this, and he thinks it means that"; it means what it means. How it is applied in the evaluation is where the beneficial discussion happens. Do not assume that knowing the concrete definition automatically leads to an easy conversation; the conversation may still bring a challenging interaction. To read a technical discussion on causality, please skip ahead to Chapter 15.

The remainder of this chapter focuses on the second group: the words and concepts that have fuzzy and varying definitions. In each of these instances, discussing and negotiating the definition are wrapped up in the discussion of how it will be applied, making for an often complicated yet much-needed conversation. Regardless of the group into which a word falls, each conversation will, at the very least, support the evaluation's transparency, credibility, and use; *at the very most*, it will contribute to an engaging, collaborative, and social equity–building process.

THE EVALUATOR'S ROLE IN CLARIFYING TERMINOLOGY

When terms have multiple definitions and/or meanings, evaluators can often find themselves in the position of needing to clarify the terminology. As such, an evaluator can serve in three roles: as an educator, negotiator, *and* facilitator, so that each concept and its application are agreed upon for that specific evaluation. An intimate knowledge of the multiple definitions for the same term, and the subtler nuances that exist, will allow the evaluator to initiate and facilitate fruitful discussions. In turn, these discussions support equitable engagement, transparency, and clear expectations among those involved in the evaluative process of how the term will be applied, and how that will influence the evaluation. As suggested above, this process ideally increases the likelihood of a useful evaluation.

Throughout this book, the evaluator is positioned as one who leads processes to untangle meanings, clarify concepts, and concretize the application of evaluation terms, which supports evaluation use. In this way, I unashamedly lay the responsibility of a clear evaluation process in the hands of the evaluator. Do not interpret this to mean that the evaluator should hold all the power in an evaluative process; rather, the evaluator recognizes who holds power, acknowledges how and why that power is held, and engages with terminology so that power is more evenly distributed. After all, language is a major form of power. For a more specific discussion of language and power in an evaluation, skip ahead to Chapter 13.

BOX 1.2. The Evaluator's Role in Clarifying Terminology

The evaluator's role is to comfortably engage with terminology and, whenever needed, to clarify it with evaluation users and those involved in the evaluation process. To do so, she needs an in-depth knowledge of evaluation, as well as facilitation, negotiation, and education skills.

I am an evaluator for a small organization. I find that sometimes evaluation words are not concrete, and I need to negotiate their meaning with the donor who provides the funding. What if the donor who provides the funding disagrees with what my internal evaluation guide says?

The uses of words that do not have concrete definitions are often determined by those who have the most power. Commonly, though not always, these individuals or groups are those who provide or control the resources or make other key program decisions. If a donor or government agency that provides the bulk of the intervention's funds (and/or is your boss) insists, "This is how we define X," this is likely not a good situation in which to have an argument premised on "My definition is right and yours is wrong, and here is the guidebook that backs this up." Rather, what is key is that there is a shared, explicit understanding of how the term will be defined and applied in the evaluation. I strongly suggest that this be written, not just orally agreed upon, and that all people involved agree that *this* is indeed the agreed understanding. The most worrisome thing about providing advice in a book is that there will always be exceptions to the rule; there may be times when bringing your definition, or a different definition, to the discussion is useful. Ask yourself, "How will having this conversation, clarifying this term, and using that definition contribute to a useful evaluation?" And ask the opposite: "If we use that definition, how could it create challenges, and to whom?"

There may be one factor that makes everything a bit tricky: the personal factor. Even if the funding source or management structure does not change (i.e., the government department or donor remains the same), the discussion of terms may still need to be revisited throughout the life of the program or the evaluation. When a new *person* fills the decision-making or funding role, they may bring new interpretations to evaluation terms and processes (often without explicitly stating this), which will leave the recipients confused and often frustrated. The personal factor influences all evaluation processes.

This last point reminds me of another trade secret I must share with you: The personal factor is one of the biggest undiscussed influences in any (and all) evaluative processes. Recognizing, and not ignoring, the fact that individuals influence an evaluation process is critical, as each person can be a tremendous facilitator, an impediment, or just a source of constant bumps and bruises along the way.

I am an evaluator for multiple interventions in a large nonprofit organization. As such, I have multiple donors who all bring different understandings to the same evaluation terms. How do I straighten this all out?

Working in an organization that is accountable to several different donors, departments, or managers, all of whom use the same evaluation terms or concepts in dissimilar ways (or sometimes with just enough nuanced differences), can cause havoc. I recommend starting by clarifying *who* means *what* for each evaluation concept or term, and how each meaning translates into practical application (even for the words with concrete definitions). Then determine in what way practically applying the different definitions and/or interpretations of the same evaluation word influences how to conduct an evaluative process. Compare how the different interpretations will influence what is done; will they look the same in practice? If not, clarify how the differences influence how the intervention will be evaluated and valued, and use that information to have an informed discussion on how to move forward.

LEARN THE MEANING—NOT JUST THE LABEL

Evaluators need to use a term or concept with the same understanding as their peers, colleagues, or clients to ensure a useful evaluation. It is with the utmost hesitation that I use the following example to support a conversation about the potential dangers of using labels without having a clear definition of what the terms mean. (Chapter 7 talks about effectively using results labels and refers to the example that follows.) The example is provided to start *our* conversation on labels; it is not a conversation to be used with anyone else on how to use and apply the terms.

Some common labels in evaluation are *input, activity, output, outcome,* and *impact.* Here is one example of how these terms may be used. Some of us monitor how much money is spent to get something (e.g., $100 for running shoes). In evaluation, we call that input, or what was put in to get something out. What the person is doing (e.g., running) is called the *activity.* The very first thing that happens because of that activity, such as how far or how often the person runs every week, is often called the *output.* Some of us may also then monitor how much weight the person loses because he runs so much, which is often what evaluators call the desired or intended *outcome,* or what happens because of the output (e.g., the distances ran). Then, because the person has lost weight, he has higher self-esteem and better overall health, which some evaluators call a *higher-level outcome* (and some call *impact*). He then decides to start a new career and adopts an overall healthy lifestyle, which brings him greater happiness, and some refer to this result as the *impact* (and some call it *longer-term impact*).

This example illustrates a common, simple, and quick way of using these labels without much concern for the dangers of doing so.

I now implore you to be patient and trust our journey. I ask you not to argue with or question what is written in the previous paragraphs (not just yet, anyway), and to not immediately use these labels mechanically as described. Rather, I invite you first to read the next section about the dangers of using labels in evaluation. If you want to jump ahead to read an in-depth discussion on sorting out the input–output–outcome–impact (and so on) discussion, go to Chapter 7 (though I encourage you to keep reading from here through Chapter 10 to see all the linked discussions). After reading *through* to Chapter 10 (or, if you must, after only reading Chapter 7 on results labels), revisit the example that starts on the previous page. You will then understand why I have asked you not to argue (just yet) or to use the labels without a deeper understanding of the questions they pose. I'll see you on the other side.

Learn the Meaning—Not Just the Label

Labels can be useful when we buy a product. For example, "Here is shampoo for babies, and there is shampoo for dogs." Or "That is dog food, and this is cat food." Or "That is poisonous." I buy cat food for my cat, and dog food for my dog. Labels are meant to be helpful. To be honest, however, my dog seems to prefer the cat food, which she always steals from the cat; as such, this provides my first practical example of how perhaps labels are not always helpful in the way we think they should be. Although my dog's eating cat food is expensive for me (as she steals copious amounts), there is little harm done from her perspective (but from the cat's perspective, he may disagree!). It would be much worse if my dog ate something labeled "poison." In M&E, some labels can be just as wily.

Do not get caught up in label-fueled arguments, such as "That is monitoring!"/"No, that is evaluation!" or "That is an impact!"/"No, it is an outcome!" These discussions will exhaust you. If someone uses an evaluative term (even when the word or concept has a concrete definition), ask them what they mean by it. *Descriptions* under the labels are important. When you are engaging with a client, colleague, or friend about an evaluation process or term, the primary goal is for everyone to have the same understanding insofar as what is needed, intended, and expected. Use a label when, and only when, the meaning is explicitly clear to everyone.

I have now talked about the importance of knowing when a word has a *concrete* definition and when it has a *fuzzy* one; about the need to be wary when using evaluation labels; and about the role of the evaluator in bringing clarity to each context. Now let's apply what we have just learned by discussing three convoluted terms in the field.

Evaluation, Evaluative Thinking, and Monitoring: What These Terms (Can) Mean

The terms **evaluation, evaluative thinking,** and **monitoring** are often used together, and sometimes interchangeably, in an evaluative process. As the next several pages illustrate, there are many "correct" definitions and understandings for each term. However, for many of these words, there is also a non-negotiable core element (or set of elements) in the definition. These elements can be described in multiple ways by various people, implicitly or explicitly, which adds to the trickiness.

Together, let's explore these three terms, and explore how to discuss and engage with them so that their meanings are clear and support straightforward evaluative processes. Facilitation and training tips are provided that can be used to promote self-reflection or to engage others in a discussion aimed at creating understanding and agreement, or simply at clarifying disagreement (the old "We agree to disagree" sentiment). Each is useful in its own way. Let's start with the word *evaluation*.

Evaluation

What is *evaluation*? The word has different meanings and associations for different people, who are informed by, among other things, their education, cultures, values, and exposure to various evaluation experiences. Add to this that organizations, evaluation theorists, social science disciplines, governments, foundations, institutes, and donors often have their own slightly nuanced definitions, and sometimes what appear to be just completely different understandings. Thus asking more than one person, "What is evaluation?" rarely results in a specific and consistent answer. An even more complicated discussion revolves around who is an evaluator, and who is not, as discussed in Chapter 11 of the book. For now, let's focus on uncomplicating the term *evaluation*.

Thomas Schwandt (2015) offers two definitions that provide one place to start a discussion. Schwandt provides a narrow definition of evaluation as a process that draws on research methods to gather information about how a program or policy is working and whether it is effective. He also provides a broader explanation by stating that evaluation is a form of critical thinking that employs evaluation-specific methodologies to judge something. That "something" is broad. I like and will use Schwandt's basic understanding of "something," and I will add a few more throughout this book, some of which are also used by Mathison (2005). When I talk about evaluating "something," I am referring to evaluating an activity, event, intervention, performance, process, product, policy, practice, project, or program. Wait, I am not done yet. Evaluation can also be used to explore and evaluate strategy, systems change, ecological sustainability, resilience, networks, and principles, to give a few additional nouns (Patton, 2015; Rogers, 2016). From this point onward in this text, all of these common nouns will not be written out; this would make the sentences too long. Therefore, when examples are provided, just one of these words is chosen, most often the word *intervention*. Keep in mind from now on that in any example in any part of the book where the word *intervention* is used, any one of these other common nouns can be substituted.

Two further definitions provided by two influential evaluation theorists, Michael Scriven and Michael Patton, involve different perspectives on evaluation, and therefore the definitions differ slightly. According to Scriven (1991), evaluation is the systematic determination of the merit, worth, or value of something, or the product of that process.

BOX 1.3. Merit, Worth, and Significance

Merit refers to the quality of an intervention—the inherent value. *Worth* refers to how others view the intervention, and determining it involves looking at an intervention in its context. For instance, an evaluator has merit if she brings strong evaluation knowledge and solid experience to an evaluation process. She has worth if those involved in the process have found her knowledge and her services useful (Davidson, 2005; Mathison, 2005; Scriven, 1991). It has *significance* if someone considers what the evaluator did to be special or to have particular meaning.

Michael Patton (2008) offers a broader, more multifarious definition, and one that brings in the idea of evaluation's having multiple purposes, uses, and users. He suggests that program evaluation focuses on three elements: "(1) the systematic collection of information about (2) a potentially broad range of issues on which evaluation might focus (3) for a variety of possible judgments and uses" (p. 39). Patton's definition suggests that different people may have different needs for evaluation. These differing needs are likely to result in the use of different questions, approaches, and criteria to value the intervention.

All of the definitions described in this section are widely acknowledged and offer commonly accepted explanations for the role and purpose of evaluation. However, Schwandt's, Scriven's, and Patton's definitions all stem from different perspectives, leading to some nuanced and some blatant interpretations of the term *evaluation*. None of the definitions provided (Schwandt's, Patton's, or Scriven's) contradicts the others per se, but they give very different understandings of evaluation's role in society, and these differences undergird the discussion about what an evaluator does. Nonetheless, at the core of each definition of evaluation, there are two inherent commonalities.

1. *Evaluation is systematic.* Evaluation draws on systematically gathered evidence. Any evaluation process must have clear, transparent, explicit approaches for collecting and analyzing data. The processes of collecting, analyzing, and interpreting the data must be logically consistent (Patton, 2015; Rossi, Lipsey, & Freeman, 2004; Schwandt, 2015).

2. *Evaluation values or in some way judges something.* The word *value* is part of *evaluation.* (Well, sort of, as we do need to add an *e.*) Nonetheless, an evaluation provides more than just findings; it gives a value judgment. Here is where one of the most complicated parts of evaluation often comes in; after all, a value is based on assumptions or worldviews, which are culturally and socially embedded, and very much otherwise context-dependent (Mertens & Wilson, 2012; Patton, 2015; Schwandt, 2015).

There is one more item that is not explicitly stated in these definitions, though it is a core part of defining and discussing evaluation.

3. *Evaluation is political.* A third core element of evaluation is that evaluation is political (Candel, 2018; Chelimsky, 1987; Greene, 2000; House & Howe, 1999; Patton, 2015; Weiss, 1987). What does that mean? Essentially, it means that evaluation can influence—and is influenced by—who gets what, who does not get what, who benefits, who does not, who is even involved, and who is not. Politics are involved in every part of an evaluative process, from the decision to have an evaluation, to how data are interpreted, to how and with whom the knowledge generated from an evaluation is shared, to how decisions are made (Bowman, & Dodge-Francis, 2018; Patton, 2008). See Chapter 13 for a more in-depth look at politics in evaluation.

*Hold on a second. Before you continue, I have a question. The word **data** is used a lot in the explanation. What's the difference between **data** and **information**?*

Data and *information* are words that are sometimes used interchangeably, yet they are not the same thing. Data are the raw facts, figures, and words that, when analyzed to make some sort of sense, become information. Information is shaped or interpreted. In academic language, the word *data* is always considered to be plural. For some reason, this is only true in academic writing. In newspapers, for example, it is acceptable to say "Data is." The word *information* is always treated as singular.

Here is an example of data versus information. My son, Rhys, is 9 years old at the time I am writing this. Some days when I go into his room, he has unceremoniously dumped hundreds (dare I say thousands?) of little colored blocks on the floor. To me, it looks like one big mess. To him, it looks like lots of potential items (data) with which to create (interpret) something. And he does. He creates cars, castles, houses, monsters, and more. He takes what looks like a big mess to me (his data) and creates meaning (information) from it, which he gives to me (his client). To state this another way, when data (the individual blocks) are formed into something through analysis and interpretation (my son's creative design process), they become information.

*Given how you have defined **data** and **information**, then what is **evidence**?*

Evidence supports a statement. So data become evidence when used to support an argument, a hypothesis, or a belief. Evidence comes from data, which most often come from one of our five senses—we can hear it, touch it, smell it, taste it, or see it. And other people can, too. I say "most often," because there are other ways of knowing that do not use these five senses (see Chapter 4 for further explanation). Another way to think about evidence is how it is used in a murder mystery. A detective identifies the murderer with her evidence; the evidence consists of the knife, the body, and the killer's motive.

Because of our acceptance of using some words interchangeably in our daily lives, the boundaries among terms such as *data, information,* and *evidence* can be blurry. Discuss the meaning of *data, information,* and *evidence* (and other similar words, such as *knowledge*) with all parties you are working with or for, and ensure that everyone has a clear and shared understanding of their meaning.

BOX 1.4. Core Elements of Evaluation

There are three fundamental answers to the question "What is evaluation?" Evaluation provides systematic, transparent, and logically collected evidence; it offers a value judgment; and it is political.

Now that we are clear on what data, information, and evidence are, and have looked at some basic definitions of evaluation, let's engage in an in-depth discussion.

Where Evaluation Definitions Begin to Differ

The core understanding we have just discussed is that evaluation is a systematic, transparent process; it values something; and it is political. Even when we agree that these are the core elements, however, differences emerge. These differences are often rooted in who provides the definition (e.g., a person's training and experiences), how evaluation is used in an organization (e.g., its formal definition and practical applications), and its perceived role in society. Thus discussing what is evaluation goes beyond providing a rote definition of evaluation to a discussion that encompasses political, social, and cultural worldviews, among others. Remember, when engaging with colleagues or clients about evaluation, facilitate a conversation that leads to an explicit understanding of what evaluation means to them, what they expect evaluation to do, and what they expect to happen because an evaluation takes place. Do not just ask for their definitions (and do not just provide one).

BOX 1.5. The Meaning of *Empirical*

The word *empirical* is commonplace in evaluation. But what does it mean, exactly? The *Oxford Living Dictionaries: English* (2018) website defines *empirical* as follows: "Based on, concerned with, or verifiable by observation or experience rather than theory or pure logic." I would supplement that definition with the statement that the means of gaining that knowledge need to be transparent and logically consistent.

To encourage learning and dialogue, activities are suggested throughout the book. The first activity described on the next page addresses the term *evaluation*. All activities draw on adult learning principles, which assert that adults' knowledge and life experience should be recognized and drawn upon in any learning opportunity. Drawing on adults' previous experience with conducting, managing, or observing evaluation through their work, or even in their daily lives, will help to ensure that conversations resonate with them, which in turn helps to ground learning. To conduct the activities, facilitation skills are critical. If you are still building those, consider working alongside a skilled facilitator who can demonstrate these skills, and from whom you can learn (i.e., a knowledgeable other).

BOX 1.6. Knowledgeable Others

As we move through the book, you will realize the many skill sets and knowledge areas that an evaluative process may require. When building knowledge and skills as an evaluator, it is often useful to draw on *knowledgeable others*. Susan Tucker, an education evaluation specialist, describes knowledgeable others as people who bring in knowledge and skills that supplement your own knowledge and skill set. These may be knowledge and skills that you have not yet acquired, or never plan on acquiring due to lack of time, differing interests, or other factors. Evaluators often (though not always) work in teams that include knowledgeable others, or subsequently draw in knowledgeable others as needed. In any evaluation process, including knowledgeable others often creates a richer, more diverse team that can bring added value not only through needed knowledge and skill sets, but also through their lived experience and perspectives.

While reading different definitions and explanations of new terms is helpful, having to apply and engage with various definitions concretizes learning. Therefore, the first teaching activity offers a structure for engaging in a discussion centered on the term *evaluation*. If you are new to the field, try applying the exercise with a few colleagues. When you feel more confident, facilitate the activity in a classroom, with clients or colleagues, or with a group of evaluators.

ACTIVITY 1.1. Learning through Discussion: Evaluation

Purpose: The facilitated discussion encourages people to think about how different evaluation definitions can influence a person's understanding, and therefore implementation and expectations, of evaluation.

Time: Allow approximately 5 minutes for preparation, 10 minutes for discussing the two questions, and 15 minutes for group discussion. Total approximate time: 30 minutes. Longer time frames are likely to encourage more in-depth discussions.

Preparation: First, select two evaluation definitions. Second, on flip chart paper, write the selected definition for each evaluation term, and put them on the wall (an option is to provide each group with both definitions). The groups need to see both definitions at the same time. Patton's and Scriven's definitions can be used, or other definitions as appropriate, such as the government department's, organization's, or donor's. Second, write the two facilitation questions, given in the next column, each on their own piece of flip chart paper, ensuring that only the first question can be seen. (Or write both questions on the same piece of paper, but cover the second question.) These two questions will be used during the group discussion.

Preparation of room: Divide the participants into small groups of three to five people, to allow for good discussions. Consider how the groups are organized. You may want to have random groups (e.g., all people with birthdays in January through March in one group, or all people wearing green), or more strategically thought-out groups (e.g., one manager, one evaluator, and one junior researcher). Consider what you want to happen in the groups. Do you want a discussion that mixes various perspectives in one group? Or a discussion among people who are likely to have similar understandings? Do you want one person to learn from another? Or do you want people to build relationships?

The exercise: Once groups are in their own spaces, ask people to silently read the two evaluation defi-

nitions. Then ask them to discuss the first question within their groups.

1. In what way are the two evaluation definitions the same? In what ways are they different?

Allow approximately 5 minutes for discussion, and then introduce the second question. It is OK if the group is still talking about the first one.

2. How might these differences influence an evaluative process or an evaluation, with regard to implementation and/or expectations?

Allow approximately 5 minutes for discussion. Then ask the members of one group to share their answers to the two questions, followed by the other groups. Facilitate a discussion that compares the responses. It is important to note that for some groups, facilitating the discussion immediately after the first question, before moving on to the second, may be appropriate; for other groups, that pace may be too slow. Some suggested probing questions during the larger-group discussion include the following:

Which definition do you prefer, and why?

What are the differences and the similarities?

Why is (or what makes) it important to have discussions that lead to shared definitions of evaluation, or at least an understanding that differences of opinion exist?

What might happen in an evaluative process if there was not a shared definition, or agreement to use the same definition, of the term?

Critical learning point: Different evaluation definitions will lend themselves to different expectations, which will likely create challenges during the evaluation. Discussing and developing a clear, shared understanding of evaluation and how the term will be applied are likely to result in shared expectations of the evaluation, which is an excellent place to start any evaluative journey.

Evaluative Thinking

Sometimes people use *evaluative thinking* and *evaluation* in the same breath. While they are indeed closely related, the terms connote different meanings. Evaluative thinking is what encourages the reflection on, and the use of, data and information. It encourages continual thinking about what can be done differently, improved, changed, or enhanced. I have heard some argue that anyone who can think evaluatively is an evaluator. For me, this argument is akin to contending that anyone who knows that it is important to brush their teeth twice a day is a dentist, or that anyone who knows that a steady diet of processed sugar is not good for the body is a nutritionist. Evaluative thinking is a critical part of being a thoughtful and engaged development worker or program manager. Thinking evaluatively means using data and information to be reflective, to learn, and to inform actions. While it is a critical element of being an evaluator as well, evaluative thinking does not by itself make someone an evaluator. (For a rich discussion of why this matters, skip ahead to Chapters 2 and 11.)

Monitoring

Now that we have discussed evaluation, and we have chatted about evaluative thinking, let's tackle the next term often associated with evaluation and evaluative thinking: *monitoring*. Monitoring is a common term used in public management that has crept slowly into evaluation books, journals, and evaluation conferences in the Western world. In the developing or emerging world, monitoring is often a familiar term.

We can all breathe a sigh of relief on how to define monitoring, as different groups tend to agree (though not always) on a common core definition. Monitoring is done on a day-to-day basis, and is the ongoing routine tracking of a program, project, intervention, or policy (or any of the other nouns mentioned earlier in this chapter). The confusion comes in when we are trying to distinguish monitoring from evaluation. Making this distinction is often a thorny conversation in the West, where monitoring can be subsumed into an evaluation process or completely disregarded as not being a part of the evaluation conversation. In developing or emerging markets, monitoring is so closely associated with evaluation that it is difficult to have a conversation that does not reference the M (monitoring) without the E (evaluation) in M&E. Speaking about monitoring as something different and separate from evaluation is practical, however, in that it allows a clearer understanding of what is done when, for what reason, and by whom. Let's take a closer look at monitoring.

Monitoring is something many people do naturally and answers a very basic question: **What is happening?** The question subsumes or includes three foci:

- What is (or is not) happening with the resources used for the intervention?
- What is (or is not) happening in terms of actions to implement the intervention?
- What is (or is not) happening as a result of those actions?

Sometimes we put in a number to gauge if something is happening: For example, did a person run 5 miles or lose 2 pounds? Setting these numbers, which evaluators have often called *targets,* helps us to specifically monitor progress, and show whether the person is moving toward or away from what he set out to accomplish. We discuss setting targets and other related concepts, such as benchmarks, more fully in Chapter 9.

Just a side note here: A critical element to remember in the evaluation journey is that staying on task is critical to untangling and focusing the process. However, because there are so many evaluation concepts and discussions that have interrelated and spin-off conversations, it is easy to get sidetracked. Sometimes a tangential term arises and causes havoc, and there is a need to stop and provide a detailed explanation. At other times, the tangential term adds a needed detail to the conversation (such as *target* above, or earlier in the chapter, when I stopped and explained the terms *data* and *information*) and requires no more than a quick, yet informative, chat. The critical part is, once the tangential term is explained, to return effectively to the core conversation. So let's go back to monitoring.

Let's assume we are monitoring an intervention. Our monitoring data suggest that the intervention is on track and moving toward where it intended to go, or maybe that it is not on track and thus requires one or more management decisions. The management decision could be to make an immediate change, do nothing and continue to monitor, or conduct an evaluation to find out why the intervention is (or is not) on track. The same monitoring data may also be used to demonstrate accountability. For instance, the data may be used in a monthly report that is presented to a board of directors.

Monitoring is a management function mainly used to determine whether an intervention is using appropriate resources and using them appropriately, doing what it aimed to do, and achieving the results it intended. Monitoring can also be used to keep an eye on external or internal factors that may influence the intervention (e.g., the economy, policy shifts, or people). Monitoring is often associated with informed decisions and accountability. Combined with evaluative thinking, monitoring provides a way to use data to learn and reflect; to improve a project, program, intervention, policy, or the like; to identify what was (or was not) achieved; and sometimes to recognize unexpected results.

BOX 1.7. Monitoring

When discussing the definition of monitoring, we need to consider four core concepts: The data collection is (1) empirical and (2) continuous, and data are used (3) to manage the intervention and (4) to provide accountability. Monitoring answers these questions: What is happening, and did the intervention do what we intended it to do? Monitoring does not ask if we are doing the right thing, or if we are doing things right; it also does not probe in any way to find out *why* the intervention did what it said it would do, or *why* it did not. Monitoring does not ask why or place a value on the results. When it starts to venture in that direction, it is more properly called evaluation.

Discussing monitoring is often more straightforward than discussing evaluation. However, monitoring also has its own nuanced definitions and various labels in different countries and in different organizations. For example, some people use the term *performance monitoring,* and others call the same process *performance management.* These terms have specific definitions that refer to tracking performance against stated targets, or goals. Earlier the term *M&E* was introduced, which can involve another fuzzy discussion, so let's talk about that next.

The Siamese Twins: M&E

My daughter, Gemma, has a book about a little girl who is told to count sheep to make her go to sleep (McQuinn, 2010). The little girl lies down and starts to count the sheep. Except the sheep do not behave and stay in a line: They play games, they swim, they hide, and they go in-line skating, all of which makes them very difficult to count. The little girl keeps running after the sheep to try to count them. Finally she exclaims, "You're exhausting!" and, ironically, falls asleep. I feel this way about how *M&E* is tossed around; it exhausts me. When someone says, "I am going to do M&E," I always wonder, "Well, which is it? Is it the M or the E?" Add to this that when I meet M&E experts, and they explain what they do, the explanations often vary considerably from one expert to the next. Oh, and then how the M&E persons define *monitoring* and how they define *evaluation* also often vary (refer to our earlier discussions on these terms). These are some of the conversations that exhaust me, and sometimes help put *me* to sleep.

When separated and defined, each term becomes useful, and then, when they are loosely linked back together, they serve a valuable role. However, when the term M&E is flung around without any questioning of what is being referred to, monitoring and evaluation become the troublesome twins indeed. Let's explore the practical link between the two terms.

The Practical Link

The link between the two terms is very practical. Monitoring an intervention should provide enough relevant data for a program manager (or whoever has the responsibility for the program, regardless of job title) to manage an intervention adequately and be accountable to those with power over the program (e.g., government, donors, community leaders). When something in that monitoring data raises a "why" question (e.g., "Why are people not coming to a training?" or "Why is that neighborhood having better results than other neighborhoods?"), evaluative thinking moves the manager toward evaluation territory, thus linking what is done through monitoring to evaluation. When an evaluator draws on monitoring data during an evaluation, it is important to verify that the data are available, accurate, precise to the extent necessary, and credible. For an in-depth discussion on data and data credibility, please skip to Chapter 5.

BOX 1.8. Monitoring, Evaluative Thinking, and Evaluation

Monitoring data raises the flag; evaluative thinking makes us go "hmmm"; and evaluation answers why and brings the valuing.

Evaluation Triplets:
Monitoring, Evaluation, and Evaluative Thinking

While the twins are troublesome, the triplets bring their own mischief. Here is a way to engage with the threesome. Monitoring is a process that answers the question about what is happening (descriptive). When we see that something is or is not happening, and we ask why, that moves us toward evaluative thinking. When we engage in further data collection or analysis processes to answer the why, and bring in a value judgment, that is evaluation. And often the processes associated with these words are all so tangled up into one exacting process that it may be difficult, if not impossible, to separate them easily in practice.

Now that we are near the end of our discussion on monitoring, evaluative thinking, and evaluation, I would be remiss not to introduce a few more acronyms that are becoming more common in the evaluation field. The newer acronyms I am seeing include MEL or MEAL (monitoring, evaluation, and learning), MER (monitoring, evaluation, and research), MERL (monitoring, evaluation, reflection, and learning), and PMEL (planning, monitoring, evaluation, and learning). And there are more. When working for or within an organization, we need to define and discuss their acronyms, what meaning each word brings, and who does what and when for whom, thus starting a conversation that leads to clarity and supports a useful evaluative process.

Alphabet Soup: The Use of Acronyms (or TUOA)

The evaluation field, and often the many technical fields it engages with (e.g., health, education, environment, community safety, climate change), seem to have a love affair with acronyms. In South Africa, nearly every day I hear or see the acronym ANC as an abbreviation for the African National Congress, the current ruling political party (often best known in other countries for being the political party of the late Nelson Mandela). When I started implementing health systems evaluations in South Africa, people talked about ANC all the time. I could not understand why the ANC played such a large role at the community health clinic level. Then one day I realized that ANC, in the health system, most often meant *antenatal clinic*—though sometimes it still meant the African National Congress. I was telling this story to a friend, and she said, "Oh, I thought it meant *antenuptial contract*." Hmm. My first piece of advice? Don't be shy; always ask what an acronym means.

My second piece of advice? Do not use acronyms if you can avoid them. First, it makes texts hard to follow, particularly for those not as familiar with the context as the evaluator or program staff. Second, in some cases, it can lessen the impact or take away the very meaning of what you are trying to convey. For instance, in a report about gender-based violence, using the acronym GBV can remove the very urgency or criticalness of the issue being addressed. It is a very different experience for the brain to read *GBV* rather than *gender-based violence*. A key point of writing an evaluation report (or anything, really) is to engage readers, not distance them.

While the term *research* is more thoroughly discussed in Chapter 2, the three words (monitoring, evaluation, and research) offer another set of triplets habitually intermingled in one conversation. Thus two activities are now provided to engage others in a discussion of these triplets and to provide foreshadowing for the more in-depth conversation about research and evaluation, and researchers and evaluators, in Chapter 2.

ACTIVITY 1.2. Monitoring, Evaluation, and Research Discussion

Purpose: The facilitated discussion brings out how the terms *monitoring, evaluation,* and *research* are often intermingled, and encourages people to think about how the three terms relate to each other in practice and how they are different. The activity works best as an introduction to the three words, not a summary.

Time: Allow approximately 5 minutes for preparation, 5 minutes for a discussion on each word in a small-group format, and 10–20 minutes for a large-group discussion. Total approximate time: 20–30 minutes.

Preparation: With a marker, write the word *monitoring* on a flip chart. On the next (and hidden) sheet of flip chart paper, write the word *evaluation*. Then write the word *research* (also on its own sheet of paper, and hidden). Thus, at the start of the exercise, the participants can only see the first word (monitoring). You may choose to write all three words on the same flip chart paper; if so, however, ensure that only the first word can be seen by the participants.

Preparation of materials: Each group needs three blank pieces of paper large enough to write a two-

or three-sentence definition with marker or pen. It is often better to use marker, as then you have the option to attach the participants' work to the wall, and it is readable.

Preparation of room: Organize groups with no fewer than three members and no more than five. This size allows for good discussions. Consider how the people in the room are divided. You may want to have random groups (e.g., all people whose first names start with A–E in one group), or more strategically thought-out groups (e.g., one manager, one evaluator, and one junior researcher per group). See reasoning and hints from Activity 1.1.

The exercise: Before providing any definitions or explanations of monitoring, evaluation, or research, explain to the larger group that it is their job to teach a brand-new colleague (or classmate or staff member) the definition of monitoring. Show the group the word *monitoring* written on a piece of flip chart paper. Provide each group with one piece of paper, and have one person in the group write down the word to be discussed (i.e., monitoring) at the top of this piece of paper. Then ask them to discuss, in their group, how they would explain monitoring to a colleague who is not at this training session. Ask the group to write down the explanation on the paper, below the word. When groups are finished, show the word *evaluation* to them, which is written on the next flip chart. Then have one person in the small group write this word at the top of a second blank piece of paper. Now that they have explained what monitoring is to the new person, ask them to explain what evaluation is to that person. Have groups discuss the term and write down how they would explain evaluation to the same colleague. When this is done, show the word *research* and repeat the steps. After each group has written a definition for each term, have the groups share how they would explain these three terms to their new colleague.

As a facilitator, listen for the distinctions made among the terms (or lack thereof). Ask the groups to provide feedback on their internal discussions, not just their definitions. After this exercise, present the more common definitions (those described earlier in this chapter, or other definitions relevant to the group) to close the session.

When facilitating, consider using these three questions:

- What were the challenges, if any, in describing these words?
- What is the importance of clarifying a distinction

among these words? Why does it matter in practice?

- What are some of the likely challenges if the words are not clarified—for example, in common usage, in a job description, at the office, or in an evaluation process?

Facilitation hint: Before the groups present their descriptions of the three terms, tell them that they may only read what is on the cards. Reading what is on the cards helps the groups to focus, and helps keep the activity to its set time.

Optional exercise: To make this activity a bit more fun, use role playing. After all groups have their explanations of the three terms, invite one person to the front of the room to "play" the new colleague. Have the members of each group present their explanations to the person, and then ask the person which one was clearer. There is no intent for a winner; rather, the reasons for choosing one description over the others should invite more discussion.

Critical learning points: Knowing the definitions for these three terms, and practically applying them, are two different things. The group should be comfortable discussing the three different words and how they are practically applied in their organization or in their work (not just providing rote definitions).

ACTIVITY 1.3. Stories about Research, Monitoring, and Evaluation

Purpose: The facilitated discussion brings out how monitoring, evaluation, and research are often intermingled, and encourages people to think about how the three terms relate to each other in practice.

Preparation: None, unless you want to create your own story.

Time: Allow approximately 2 minutes to read the story, 5 minutes for individual thinking time, and 15 minutes for group discussion. Total approximate time: 22 minutes.

The exercise: Read the example. Here is an example that can be used: "When baking a cake, I first **research** what kind of cake I want to make—say, a chocolate layer cake or plain vanilla. I research different recipes, and I choose one. I then set about making the cake, and I **monitor** what I put into it, such as how much flour or salt. I also **monitor** the cake to tell me how brown the top becomes, so that I know when to remove it from the oven. When **evaluating** my cake, I decide if the cake is good or bad, based on my preference, and sometimes I even listen to what others think of my cake." In my example, I have talked about using research, monitoring, and evaluation.

Now ask individuals to develop short examples (one per person) from their everyday life, and provide 5 minutes for the short examples to be written down. Ask for a few participants to share. These are some facilitation questions you can ask:

- What are the practical differences among the three terms?
- What challenges did you have in describing the three different processes, if any?
- How do these critical differences translate to your work?

Critical learning points: Again, knowing the definitions for these three terms, and practically applying them, are two different experiences. The group should be comfortable discussing the three different words and how they are practically applied in their organization or in their work (not just providing rote definitions).

Here are the more common conversations I have with regard to M&E. Reading these dialogues will build your confidence about engaging in these and similar discussions.

If someone holds the job of an M&E officer, or they say they are an M&E expert, what does it mean?

It can mean many things, so take the time to inquire what someone means when they use this term. While some organizations or governments may specify requirements associated with these job titles, there is no accepted or general job description for an M&E officer or an M&E expert. Someone holding this title or position (or self-labeling) may have extraordinary experience and knowledge of M&E, or may have little to no knowledge of either monitoring or evaluation.

Consider when someone takes a position as an M&E expert, and brings substantial knowledge and skills with monitoring to this position, but little to no evaluation knowledge or experience. This creates awkward situations for the M&E expert, who is then asked to do or manage work for which they have no background, training, or experience. At best, the M&E expert recognizes this challenge and seeks advice, training, knowledgeable others, or mentoring. At worst, the person's lack of knowledge and experience damages an intervention, gives a poor name to evaluators and evaluation, and frustrates key stakeholders and others who are negatively affected by a poorly implemented evaluation. So when people say they "do M&E," always ask them, "So tell me, what do you do, exactly?"

Finally, be aware that the same conversation may also happen when someone says they are an evaluator. Being an evaluator can mean many things—as described in Chapters 2 and 11 of this book.

I am not sure if I can ask an M&E person to do an evaluation. What do I do?

Clarify what skills, knowledge, and experience the person has with evaluation. Here are a few questions you can ask to determine the person's likely ability to do an evaluation that will meet your needs:

- What would be the steps that you would use to conduct the evaluation?
- What are your favorite evaluation approaches, theories, or models? Can you tell me about some you have used in the past?
- What are the ways in which you will determine the valuing criteria (i.e., determine their merit or worth), or what processes will be used to value the findings?
- Please tell me about the last evaluation that you conducted (or the most interesting, or the most challenging). What were some of the challenges? What worked well?

Answers to these questions will encourage a dialogue that provides insight into the M&E person's level of evaluation knowledge and experience.

Is a program manager expected to be an evaluator?

While the response to this question will depend on the organization, in general the answer is no. Program managers need "enough" evaluation knowledge to be able to engage with an evaluator, an evaluation unit (internal), or an evaluation team (external or internal), and/or to manage an evaluation. Here is another way to think about answering this question. I do not expect a program manager to be an auditor, or therefore to conduct a financial audit. However, I do expect a program manager to understand his budget, and to know if the intervention is over- or underspending. Similarly, I do expect a program manager to be able to use monitoring data. He needs to know enough to interpret the data and understand what the data are saying—for example, to take action (or not). For instance, in a high school tutoring program, the program manager should be able to answer questions such as these: Do children show up for tutoring (and, if so, how many)? Do children who show up for tutoring have better grades (if that is the intended result)? How many tutors are there who can cover advanced math, and does that number meet the current students' needs? Thus, just as a program manager is not (often) an evaluator, an evaluator is (in most circumstances) not an auditor or a program manager. A program manager needs to understand how to engage with monitoring and evaluation so that it is useful. Please see Chapters 2 and 11 for an in-depth look at the role of an evaluator.

INTERVENTION, ACTIVITY, PROJECT, PROGRAM: DOPPELGANGERS OR DIFFERENCES?

I like the word *doppelganger*. It has a specific meaning that is exactly what I am trying to convey. Vocabulary.com (n.d.) provides a nice explanation: "Someone who looks spookily like you, but is not a twin, is a doppelganger. Originally, this was a type of ghost. The word doppelganger is German and literally means double walker—as in a ghost or shadow of yourself."

Doppelganger is a wonderful word to describe how the labels *intervention, activity, project,* and *program* are used. For example, *intervention* and *program* are sometimes used interchangeably to discuss the larger picture (e.g., "We have an environmental program," or "We have an environmental intervention"), while *project* is sometimes but not always used to describe a collection of smaller activities (e.g., "Our program focuses on projects that address fish and wildlife conservation"), and *activities* are often specific (e.g., "Our project has several activities, one of which is to issue licenses to fish farmers"). And sometimes not. When you are working with any organization, ask them to describe how they use these labels and terms, so that everyone is clear about what is what, and which label is attached to what description.

Here is an example of how these words may be used in Organization A.

Intervention	Activity	Project	Program
The nonprofit is teaching high school students how to study for exams.	One tutor works with one student for 2 hours per week.	Each site (and there are 450 sites) has five tutors who work 5 days a week for a total of 20 hours.	It is a national program for inner-city youth.

Here is an example of how these words may be used in Organization B.

Project	Intervention	Activity	Program intervention
The nonprofit is teaching high school students how to study for exams.	One tutor works with one student for 2 hours per week.	Each site (and there are 450 sites) has five tutors who work 5 days a week for a total of 20 hours.	It is a national program intervention for inner-city youth.

VISION, MISSION, GOAL, OBJECTIVE: MANAGEMENT SPEAK TRANSLATED INTO M&E SPEAK

For *mission, vision, goal,* and *objective, doppelgangers* is an appropriate term to reuse here, and let me just say "ditto" to what I have written in the previous section. The management language and the M&E language can be thought of as distant cousins (perhaps second cousins), or we can view them as terms that live in their own separate yet parallel universes. When you are working with management terms, identify what should happen or be achieved when, and to what extent, the organization is held directly accountable for which achievement (i.e., which result). Knowing both (what is intended to be achieved and what the organization is held directly accountable for) will clarify what *needs* to be monitored and evaluated (there are many things that can be monitored, and we delve into this in Chapters 3 and 4), and what is the far-reaching but necessary dream (e.g., a better world, equality for all), which is not (often) assessed in the lifetime of the intervention. I say "necessary," because most interventions are aiming for something just beyond their reach, and this dream guides the work in the present, like a guiding star. When M&E words are mixed and matched with management words, they tend to (though they do not always) have corresponding levels. It is with trepidation that I note the following common equivalents:

- Vision, mission, goal = Impact
- Objective = Outcomes

Again, these are often somewhat similar levels—but not always. Please jump ahead to Chapter 7 for a more in-depth look at why these examples are provided with some trepidation.

Discussing Concepts, Terms, and Labels

Do not assume that everyone engaging in an evaluation discussion has the same understandings of concepts, terms, and labels—even those that have concrete definitions. Here are three pieces of advice:

- Discuss each concept or term.
- Define and describe how it will be applied.
- Write it down and get physical sign-off on it.

WRAPPING UP

Common evaluation concepts and terms, even when they have concrete definitions, can be defined, interpreted, and applied by different people, groups, and organizations with nuanced or astronomical differences. Knowing the difference between concepts and terms that have specific definitions and uses, and those that do not, is important. An evaluator needs to know when she can say, "That is indeed the definition; let's discuss how we will use it," and when she needs to negotiate a concept's or term's definition, meaning, and application. When an evaluator ensures that those who need to be on the same page with regard to a term or concept's meaning are actually in agreement, she avoids mayhem, misunderstandings, frustration, and likely major disappointment in the evaluation and its process. An evaluator who explicitly engages with evaluation words, concepts, and their meanings (whether through a 2-minute conversation, a written clarification, or a longer process) is more likely to have a useful evaluation. Some side benefits of clarifying language (evaluators call these "unintended results") may include building capacity, strengthening relationships among those engaged in the process, and leveling the playing field among stakeholders.

The next chapter moves us from talking about monitoring, evaluative thinking, and evaluation to another topic that is often as intensely discussed: the differences between evaluation and research, and between an evaluator and a researcher. Before you leave this chapter, however, join me in a conversation.

Our Conversation: Between You and Me

Here are two types of situations that you may encounter with regard to the concepts and terms just covered. Practicing with these common scenarios can be a great help as you deal with these kinds of situations in the real world.

1. **Your clients (or boss or colleagues) have asked you to do the M&E for a program. You have no clear idea of what they want you to do.** Start at the beginning, as we have done in this chapter. Encourage a dialogue to get clarity about what they expect from M&E. To prepare, identify the organization's or client's definition of *M&E* (or its component terms, *monitoring* and *evaluation*), or any description of how the acronym is used in the organization. Reading the organization's information will help you identify a basic place to start asking questions. Here are some general discussion guidelines:

- Be clear about what is within your boundaries and what is outside them, with regard to what you are capable of doing in terms of your own knowledge/skills and the resources that are provided.

- Move the initial conversation away from labels. For example, if the request is "We expect you to do monitoring," a good follow-up question would be "Could you explain a bit more what you mean by *monitoring*, perhaps with some examples?" If they seem hesitant or unsure, offer some suggestions or examples of types of activities often associated with monitoring.

- Seek to understand how the data that you collect, and the processes that you engage in, will be used by whom to do what.

- Once you think you have a clear understanding of what is wanted, provide some concrete descriptive examples of what you are going to do, and have them react to those examples. Provide some examples as well of what you will not do, and have them then react to those examples.

Draw on the definitions, discussions, and exercises demonstrated in this chapter to engage your clients (or boss or colleagues).

2. You are working in a place where English is not the first language, and there is confusion about how to translate or how to use the terms *monitoring, evaluative thinking,* and *evaluation*. A discussion of the distinctions among *monitoring, evaluative thinking,* and *evaluation* is not always a useful conversation when terms are translated. Or the terms may simply not be useful in the culture in which you work, even if English is the dominant language. So remove the labels. Facilitate a process that draws from how monitoring and evaluation are described in this chapter, without using the terms. For instance, ask the person, "How will you know if the intervention is doing what it is supposed to do?" What *is* needed is a clear understanding of what data are collected when, by whom, how, and for what reason, and how those findings will be valued and by whom. Once all that is clear, you can then discuss who does what in that process. Then and only then, choose appropriate labels (e.g., "We will call this X and that Y"), *if* labels are needed. For example, labels may be needed for the group to engage with their donor or others outside the organization. Or perhaps no labels are needed.

The other day my neighbor said to me, "Tell me again what you do for a living. You are a researcher, right?" Sigh. Please come join me in Chapter 2.

CHAPTER 2

The Tale of the Researcher and the Evaluator

I am a researcher; therefore, I am an evaluator.

The conversation that informs the evaluator–researcher debate is rooted in the "research versus evaluation" debate, so let's start there. Sometimes it is a deliberate and enjoyable conversation, and sometimes it is a subtler, strained one. Either way, the extent to which differences between research and evaluation exist influences several key decisions, such as what to study to be an evaluator, or whom to hire to design, implement, or critique an evaluation.

Before we embark on a somewhat dizzying journey, keep in mind that the basic aim of social science research is to produce or generate knowledge. Patton (2008) says that evaluation aims to influence actions; it is action-oriented. He notes that some evaluation texts mingle these definitions, such as Rossi and colleagues' (2004) popular text *Evaluation: A Systematic Approach,* which is in its seventh edition and is used in many social science graduate programs. In their book, Rossi and colleagues define **program evaluation** as "the use of social research methods to systematically investigate the effectiveness of social intervention programs in ways that are adapted to their political and organizational environments and are designed to inform social action to improve social conditions" (p. 16).

Some people put the two terms together and talk about **evaluation research.** Kelly (2004) describes evaluation research as an approach in which the purpose is to "solve practical problems" (p. 522), suggesting that the focus is not on judgment or improvement of interventions. Babbie (2017) notes that the purpose of evaluation research is to "determine whether social interventions or programs have had their desired effects" (p. 387). Here, the word "value" is noticeably absent. At the same time, other evaluators use the same phrase, *evaluation research,* to mean research that is done *on* evaluation. And let's not forget basic and applied research. McBride (2013) tells us that basic research aims to address "fundamental processes of behavior," while applied research aims to "solve real-world problems" (p. 10). Hmm. Obviously, distinguishing between an evaluator and a researcher can be a bit mystifying—so I will make it as clear as I can. Keeping Patton's understanding of evaluation (its aim is to influence actions) and the core meaning of social science research (its aim is knowledge generation) in your mind, let's take a closer look at the differences between researchers and evaluators.

WHY IT IS IMPORTANT TO UNDERSTAND THE DIFFERENCES BETWEEN RESEARCHERS AND EVALUATORS

Understanding the difference between evaluators and researchers can inform your career path in terms of which one you may like to be and therefore what to study. It can also clarify for you which types of positions to apply for, or whom to hire. While I was writing this book, an international development agency advertised for an evaluator to review evaluations of development programs in education and health from an external perspective, and to provide critical feedback. The job description asked for a person with strong communication skills, strong qualitative and quantitative research skills, and knowledge of the organization—all of which gave me pause. What about knowledge of evaluation methods, theories, or approaches? Or practical experience in designing or implementing evaluations? Or knowledge of how power, politics, culture, and language influence an evaluation approach? I was a bit aghast; surely they did not want a researcher to review an evaluation and provide feedback? Or maybe, just maybe, they did not know the difference between a researcher and an evaluator?

RESEARCHERS AND EVALUATORS: COMPATRIOTS OR COMPETITORS?

Having a conversation about the differences between evaluators and researchers can be enlightening and uncomfortable at the same time. Sometimes the conversation is sensitive, such as when a researcher considers himself to be an evaluator. Or, awkwardly, you are a researcher and are wondering, "What does an evaluator have that I do not?" At other times, it is frustrating, such as when an evaluation commissioner hires a researcher to design an evaluation. So should you ever find yourself engaged in these kinds of ponderings, conversations, or situations, either with yourself or with someone else, consider these three essential conversation points: **valuing, purpose,** and **approaches.**

- *Valuing.* Valuing findings is at the core of an evaluator's work. Evaluators determine criteria (which can be done in multiple ways; see Chapter 12) to value evaluation findings. Researchers are not asked to value their research findings.

Wait, stop on that first point. I find some research to be very valuable.

I agree that some research is very valuable. Researchers use data to support a claim about something; however, they do not follow up that claim by valuing it. Here's an example. All females on my mother's side of my family suffer from migraines. Research has shown that certain so-called "trigger foods" may bring on migraines, and research also shows that certain types of drugs alleviate the pain. The females in my family are delighted about the research findings. While the researchers did not value their findings, my female family members found the research to be very valuable. For the evaluator, valuing a process or result is at the heart of her work.

- *Purpose.* Researchers ask questions on behalf of the larger scientific community. Basic scientific research seeks to uncover new knowledge, investigate and test theories, identify findings, and generalize them. Evaluators aim to provide information to a specific group on a particular intervention. The information is intended to be used to improve or judge that intervention—to learn more about that particular intervention, in a particular context, for a particular group of people, in a particular time frame.

- *Approaches.* Evaluation uses research methods, and then also brings its own approaches, theories, and models that are specific to the evaluation journey (see Chapter 15). Because evaluation approaches, theories, and models guide the evaluation process and its valuing framework, an evaluator needs to know them; a researcher does not.

BOX 2.1. Research and Evaluation: Some Distinct Differences

While the aim of applied research (and researchers) is often to generalize the results to the larger population (McBride, 2013), the aim of an evaluation (and therefore evaluators) is more commonly to look at a specific intervention, program, process, or policy and to judge its merit, worth, and significance, with the intent that the findings will be used by a specific group to make management decisions. A researcher fills the role of methodologist; an evaluator can often fill the role of methodologist, evaluation theorist, facilitator, negotiator, educator, and more. See Chapter 11 for further elaboration on an evaluator's potential roles.

Let's take a moment to look at what a conversation between a researcher and an evaluator might look like.

I am a researcher.	I am an evaluator.
I seek to generate knowledge, and I answer questions. I contribute to broader scientific knowledge.	I seek to generate knowledge, and I contribute knowledge to use in making decisions or improving an intervention or policy, for a specific group of stakeholders.
I use research methods of inquiry.	I use research methods of inquiry. I also use evaluation frameworks, theories, and approaches.
I identify results.	I identify results, or sometimes I use a researcher's results. And then I often work with diverse stakeholders to determine criteria on which to value those results.
My work is researcher-centric. I get to decide what I research and how to focus the research, though sometimes others, like those who fund me, also influence the decision.	My work is stakeholder-focused. Sometimes I help to shape stakeholders' questions. I shape them so that answers are likely to be useful to the stakeholders.
I publish my results in journals and books, and I also share my research at conferences so that the knowledge generated can be used.	I provide my reports and findings to the key stakeholders, so the findings can be used by them. Sometimes I publish, although publishing is not key to my evaluation work. Sometimes I give presentations at conferences on the work that I do.

Both Chapter 1 and this chapter may appear to suggest that conversations to clarify words and how they are used (e.g., **evidence** or **data, evaluator** or **researcher**) are easy conversations. They can be. At other times, however, to say that they become more antagonistic is to put it nicely. Knowing how to facilitate these tense conversations is a skill essential to being an effective evaluator, as difficult conversations can arise in all parts of an evaluative process. Let's stop for a moment and talk about facilitating useful conversations.

How to Facilitate Useful Conversations

In most evaluative processes, there will be times when people are on opposing sides, such as when I say "researcher" and you say "evaluator." Practicing how to manage these discussions in often less sticky situations (e.g., evaluation vs. research) can prepare you for occasions when you will need to engage with facilitating more challenging ones. Here are some other likely examples: (1) In an evaluation, there are data to answer a question that are as convincing for one side as another (e.g., "Yes, do it" vs. "No, do not do it"); (2) two groups (or more) analyze the same data and reach different conclusions; (3) there is agreement on the conclusions, but a difference of opinions on the recommendations; and (4) there are people who just plainly have different opinions or understand a situation or word differently, and to whom the group needs to listen.

The approach described next describes how to facilitate a process that encourages people to listen to opposing viewpoints. There are three reasons to consider using this approach. First, when people know that others will listen to them, they are more likely to engage and work with these others, even when they have different opinions or assumptions. A second, and somewhat related, reason is that it can be very frustrating to perceive (rightly or wrongly) that no one is listening. This can cause a person or group to "shut down," and thus can cause an evaluator to miss important perspectives in the discussion. Third, truly listening to what others have to say who think differently opens new ways of understanding.

ACTIVITY 2.1. Listen–Speak–Listen

Purpose: A useful approach to engage groups who have very strong and clearly very different viewpoints is to facilitate a discussion where people *must* listen to other ways of thinking and other ideas. The purpose is to ensure that each idea, thought, or fact is spoken (or signed, as in sign language) and that people listen to each other; the purpose is not (necessarily) to reach agreement.

Time: The time will vary considerably, depending on the number of people in the room, and the number of ideas, thoughts, and/or facts that people want shared. I recommend, however, that groups be allotted 10–15 minutes to write down their key ideas or thoughts. While topics and the size of the group will further determine the time frame, keep in mind that it is hard work to listen. Limit the discussion, if possible, to 15–20 minutes. A longer-drawn-out listening session can be counterproductive, as people tend to stop listening when they are tired. Total time is approximately 25–35 minutes, though it can vary.

Preparing: Prior discussions inform the debate topic. Prepare small pieces of paper (with space to write one or two sentences) for each group; there should be at least one piece of paper per person, though more

pieces of paper are recommended (should there be more ideas). Gather pens or pencils.

The exercise:

1. Summarize the question or debate on a piece of flip chart paper, and place this sheet at the front of the room. Summarize the two (or more) sides as equally as possible. Read these to the group.

2. Have people choose the side of the debate that they support more (or most) strongly, and form groups. If any persons are truly neutral or undecided, or just uncomfortable with the exercise, they stand off to the side as observers. During the activity, they are not allowed to speak or sign.

3. Read the rules to the group (see "The rules" on page 34).

4. Provide each group with pieces of paper and some pens or pencils, and ask them to write *one* key idea/point per piece of paper. Each person in the group should have *at least* one slip of paper to present, if possible, though each person may have several pieces (i.e., several ideas).

5. When the groups are ready, have them form a circle, with an opposing group member on either side of each person, so that every other speaker is on the same team. To decide who goes first, flip

a coin and choose a person from that group. He reads his statement, and then the person to his left reads hers, and so on, until all the points are made. Sitting in a circle encourages a discussion-like format. The process continues until all people are heard.

The rules: There are six simple rules.

1. People must show respect at all times (i.e., no yelling; no disrespectful words or body language).
2. Only one person speaks at a time.
3. Each person may only read what is on the paper—no more, no less.
4. Once an idea, thought, or fact is shared, it cannot be repeated, even if different words are used.
5. There is to be *no response* when the idea is presented, from either the other team or the observers.
6. Everyone must agree to the rules before the discussion starts.

This exercise encourages listening that enables engagement with other points of view. Such engagement has the potential to inform deeper thinking, promote stronger conclusions/more focused recommendations, or lead to agreement—although, of course, it may not. The Listen–Speak–Listen discussion is an example of a situation where an evaluator fills the role of negotiator and facilitator. (Again, for more on an evaluator's roles, see Chapter 11.)

Here is a specific example of when to use the Listen–Speak–Listen activity. Empirical data sometimes provides two opposing answers to the same evaluation question. While the evaluator can present both empirical findings to the evaluation user (and sometimes it is acceptable to do so), it can sometimes leave the evaluation user confused at best, or annoyed at worst. After all, an evaluator was brought in to provide information to inform management decisions, not a response much akin to "Well, sometimes it does, and sometimes it does not." While both sides can still be presented in the report, reasons (drawn from the Listen–Speak–Listen discussion) can now be given for why one answer is likely to be more appropriate than the other (through the depth of additional detail and explanation), or at the very least the evaluator can provide more information that management can use to make a decision.

 EVALUATION VERSUS RESEARCH

- *Have a minute?* If you want a good giggle, peek at a blog by Patricia J. Rogers and E. Jane Davidson called Genuine Evaluation (*www.genuineevaluation.com*). For example, Rogers and Davidson provide a funny, realistic take on the difference between evaluators and researchers with their May 25, 2012, list of "Top ten things you'll never hear from the researcher you hired to do an evaluation."

- *Have a few hours?* Read an article by Levin-Rozalis (2003), "Evaluation and Research: Differences and Similarities," which can be found online in the *Canadian Journal of*

Program Evaluation. Or read a chapter by Mathison (2008), "What Is the Difference between Evaluation and Research—and Why Do We Care?" in N. L. Smith & P. R. Brandon (Eds.), *Fundamental Issues in Evaluation*, pp. 183–196.

- *Have some more time?* Read Chapter 2 in Michael Quinn Patton's (2008) *Utilization-Focused Evaluation*, fourth edition.

Researcher or evaluator? Research or evaluation? As we have reviewed in the chapter to this point, there is a difference. Understanding this difference should influence many things—from what knowledge and skills to pursue, to who is hired, to how something is shaped and used. The differences are confounded when researchers self-identify as evaluators, or when evaluation is mislabeled as research (and vice versa). And more mixed signals are sent when, for an example, an economist does an evaluation, yet labels herself as an economist rather than an evaluator. Knowing and understanding the differences (and the points where research overlaps into evaluation) is critical for evaluators, and those who commission them, to ensure that persons with the right knowledge and skills are present to conduct an evaluation.

The evaluator-versus-researcher conversation has opened up a space to confess that in the real world, some conversations may not go smoothly. It has also suggested a practical solution: the Listen–Speak–Listen activity, which provides a technique for facilitating lively conversations and active listening. This approach can be used at any point in the evaluation process when, for example, different opinions arise, where data do not provide clear answers, or when different interpretations of the data offer useful but opposing insights.

Now that we have covered some basic differences between evaluation and research (and evaluators and researchers), and have learned a practical facilitation technique, it is time to commence our evaluative journey. Before we let the adventure continue, however, I invite you to have a conversation with me.

Our Conversation: Between You and Me

Here is a situation that you may encounter with regard to the concepts and terms we have just covered. Practicing with this common scenario can be a great help as you deal with this kind of situation in the real world.

If someone asked you the following, how would you answer: "Are you a researcher or an evaluator?" Think about how you might respond so that a nonresearcher or non-evaluator would understand you—that is, without jargon, technical terms, or abbreviations. For example, most people would probably start drifting off if you were to say, "Well, I am an evaluator, and I do empirical research that then draws on evaluation theory to value findings—and a researcher, well, a researcher uses social science theory to . . ." If we met at a cocktail party, and I asked you that question, what would you say to me?

DESCRIBING THE EVALUATIVE JOURNEY

The next eight chapters illustrate the iterative logic of monitoring and evaluation, and suggest a process that is appropriate for nearly any monitoring or evaluation exercise. There are challenges to writing a book about an *iterative* process (i.e., one involving repetition to achieve a series of outcomes). First, it is nearly impossible to write iteratively without sounding redundant or having too much repetition for a reader. Although an iterative process works well in a workshop or discussion, and in real-life evaluative processes, it does not work so well in a book. The second challenge is that sometimes what logically seems like the beginning, or the place to start, is not. Sometimes it is better to dive into the middle of the process, in order to untangle the beginning and sort out the end, which brings us back to the beginning and then back to the end, and then back to the middle. And so on. Related to this is that your evaluation journey may start in a different place than where the book starts the journey. The third challenge is that there are often concepts, ideas, and definitions buried in each step that need to be discussed. So you see my dilemma: how to present the next several chapters—which by nature are iterative, with different potential starting places that can spiral off in multiple directions (depending on the evaluator and the context)—so that the steps make sense to you, my readers.

The Suitcases for Our Journey

The solution is to organize our journey into a trip where I bring along suitcases that keep the process organized by themes. The suitcases represent the themes that will be covered in each chapter; thus you will know what I am covering, in a broad sense. We will carry our suitcases with us, unpack what is needed, and then tuck them away until, once again, we need something that is inside. For instance, the suitcase labeled "Assessment" is packed to the brim with ideas, discussions, and definitions of such terms as *indicator, facts,* and *methods.* However, I will only take out of the suitcase what is needed at that point in the evaluative process; thus the same suitcase will show up multiple times, and each time something else may be pulled out, or quite possibly the same concept or term will be reframed as needed for that part of the journey. The journey can be used to:

- Reconstruct what happened (backward-looking).
- Construct what we hope will happen (forward-looking).
- Support implementation or innovation as it happens (real time).
- Inform the completion of a practical M&E framework.

The journey is thus used to provide answers to, and inform decisions about, what and how to assess and value an intervention—in other words, how to monitor *and* evaluate. All the topics covered during our evaluative journey are depicted on the next page.

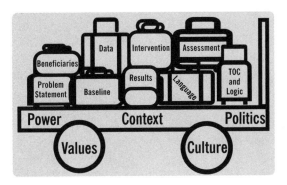

The Journey's Illustrative Example

Throughout the remainder of this book, an example of a girls' education intervention is used repeatedly, to provide a consistent demonstration of how to apply concepts, terms, and processes. The girls' education intervention will unfold along with the journey, and will continue to be refined in each step, as an intervention would in an actual evaluative process.

POTENTIAL USERS OF THE EVALUATIVE JOURNEY

The rest of this book describes a journey through an evaluative process that is mindful of how power, politics, language, culture, and values shape that journey. The process has many iterative, interconnected, and interreliant steps. These include describing and understanding the intervention, defining and interrogating the reason for the intervention, determining what to assess, and gathering data (the monitoring). The information is then used to reflect and learn and to inform an evaluation design and process that increases broader knowledge, aids in judgment, supports learning, and/or otherwise informs decisions. The evaluation journey is designed to have multiple uses for six specific groups:

- *Students of evaluation and emerging evaluators.* Students of evaluation and emerging evaluators can use the thinking and process in the remainder of this book to improve their practical understanding of evaluative processes. Immersing themselves in the book will enable them to understand how and where evaluative thinking starts (and that there are various starting places), how the intervention's logic and theory are intertwined, and how that relates to and informs evaluation. The book grounds students' and emerging evaluators' understanding in how to engage with and construct effective monitoring frameworks, and ultimately how to design and implement useful evaluations.

- *Implementers of interventions.* Implementers are encouraged to make informed decisions that support achievement of an intervention's goals. The thinking and its processes can be used so that implementers and their colleagues have a clear, holistic description of an evaluable intervention, and can use that understanding to engage in the M&E process in a practical manner. Furthermore, the process supports implementers as they engage with evaluators, donors, and others to whom they are accountable or with whom they otherwise interact.

• *Managers of interventions.* Managers of interventions can gain clarity on the intervention and the evaluative process. This clarity can support needed insight into how and why stakeholders with different perspectives may have different expectations regarding what is assessed, how it is assessed, and how findings are valued. This understanding can then be used to encourage constructive and mutually beneficial dialogues with implementers, donors, evaluators, and others to whom the managers are accountable or with whom they otherwise engage.

• *Evaluation teams.* Evaluation teams can use the process to clarify an intervention, which then informs refinement of evaluation questions, the evaluation design, and its valuing framework, and helps determine how and to whom to communicate the findings. Importantly, the process encourages teamwork with a shared understanding on all aspects of an evaluation process.

• *Lone evaluators.* A lone evaluator can use the process to think. When there is no one to engage with, and the evaluator needs to think about how to engage in an evaluation, going through the process will help keep her thinking organized and her decision making explicit—both of which are needed in an iterative evaluation process.

• *Confused evaluators.* The confused evaluator is provided with a way to untangle, engage with, and sort out confusion. Nearly all of us have all been there—perplexed, flummoxed, or mystified by the evaluation process. It happens. For example, someone says, "I need you to look at second-level outcomes and also assess the broader impact, and consider the immediate outcomes, and also look at efficiency, effectiveness, impact, and sustainability. And gender. For the capacity-building program." Our immediate response may be, "Say what?"

WRAPPING UP

We have begun the evaluation journey in Chapter 1 and this chapter by clarifying the critical use of language in evaluation, and distinguishing between an evaluator and a researcher (and research and evaluation). Chapters 3–10 present an iterative process that can have different uses for different people. A girls' education intervention, the suitcase symbols, and the clarifying icons will guide the iterative evaluation journey for all its different users. Grab your hat and shoes; we're off on our evaluation adventure!

CHAPTER 3

Starting the Evaluative Journey

We often forget to draw a new picture because we are so busy criticizing other paintings.

—DEBASISH MRIDHA, American physician, philosopher, poet, seer, and author

Now that we have clarified some basic evaluation terms, and have taken our suitcases in hand, let's talk about one place to start an evaluative process. And no worries: A conversation about monitoring will naturally be wrapped into the discussion. Whenever we are serving as evaluators or working with an evaluative process, it is critical for us to thoroughly grasp and explain the intervention with all its complexities, obscured and otherwise. While each chapter delves deeper into, and continues to untangle, the intervention and the evaluative process, Chapter 3 provides one place to start: the reason(s) for the intervention's existence.

I am going to share a trade secret with you: Most evaluators do not instinctively understand an intervention in its entirety, or in all its intricacies and nuances. Even if an evaluator is an expert in a technical field within evaluation (e.g., a specialist in education evaluation), she rarely (if ever) knows automatically, and immediately, exactly what or how to evaluate an intervention. Evaluators are not omniscient (and be very wary of ones who claim to be!). Evaluators need to have a clear understanding of *exactly* what an organization is doing or planning to do (the **intervention**); to fix, change, or make "it" better ("it" being the **problem statement**); and for whom, exactly, the intervention is intended (the **beneficiaries**). And that is just the *start* of what evaluators need to know. Now that this trade secret has been shared, let's delve into these three concepts, starting with the intervention.

INTRODUCING THE INTERVENTION

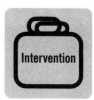

Despite what seems to be a common belief, an evaluator cannot magically answer the question "How do we evaluate it?" or "What did it accomplish?" without first knowing what "it" is that is being monitored or evaluated. The clearer "it" is, the easier it is for the evaluator to answer these and other questions.

BOX 3.1. Using the Term *Evaluative Process*

The term **evaluative process** is used to describe the entire flow from inception of the intervention, to what happens, to the valuing of what happens or does not, to the sharing and use of that information, and everything in between. The process and discussions described in the book can occur before an intervention starts (forward-looking, the planning phase); as the intervention unfolds (in real time, or for an innovative or developmental process); or after the intervention or components of the intervention have taken place or ended (retrospective).

What Is the Intervention?

Whether designing an intervention so that it is evaluable, monitoring an intervention as it is being implemented, or conducting an evaluation of the intervention, an evaluator first needs to understand what the intervention *is*. (See Chapter 1, pages 11–12, for a full listing of other nouns that can be substituted for *intervention*.) There are a few exceptions, such as in developmental evaluation, where the purpose is to inform and document the intervention as it unfolds; see Chapter 15 for specifics. The basic details that are often needed to understand an intervention, and therefore the basic questions that are usually asked, focus on (1) what it does, (2) what it aims to fix, change, or otherwise improve, (3) what it aims to accomplish, (4) how it intends to accomplish that, (5) where, and (6) for whom. Additional useful information could include (7) who provides the funding, (8) how long the intervention has been in place and for how long is it likely to be in place, and (9) who implements the intervention. These questions guide the early search for information about the intervention.

Ways to Obtain Data about the Intervention

Having conversations, reading documents, and observing (i.e., going to see something), are initial ways to obtain data describing the intervention. While the following pages provide a *brief* introduction to the types of data collection often used to learn about the intervention, Chapter 5 offers a more detailed discussion on data collection.

Reading Documents (Conducting a Document Review)

One way to obtain data describing the intervention is to read documents. The purpose of this process, also called a *document review* or *archival document analysis*, is to help inform an understanding of the intervention or answer a question in the evaluative process. The documents can contain words, numbers, or pictures (e.g., videos, drawings, or photos). Documents can be sourced from those who fund the intervention, obtained from implementation staff, requested from managers, or found on the internet, to name a few sources. Types of documents may include (to name just a few examples) pamphlets, funding proposals, meeting notes, business plans, quarterly or monthly reports, newspaper articles, promotional videos, theories of change (see Chapter 8 for a description of such theories), monitoring frameworks, or previous evaluations. An organization or intervention's website or webpage is often a very useful place to get started, as it likely provides a short description that gives a sense of the intervention, as well as other documents. However, the website or webpage should not be the sole source of data or information. Although it may provide easily accessible information or data, these may also be outdated or may only provide a partial picture.

Having Conversations (Interviews)

One way to understand what the intervention is, and why it exists, is to ask different people who probably have different perspectives on and insights about the intervention. As a starting place, consider talking to people who implement the intervention (perhaps those who designed it) and those who manage it, either individually or as a group. You can also talk to those who benefit, receive services, or otherwise take part in the intervention. These conversations are called *interviews*. Interviews can use open- or closed-ended questions.

An open-ended interview question is one that has no preselected answers. An example of such a question is "Tell me about your experience of reading this book." The upside? A person can say anything, thus providing a wealth of information. The downside? A person can say anything, thus providing broad and perhaps haphazard (and not useful) information. A more focused yet still open-ended question can also be used, such as "Describe what you like about how M&E is discussed in the book." That question guides the person to talk about what they liked about how M&E was discussed, not just any topic in the book. There are advantages and disadvantages of using more focused (sometimes known as leading) questions. The advantage is that it increases the chance of obtaining usable answers for description. The disadvantage is that respondents may be more likely (either consciously or unconsciously) to provide an answer they think you want to hear, and perhaps not mention another topic that would have proven informative.

An interview can also use closed-ended questions, which may or may not have predetermined answers. An example of a closed-ended question is "Do you consider yourself an evaluator?" which can be answered "Yes," "No," or "Not yet." Advantages of closed-ended questions are that they are often easier and quicker to ask and answer. A potential glitch is that someone who brings no knowledge can still answer the question, even if the person asking the question does not realize that; similarly, a person who does not understand the question can still likely provide a response. Furthermore, if there are preselected answers, the *actual* answer a person wants to give may not be a choice.

The evaluator can mix question types as needed. Finally, an evaluator can ask follow-up, open-ended questions to either an open- or closed-ended question, which are called *probes*. An example would be "Tell me, what makes you think that?"

Going to See the Intervention (Observation)

Observing the intervention can be a good way to begin to understand what the intervention does. Before an observation can take place, however, an evaluator will need to ask about and adhere to any applicable guidelines, such as obtaining ethical or legal permission, understanding what is culturally appropriate, and considering practical things such as determining appropriate times for visits. Observation can be done with a checklist that will provide focus (e.g., a set of closed-ended questions as described in the previous section); a partially structured guide that gives some guidance on what to observe, such as thematic areas (e.g., male–female interaction, use of cellphones); or an exploratory approach that provides no guidance (the evaluator uses just a blank journal or the electronic equivalent to take notes). Typically, an evaluator will observe how participants and staff interact, what the intervention does (e.g., tutoring, training), or how participants gain access to the intervention (e.g., is it near a bus stop or in a central location?), though observations can be broader. The chief advantage of observation is that it immerses the evaluator into the field, providing a sense of the intervention (e.g., its context and meaning) that often cannot be derived from interviews or document reviews. A disadvantage, however, is that when people know that an evaluator is coming, a different picture may be presented from what happens normally. In addition, observation can be costly and time-consuming.

Gathering and Organizing Data for a Nutshell Description

In interviews, when people respond, their words (their own or preselected ones) are called **data.** In the document review, the words and pictures gathered are also called *data*. In observation, what is observed is also called *data*. (For a reminder of the distinction between *data* and *information*, see Chapter 1, page 13.)

Here is one example of the steps to consider when you are starting an evaluation and you need to learn about an organization or an intervention. Visit the webpage or website (if one does not exist, move to the next step). See what kinds of program descriptions and documents exist. Then call the organization and ask for additional documents not currently on the website that would be useful in understanding the intervention. Give some examples from the list provided on page 41 (e.g., newspaper articles, quarterly reports, evaluation reports). Read the documents, and sketch a description of what is known thus far. Then write down any areas that need clarification, and use these to inform the interview questions. Share the questions with the organization (by phone or email); then ask who is best situated to answer these questions, and organize the interviews. The interviewees (also called *respondents*) may or may not be able to answer the questions. If not, that is fine; continue to ask the unanswered questions throughout the evaluative process. Your initial sketch of the intervention is what is called the *nutshell description* (defined in the next section). This is just one approach of many that can be used to grasp the initial understanding of what "it" is that we are seeking to monitor or evaluate.

The Nutshell Description

Synthesizing data from interviews, document reviews, and/or observation provides a broad initial understanding of the intervention, called a *nutshell description*. Such a description is needed to begin to understand what the intervention is aiming to accomplish, how it intends to accomplish that, where, when, and for whom. It is called a *nutshell description* because of its brevity; ideally, the description would fit into a proverbial peanut shell. In the early stages of the evaluative journey, it is not likely that all the intervention's details will be clear (and that is fine). For example, the funding document, a recent monitoring report, and several interviews may all suggest that the intervention aims to address troubled youth; however, the details are not consistent regarding exactly what is being done, or specifically for whom (e.g., the term *troubled youth* is not defined). Thus the nutshell description provides "enough" of an understanding about the intervention to enable the monitoring or evaluation process to move forward. A clearer, more detailed intervention description will iteratively emerge through the evaluative journey.

Identifying gaps, inconsistencies, or conflicting descriptions generates *clarifying questions* to be asked during the monitoring or evaluation process (questions the evaluator asks to clarify the intervention); the answers to these questions will then inform further interviews, document reviews, or observation. Exposing inconsistencies between stakeholders' perspectives and experiences can be particularly important to engaging with realities, as opposed to what is on paper. For instance, an evaluator could ask, "Your documents say that the intervention is aimed at troubled youth. However, my interview notes suggest that you only work with youth who have drug addictions. Can you tell me a bit more about the beneficiaries?" These kinds of details affect how and what to monitor and evaluate. For instance, both interventions may be aimed at youth who regularly skip school and have failing marks; however, one intervention would also address drug addictions, while the other intervention would not. Each intervention then suggests different kinds of results (some of which are likely to be overlapping), which will affect, for example, decisions about what to monitor and evaluate.

Depending on the timing of the evaluation process, the nutshell description may describe what the intervention is designed to achieve, what is happening, what did happen, or a mix of all three (i.e., some parts have been implemented while others have not). What follows is an example of a useful nutshell description for the girls' education intervention. This example is followed throughout the next several chapters.

> **Girls' Education Intervention: Nutshell Description**
>
> The intervention started 3 years ago and will be funded for 2 more years. It focuses on helping school-age girls access education that is freely given in their community. The intervention mostly focuses on convincing fathers who currently prevent their daughters from attending to support their daughters to get an education. Local knowledge suggests that fathers or father figures often prevent girls from attending school. The intervention also addresses some contextual issues, such as the safety of the girls as they go to and from school. The intervention's theory is based on literature drawn from education, development, and gender studies, as well as local cultural knowledge.

The purpose of the nutshell description is simply to provide a place to *start* a more in-depth conversation about the intervention. With the nutshell description in hand, we now seek to understand *why* the intervention exists. The answer or answers to that question almost always offer a gold mine of information to be used during the entire evaluative process.

INTRODUCING THE PROBLEM STATEMENT

Now that we have a very broad understanding of what the intervention is, we (the evaluators) need to understand the *reason* for the intervention. An activity, policy, program, or intervention is put in place for at least one reason. It exists to fix, improve, or otherwise change something, for someone. This "something" is labeled the **problem statement.** There may be one problem or multiple problems. It may be a well-documented problem or a hidden one. Furthermore, different people may describe the problem differently, based on their knowledge, experience, beliefs, or position in society. And some people may not describe it as a problem at all.

Uses for a Problem Statement

Although an evaluation journey can start in multiple places, addressing the problem statement always occurs near the beginning, as it provides a critical foundation for the evaluative process (and it may be the beginning of an evaluator's engagement if he has been asked to help inform the design of an intervention). There are four key uses for a well-researched and clearly written problem statement:

- *It informs how to design an intervention.* Since the intervention aims to fix the problem, whoever designs the intervention needs to know what to fix (improve, enhance, influence, or change).
- *It identifies how the intervention is relevant.* If someone asks a question about the relevance of an intervention, one answer lies in the problem statement: The intervention aims to produce results that fix an identified problem. This is what makes it relevant, and it is also how potential results are identified.
- *It identifies who aims to benefit.* You are probably thinking, "Relevant to whom?" The problem statement helps to clarify who, or what, is intended to benefit.
- *It clarifies what to assess.* When an evaluator is determining what to assess in terms of progress toward results or achievement of them, information is found in the problem statement because the intervention has aimed to fix something. If the problem is fixed or is moving toward being fixed, then the intervention is likely to have been effective (here, *effective* means that the intervention did what it aimed to do).

While these four areas (how to design an intervention, how the intervention is relevant, who aims to benefit, and what to assess) are further informed through other parts of the evaluative process, a good problem statement offers a useful place to start to find some answers (see Figure 3.1).

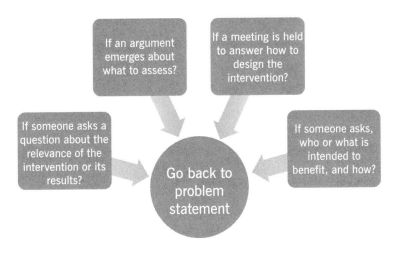

FIGURE 3.1. Problem statement: The questions it can answer.

When Labeling a Problem Statement Can Be a Problem

Sometimes a challenge to working with a problem statement is its label. Sometimes the word *problem* can be found to be abrasive or too negative. When people find the word offensive, it can become a problem in itself—mostly because when people are offended or uncomfortable, they tend to focus on the word they do not like, instead of answering the gist of a question. Thus the question does not get answered. Also, offending a person through word choice does not encourage a person to engage with you. In fact, having a person shut down in the first part of an evaluative process is likely to have a ripple effect throughout, particularly if that individual is in any way influential in the process. (To read more on language, see Chapter 13.) If the word *problem* is not appropriate, do not use it; simply substitute another word, such as *challenge*. For an evaluation to be useful, reflect constantly on how to choose words and frame questions to make the best fit with your clients, stakeholders, beneficiaries, or other actors (for more discussion of these words, jump ahead to pages 60–61). What is defined in this chapter as a *problem statement* can be relabeled to be more culturally or contextually appropriate; it is the information under the label that matters. If the label offends, replace it. Words matter.

Words Matter

How we communicate matters, what we say, and how we say it. Something we say in one situation may be appropriate, and in another it may be offensive or just confusing. Changing a word or a sentence, or an accent or emphasis on a word in a sentence, may elicit a completely different response. A colleague sent me a link to a YouTube video that provides a striking illustration of how words matter (*www.youtube.com/watch?v=WgiOt2ap-us&feature=youtu.be*).

Identifying the Problem Statement: The Questions to Ask

Now that we know what makes the problem statement useful, and now that we realize we can call it something else if that is helpful, let's talk about how to identify one. An evaluator can ask one or more of the following questions, which are all variations of the same question, to initiate the problem statement conversation:

- What is the problem that the intervention aims to address?
- What does the intervention intend to fix, change, or improve?
- Tell me about the reasons the intervention was developed.
- What gap (or gaps) was this intervention intended to fill?

BOX 3.2. Answering Questions or Asking Them?

Answering evaluation questions is often what evaluators are asked to do—yet knowing how, what, when, where, why, and with whom to ask good questions is an essential part of being an evaluator. Throughout the book, I provide examples of questions that can be used to elicit information. However, these questions will need to be modified, adapted, or otherwise cultivated to support each unique evaluation journey. For example, you may need to use words that may be more specific or more appropriate to the context, or to change the wording of a question from present to past (or past to present) tense. Or you may need to change the common noun (e.g., *intervention*) to the most appropriate one (e.g., *program, organization, policy, activity*).

These questions can be explored by using data-gathering techniques similar to the ones used to generate the nutshell description: document reviews, interviews, observation, or all three. If the questions are used to guide an interview, consider carefully how each question is worded. These questions are written as open-ended questions, meaning that they are intended to encourage wide-ranging responses. Unless you have narrowed down the answers needed, or you only require brief answers, avoid asking closed-ended questions. At this stage in the process, you will want to encourage an in-depth discussion about the problem statement because there is so much to learn about one, and from one.

Sometimes the four questions listed on the previous page may not elicit useful responses (i.e., data). If this happens, consider one (if not more) of the following options, which take different approaches to identifying the same information.

- Your organization/intervention exists because . . . ? (Rather than have someone answer a question, have the person complete a sentence.)

- Can you tell me a bit more about the background of this intervention? (Asking for a general history often encourages a nice, easy dialogue.)

- In the next 5 years, what do you expect to see change or improve, or just be different, because of the intervention? (A time frame sometimes helps people focus.)

- Tell me a bit more about what makes the intervention critical or necessary. Who thinks this? What makes them think that? (A more informal and general conversational approach may be helpful.)

- What do those of you involved in the intervention want to accomplish? (The person states what they want to achieve. You then take the answer, and restate the flip side or opposite of that, and it becomes the problem. I demonstrate this "reverse" tactic a bit later in this chapter.)

These questions can be mixed with the first set of questions; each set is not exclusive. At this point in the process, a problem of any size can be identified; this is the starting point of the conversation. These questions can be supplemented with probes as needed, such as "What makes you think that?" or "Can you tell me a bit more?"

Different-Sized Problems: Breaking Down the Problem Statement

The problem statement can (and should) be separated into two categories: the **grand problem(s)** and **pocket problems.** The words are not intended as labels per se. Rather, they are organizing concepts to guide a discussion that will allow an evaluator to explore how an intervention addresses *what* problem, which then leads to *what* specific, intended result. Eventually, the process will link the problem statement to the intervention to the results, all at the same levels (i.e., a grand problem is linked to a grand result; a pocket problem is linked to a pocket result). I describe the process in an iterative manner in Chapters 4–10. Here we are starting to lay the groundwork.

The Grand Problem

The grand problem is the larger problem, such as gender violence, pollution, or obesity. Sometimes it can be described at a lower level or with more specificity, such as "Children have poor nutrition in Town G." In other words, the grand problem is the largest problem the intervention is aiming to address, put a dent in, or use as the "guiding light" (the light that all can see, yet realize that it may not be reached in the foreseeable future).

The Pocket Problems

All the pocket problems, when combined, form the grand problem; the reverse is also true (i.e., the grand problem can be broken down into the pocket problems). Figure 3.2 shows an example. The pocket problems can be broken down further into mini-sized ones if we continue to ask the never-ending "why" questions (e.g., in the Figure 3.2 example, "Why do few healthy food choices exist in the elementary school?"). Essentially, the problem statement needs to be broken down as far as needed to inform these three kinds of understanding:

- *Before implementation.* To understand how to design the intervention so that it addresses specific problems, and in doing so to identify where expected results will happen, and for whom.

- *After implementation.* To understand why the intervention did what it did, where, and for whom.

- *After implementation.* To understand why the intervention had (or did not have) the results it did, where, and for whom.

Additional information gathered throughout the evaluative process will also inform these understandings. In addition, how an evaluator engages with and uses the problem statement will vary, depending on when she enters the process: either forward-looking (planning an evaluable intervention), in the moment (as when supporting innovation), or backward-looking (evaluation).

BOX 3.3. Using Pocket and Grand Problems

When people respond to initial questioning about the problem statement with a grand problem, ask questions to break the grand problem down into pocket problems. If they respond with a pocket problem, build the pocket problems up to a grand problem. This is an iterative process, and the discussion is likely to go back and forth between the two. In the process, gaps may be identified, such as when the pocket problems do not build up to the grand problem, or there is no awareness of what pocket problems form the grand one. These are all part of the evaluative findings.

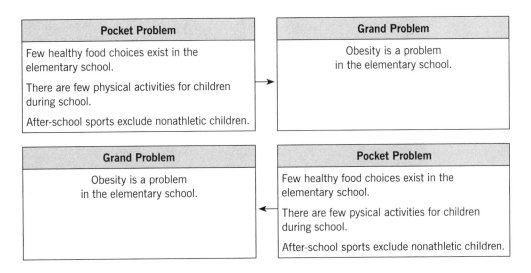

FIGURE 3.2. Pocket and grand problems.

There are no concrete definitions of grand and pocket problems, or even specific ways to write them; the terms are not intended to constitute a formula or to be used to squish problems into a predetermined check/tick box. Rather, what is offered is a loosely structured way of thinking. The thinking allows a person to conceptualize, explore, and facilitate a detailed discussion that organizes thoughts on how, and which, problems are addressed by what parts of an intervention, and how all this relates to intended (and/or actual) results. If this approach seems a bit messy, or if it is not clear how it is used in practice, skip ahead to Chapter 6 to see the concepts in action—then come right back.

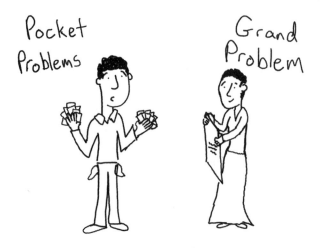

A warning is in order at this point: Do not rush to finalize the problem statement. The fluid evaluation process systematically, iteratively, and repeatedly interrogates it, and in doing so, identifies the pocket and grand problems, which creates a strong foundation for any type of planning, monitoring, or evaluation. To refer to Aesop's fable of the Tortoise and the Hare (see "A Conversation with My Readers" at the start of the book), the evaluator's aim is to be the Tortoise, not the Hare—that is, to win the race with slow, steady effort. With that in mind, let's explore the problem statement from a slightly different perspective (which may overlap with the one we have just discussed, or may bring new insights): separating what causes the problem from what is a symptom of that cause. Knowing the difference, and then clearly identifying which (if not both) the intervention aims to address, will influence expected results and help determine what to assess. Curious? Read on.

BOX 3.4. A Problem Statement, Revisited

An intervention addresses something that someone considers a challenge, a problem, or something that needs improvement, fixing, or change. A statement summarizing that "something" is called a *problem statement*, which is made up of *grand* and *pocket problems*. We evaluate interventions to see whether, or to what extent, how, and for whom the intervention has addressed (or is currently addressing) the entire problem statement, or just elements of it.

Clarifying Different Kinds of Problems, and Why It Matters

We have just noted that the problem statement has two parts: grand and pocket problems. Once those are established (or sometimes as they are being established), another perspective provides useful information: identifying whether the problem is a root cause or a symptom of that cause.

Distinguishing the Root Cause versus a Symptom

Here is an example of a root cause versus a symptom. Sometimes I have a headache. I take some aspirin, and the headache goes away. Maybe it never comes back. Maybe it does. Maybe the headache is a sign of a lack of caffeine, which is the sign of another problem (drinking copious amounts of caffeinated coffee or black tea and caffeinated diet soda can cause a caffeine addiction). Or maybe the headache is a sign that I need stronger reading glasses. Or maybe it is a sign of something more serious.

Let's say that I have another headache. Someone gives me one bottle of aspirin. When I take my aspirin, I have no headache. If I were asked at that point in time, "Does the intervention work?", my answer would be a gleeful yes. Problem solved. Or is it? When I run out of aspirin, my headache returns. Sometimes treating the symptoms (removing the pain) will not have longer-term intended results because it has not addressed the real reason (root cause) for the pain. Furthermore, the headache may result from multiple root causes, such as a need for glasses *and* a lack of caffeine. For now, let's keep it simple and assume one root cause; then I will complicate it.

Let's say the person who gives the aspirin to me digs a little deeper about the cause of my headache before he provides an intervention. Perhaps he then identifies the root cause (caffeine addiction), and provides an intervention to cure my caffeine addiction. During the intervention, the headaches grow worse (they need to get worse before they get better). If there is an evaluation at that time, I probably will provide negative feedback. And furthermore, if the funding is stopped at that point (e.g., because the evaluation says the intervention is not working), I will still have headaches, and likely my caffeine addiction as well. However, let's now say that when the intervention is fully implemented, it solves my addiction (I now drink herbal tea) and achieves my intended longer-term results of not having headaches. Now let's add back in the more complicated situation mentioned above—that the headaches are results of multiple root causes (not only a caffeine addiction, but also a need for glasses). And this is where evaluation becomes a bit more complicated. There may be no result from my drinking herbal tea and breaking my addiction because another root cause needs to be addressed at the same time (the root problem being reading without proper glasses). Problems can be simple to address, or they can be complicated, and that is why they need to be broken down to be understood.

Assumption Infestations

Beware: Discussions that clarify root causes and symptoms can be infested with assumptions. See Chapter 4 for an in-depth look at assumptions and facts and their importance to the entire evaluation process.

There are two lessons in the headache example.

1. When an evaluator is informing the design of an intervention (forward-looking) or conducting an evaluation (backward-looking) she needs to clarify what the intervention is aimed to change, fix, or otherwise address: root cause(s), symptom(s), or both.

2. The evaluator needs to identify at what point the evaluation happens during the intervention's implementation. This second lesson is only foreshadowed here; it is discussed more fully in Chapter 6.

Why is knowing that the root cause has not been identified, or maybe just not addressed, or that only symptoms have been addressed, important for evaluators?

Identifying the root cause and symptoms can be useful to an evaluation process for two reasons:

- *The discussion of root cause and symptoms clarifies the intended results.* Knowing which problem the intervention is aimed to address clarifies the expected results. As such, it provides insight (not often *the* answer, but insight) into what to monitor and evaluate in order to understand if results happened, or why intended results did not happen.

- *It provides insight into questions on sustainability. Sustainability* is a "suitcase word" of note (i.e., it needs to be unpacked). For more on suitcase words, their dangers, and how to mitigate them, skip ahead to pages 138–140, and we dig into the concept of sustainability in Chapter 7. The key point here is that the discussion about root causes and symptoms generates a wealth of information that may support at least part of an explanation as to why something is sustained (it addresses a root cause) or is not sustained (it addresses a symptom).

Looking for the root causes and symptoms of a problem, and which of these the intervention aims (or aimed) to address, should be on your radar screen.

Avoiding the "Why" Question by Asking a "What" Question

Starting a question with "Why" can be difficult to answer, as it is essentially asking a theoretical question. Switching the "Why" to a "What" allows for a more concrete descriptive answer. Paula Bilinsky, an evaluator who introduced me to evaluation, once told me, "It is often better to handle a 'why' question with a 'what' question." For example, if you want to know why a person is attending a program, it can be challenging for many to answer the question "Why are you here today?" Asking the person, "What made you choose to come to this program today?" is likely to result in more concrete answers, as it is a more direct question.

Why—I mean, what are some examples of what happens when an evaluator identifies that the intervention is not addressing, or has not addressed, the root cause?

Consider these three evaluation scenarios in which the evaluator identifies that the intervention has not addressed the root cause, and notice how that influences evaluation use.

1. *Evaluation finding is used.* The implementer is aware that the initial research used to design the intervention was poorly done. Although the symptom was addressed, and results have been achieved, the implementer is concerned about the potential of the result lasting (the sustainability of the effect). The implementer welcomes the evaluator and his finding that the intervention has not addressed the root cause, and uses that information to make substantive changes to the intervention. Thus the evaluation is used to influence the intervention.

2. *Evaluation finding is rejected.* The program implementer has effectively addressed a symptom that is of critical importance to the donor, and has achieved the intended results. The evaluation, however, shows that the root cause was not addressed, and therefore there is a high probability that the results will not last. Both the implementer and the donor reject that evaluation finding and claim success. No changes are made to the intervention.

3. *Evaluation finding is quietly ignored.* The implementer has been under tremendous political pressure to "get going and get results." The evaluation finding that the symptoms are being addressed but not the root cause is of little interest to the implementer, who is dealing with continuing pressure to keep moving ahead. The report is shelved.

Even when an evaluator understands the importance of addressing the root cause, or at the very least of knowing that the root cause is not being addressed, evaluation clients may not bring the same appreciation. It happens. At the same time, the evaluation may be very much appreciated, and provide useful information that is used to inform the program.

Our intervention has been implemented extremely well, but the results are dismal. Could something be wrong with the problem statement?

Absolutely. There could be many reasons why the results are dismal, which should be explored (see Chapters 4–8 and 12–13 for additional potential reasons). However, for now, let's look at some common ways a problem statement may contribute to poor or unexpected results.

- *The problem statement only addresses one key root cause, when several exist.* See the headache example starting on page 51. If only one key root cause is addressed, but not the others, there may be no, or few, intended results identified.

- *One or more pocket problems did not exist when the intervention was designed.* Another reason is that at least one new pocket problem has arisen since the intervention was designed. This is often quite likely, considering that communities, people, politics, policies, or other **variables** (i.e., things that can change) may be constantly changing. For example, while childhood obesity may have been a problem 5 years ago and remains a problem today, the pocket problems, or the factors causing obesity in children, may now be different. In other words, what was *not* a problem 5 years ago may be a problem today, which then influences the intervention's ability to achieve the intended results (i.e., it is likely the wrong intervention).

It seems like asking questions about the intervention and developing the problem statement are good places to start an evaluative journey. However, these are not the questions I am usually asked at the start. In fact, no one has ever asked me to sort out the problem statement. My clients usually ask me to "just" assess results and the effectiveness of their intervention. Can you explain a bit more how to convince my clients that I need to clarify the problem statement?

Even when your clients, boss, or colleagues ask you to start in a different place, such as assessing results or identifying indicators (indicators are explained in Chapter 9), an evaluator first needs to have a basic understanding of the intervention and of what problem it aims to address. Rushing forward and trying to assess results, and linking those results to the intervention without first understanding how the intervention is linked to a problem, are likely to be challenging if not impossible. After acknowledging your clients' needs, explain the following logic (you may want to jump to Chapter 4 to read about facts and assumptions before using the following example):

A problem statement describes what needs to be fixed, changed, or improved (it is a fact). An intervention is implemented to fix it (it is an assumption, sometimes with a few facts mixed in). If the intervention works, it will have intended results (assumptions) and perhaps unintended ones. The results should erase the problem statement, or at least put a dent in it. Thus, to understand if the intervention is effective, we first need to understand what the problem is, how the intervention aimed to influence that, and what results were expected. Understanding each of these three items informs assessment decisions—and, indeed, a monitoring framework and evaluation design.

A follow-up to that suggestion is to select one or several of the questions listed earlier in this chapter (see page 47) and engage in a discussion. For example, "Tell me a bit more about what makes the intervention critical or necessary. Who thinks this? What makes them think that?" The responses to those questions may start the necessary conversation that leads to exploring the need for a clear problem statement.

I would be remiss not to mention other real-world possibilities for engaging in problem statement discussions. Challenges may arise when an intervention has been aimed to fulfill a political or personal agenda, "fit" within what the donor wants to do, or spend down a budget, and has never been intended to address a fact-based social problem. (A problem statement needs to be fact-based, not an assumption of a fact. As noted above, to read about the need for fact-based problem statements, go to Chapter 4.)

Wait. What if I find out that the reason for the intervention is to fulfill a political or personal agenda, fit what a donor wants to do, or spend down a budget, and I need to conduct an evaluation? What happens then?

This is a tricky situation, that's for sure. Let me provide some guidance. First, tread carefully. Second, just being aware is beneficial, as it helps you to navigate the situation. Third, consider how the evaluation *process* may be useful to someone, at some point, in some way. This is called process use. To understand more about and engage with evaluation process use, see page 229. Fourth, realize that even if the intervention was to fulfill a political agenda, for example, it may still be an intervention that aimed to do some good for something or someone, and would benefit from evaluation; or maybe not.

Admittedly, the proverbial monkey wrench is thrown into the process when the real reason for the intervention is based purely on a political or personal agenda. Even so, engaging in reality, and knowing that other reasons can exist, can bring useful insight to the evaluative process. Here is an example.

A small town (let's call it Town A) has well-maintained primary schools that have consistently good academic results. Town A is affluent. The adjacent town, Town B, lies within the same political zone (i.e., the same elected officials represent both areas). However, Town B schools have consistently poor primary school results, specifically in math and science. Most families in Town B live at or just below the poverty line. The government provides a free math and science tutoring program in Town B. Residents of Town A hear about the program and demand the same intervention for their town, where most children score average or above average on the same exams. The officials, who are concerned with re-election, decide to provide Town A with the same academic program. An evaluator is asked to evaluate the intervention (with no knowledge of these circumstances). While he finds no significant academic improvement in Town A, in Town B he identifies substantial increases in math and science scores. He may conclude that the intervention has worked in Town B but not in Town A, or that it is not necessary in Town A, and recommend that the intervention only receive further funding for Town B. Uh-oh.

Imagine, however, that the evaluator stops and asks this question: What problem did the intervention intend to address? He finds out that in Town A, the intervention has been provided to solve a political problem, and in Town B, it has been aimed to address an educational one. What *needs* to be evaluated is if Town A residents have been pleased to receive the intervention, and if so, whether they have voted for their local representative to serve another term. After all, in Town A that has been the intervention's actual goal. What is assessed in Town B should remain the same: measuring the math and science achievement of targeted children. In the real world, it is highly unlikely that an evaluation will assess how people from Town A vote, and link that to the intervention; however, knowing that alternative reasons exist for an intervention to exist (as opposed to an actual social problem) will keep an evaluator sane when he exhausts all other logical reasons, or his recommendations are rejected. (Cut funding from Town A? Um. No.) All I can say is that it is the real world out there, people, and not sweeping reality under the rug is one of the many tough aspects of being a good evaluator.

Who does the problem identification, and who does the rest of the evaluative process— the researcher, evaluator, program manager, or someone else?

Here is a very nice example of how a researcher, evaluator, and program manager can work together in harmony, which elaborates on our discussion in Chapters 1 and 2. The researcher (or the evaluator, using her research skills) identifies the problem that needs to be addressed through using a research design that provides facts; the program manager reviews these facts and designs the intervention to address one or all of the problems, noting specific results for certain people, animals, or the environment. The evaluator works with the program manager to ensure that the intervention is evaluable, and identifies the criteria that will be used to determine the intervention's value, merit, and worth. In rare cases, the three roles may be performed by one person. In more common scenarios, each role is carried out by multiple people. Note, however, that the evaluator often arrives after the problem is identified, and often after the initial intervention is designed (though not always).

I thought that the place to start engaging in an evaluation process was to focus on the intervention's theory. Can I start there instead?

Sometimes people consider the starting place of an evaluative journey to be discussing the program's theory. I find that a more difficult and less tangible place to start. The main problem is that it *is* theory—which often does not provide a concrete enough starting place for the evaluator or for those with whom she needs to engage. Rather than discussing program theory first, I focus on untangling the logic (which is what we are doing here in this chapter, starting with the problem statement), which then provides a scaffolding for a move to a theory discussion (the process is still iterative, though; discussion on theory is just brought in later). To learn more about (and be able to facilitate a concise discussion of) theory and logic, or if you would like to start an evaluation journey by discussing intervention or program theory, please jump ahead to Chapter 8. For now, let's look at the evaluator's role in facilitating and describing the problem statement.

The Evaluator's Role

The evaluator can fill many different roles with regard to the problem statement. If she is there when the intervention is conceptualized, she can play an active role in identifying and confirming that there is indeed a problem. If she arrives after the intervention is designed or implemented, she can then facilitate a process to identify the grand problem and then unpack it into pocket problems, or the reverse. Sometimes the evaluator must sort out what the intervention is aiming to address on her own, or with her team, often through a document review. Regardless of the process, remember that an iterative interplay exists among the discussions of the problem statement, intervention, and results, and that each discussion helps to clarify and refine the others. While facilitation skills prove useful in this process, logical thinking and patience are necessities.

> ### BOX 3.5. Facilitation
>
> If you are using this book to learn about working in the field of evaluation, or to guide self-reflection, then facilitation skills are not yet needed. If you are using this book to engage others in an evaluative process or teach others about being an evaluator, then facilitation becomes a critical skill. Facilitation skills are developed over time, and are not something that one can learn effectively in an afternoon, in one course, or by reading a book. Strong facilitation skills demand a combination of reading, practice in a variety of settings, and self-reflection.

Learning to Be a Facilitator

If you know someone who is a good facilitator, ask to observe him in action. If you know more than one facilitator, this is even better, as different people have different facilitation styles, processes, and games. Observe, practice, reflect, observe, and practice again. If you are not fortunate enough to know at least one good facilitator, think back to a well-facilitated class, workshop, or seminar: What made the facilitation strong? What did not go well? How would you do it differently? Then practice, reflect, and practice some more.

FACILITATION

- *Have a minute?* Take a look at the website of the International Association of Facilitators (*www.iaf-world.org/site/index.php*), which provides various types of resources.

- *Have several hours?* If your interest is deeper, consider reading *Facilitating Evaluation: Principles in Practice* by Michael Quinn Patton (2018a).

- *Want to have some fun?* Check out Chris Lysy's blog (*https://freshspectrum.com/blog*), where he provides cartoons depicting everyday evaluation conversations that bring touches of levity to facilitating evaluation processes.

The world is messy. Where I work, defining what my intervention is attempting to change is complicated. I see problems (and other influences) all over the place that likely affect what my intervention is trying to address and achieve. What about those other problems and influences? How do I sort this out, in terms of monitoring and evaluation?

The world indeed seems *simple* at times, *complicated* at other times, and *complex* at still others. These terms are associated with the Cynefin framework, which includes two more categories, *chaos* and *disorder* (Kurz & Snowden, 2003). Using these words brings in language that specifically acknowledges systems thinking in evaluation, and thus addresses the issue raised in your first statement: The world is a messy place. The evaluative process described in this book provides one basic starting place for understanding an intervention, what it aims to achieve, and what can influence it. The process slowly builds, and eventually different elements that complicate the world around us are added and bring the needed level of complexity to the discussion. We will get there, all in good time. When faced with a complex or complicated problem, I often feel overwhelmed (which throws my brain into chaos and disorder), and thus I break down the evaluative process so that it is graspable (before I have a breakdown myself). I begin just by trying to simplify, clarify, and focus. And then, and only then, do I start to bring in the complexities that I need to engage with, in order to understand what else may be influencing the program and its results.

I have just mentioned the usefulness of the Cynefin framework. I recommend an article by Snowden and Boone (2007) on applying the Cynefin framework, where they provide real-life examples of its usefulness. Two other great thinkers in the systems field are Donella Meadows (*http://donellameadows.org*), whose approach to systems is user-friendly and easily accessible, and Bob Williams (*www.bobwilliams.co.nz*).

The perception of a problem can be just as much of a problem as the problem itself, right?

The perception of a problem is indeed a problem to be discussed. However, exploring people's perceptions is different from engaging with what they perceive to be a problem. Clear as mud? If there is a fact-based problem that girls do not go to school because they do not have access to school uniforms, then one intervention would be to provide the uniforms. However, if that is only a perception (it is not actually true, people just think that), then providing the uniforms will not solve the problem (because the intervention is addressing a perception of a problem). In this case, an evaluator needs to find out why that perception exists and address that perception. An evaluator needs to know how, or to what extent, that perception has the potential to negatively affect the intervention or its results.

Is a situational analysis the same the thing as identifying a problem statement, or a root cause and symptoms?

A situational analysis is often broader than simply identifying a problem statement. A *situational analysis* is a process that looks at a situation to understand what is happening, why, and what needs to be addressed. The analysis helps to ensure an intervention's relevance. There are several elements to a situational analysis:

- Defining the extent of the problem in that context.
- Identifying the perceptions and experiences of key stakeholders in relation to the problem.
- Identifying what already exists to address the problem, and the gaps in those already existing strategies and/or interventions.
- Identifying possible partners.

Ask if a situational analysis was done at any point in time, as it has the potential to provide a wealth of data for any evaluative process.

Wait, what about a needs assessment? What is that?

A needs assessment identifies what is needed by a specific group of people, is used in many professions, and can be conducted via many different methods. For example, a needs assessment can be used to identify what specific knowledge and skills exist, and what skills and knowledge are needed, thus identifying the gaps where training needs to take place. Needs assessments are also conducted in a broader sense, for determining what the needs are, for example, in a community. See below for further reading.

BOX 3.6. The Reasons for Developing a Clear Problem Statement

Without an exact understanding of what an intervention is trying to change, address, fix, or make better, it is nearly impossible to be clear about anything else in the evaluative process. A clear problem statement, and the facts that support the statement, are vital for designing and focusing a relevant intervention, for assessing its progress toward or achievement of results (or lack thereof), and for understanding who is intended to benefit.

We now have a *general* idea of what the intervention is (nutshell description) and a general understanding of why the intervention exists (problem statement). We now need to understand who (person) or what (place or thing) is intended to benefit or in some way receive services from the intervention.

USEFUL TOOLS FOR IDENTIFYING ROOT CAUSES

- *Have a few minutes?* Check out this summary of the Five Whys tool (*www.betterevaluation.org/en/evaluation-options/five_whys*).

- *Have a few hours?* Check out what is called the *fishbone* or *herringbone* analysis, among other names (*www.mindtools.com/pages/article/newTMC_03.htm*).

- *Have a day?* Use one of these two websites to work through an example; each one provides guidance in a step-by-step process (*http://web.mit.edu/urbanupgrading/upgrading/issues-tools/tools/problem-tree.html* or *www.sswm.info/content/problem-tree-analysis*).

- *Have a few hours a night?* If you are interested in learning more about needs assessments, check out this online publication: *A Guide to Assessing Needs: Essential Tools for Collecting Information, Making Decisions, and Achieving Development Results* by Ryan Watkins, Maurya West Meiers, and Yusra Laila Visser (2012; go to *www.openknowledge.worldbank.org/handle/10986/2231*).

INTRODUCING BENEFICIARIES AND SIX RELATED TERMS

Beneficiaries is a common term for the persons or groups an intervention is intended to benefit. **Stakeholders** are not necessarily beneficiaries, but can be. Stakeholders are literally those who have a "stake" in the intervention and its results; in other words, the intervention and its results matter to them, in some way, for some reason. Stakeholders may or may not benefit, directly or indirectly. *A beneficiary is always a*

stakeholder; however, a stakeholder is not always a beneficiary. Stakeholders can be powerful allies or detractors in an evaluative process, or even nonentities (although this is unlikely). A **gatekeeper** is someone who has the power to block or influence access to information, people, or places; a gatekeeper can be either a stakeholder or a person who is not obviously or directly related to the intervention or evaluation. Another related term you may hear is **audience.** An audience is anyone likely to use the evaluation. The reality on the ground is that most often beneficiaries are the least likely group to read an evaluation report and use it; often the donor, manager, or implementer will use the evaluation findings to inform the intervention, which then affects the beneficiaries, though there are definitely exceptions. Knowing the audience informs how to communicate the evaluation findings. The audience is sometimes a **client,** and the term *client* is most often referring to those who commissioned the evaluation. The person who commissioned the evaluation can be called the **commissioner.** The term **actor** can also be used, particularly in evaluations that draw on a systems approach. *Actor* is an encompassing term that includes those who are interested in or likely to influence the intervention and its findings, and it can refer to more than people, such as the economy or a policy. An evaluator needs to know whom the intervention is intended to benefit; who has a stake in, or is interested in, the evaluation process and/or its findings; and who needs what information communicated to them in what way, for what reason, when, and how. For now, let's get back to discussing beneficiaries.

FOCUSING ON THE INTENDED BENEFICIARIES

The entire reason why an intervention exists is to make something better for someone or something. Thus "Who or what is going to benefit from the intervention, and in what way?" is a pretty darn important question.

When you are reading through documents or conducting interviews, ask three questions (see Figure 3.3):

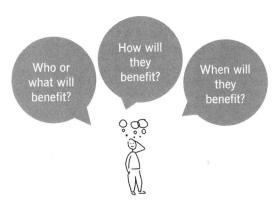

FIGURE 3.3. Considering who or what benefits.

- Who or what will benefit from the intervention?
- How will they benefit?
- When will they benefit?

The answers to these questions will provide insight into the relevance of each part of the intervention. More specifically, the answers provide information that further elaborates on the problem statement, the intervention, and the results.

- *The problem statement.* The answers to these questions identify who thinks the problem is a problem for whom. (This provides insight into who values what.)
- *The intervention.* The answers illuminate who is intended to benefit from what parts of the intervention, and how. (This conveys insight into how to design the intervention.)
- *The results.* The answers sort out who (e.g., a person or group of people) or what (e.g., a forest or an animal shelter) is intended to benefit from the intervention in what way (how does who or what benefit) and when that is intended to take place. This further clarifies the intended results (see Chapter 7 for a specific discussion of results).

Defining the Intended Beneficiaries

When evaluators ask who (or what) are the intended beneficiaries, people often tend at first to give very broad answers, listing groups or thematic areas like "children," "the environment," or "animals." It is important to probe the answer and gather as much descriptive, specific detail as possible. When "something" (or anything) is being evaluated, the more specific the "something" can be made, the clearer it becomes *what* to assess and *where* to gather information, and the lower the chances for misunderstandings become. For example, if the thematic answer is that children will benefit, probe for a bit more detail: Children who live where? What age groups? Children with siblings? Children with single parents? *These kinds of differences are important—to the beneficiaries, the design and implementation of an intervention, its intended results, how they are valued, and what to evaluate.* For this reason, the conversation should end with a rather precise (e.g., "children under the age of 12 who have unemployed parents and live under the poverty line"), and less thematic (e.g., "vulnerable children"), understanding of the beneficiary group(s). Information on the beneficiaries critically informs every part of the evaluative process.

When who or what is intended to benefit is made clear (there may be several groups of beneficiaries), there are three important follow-up questions to ask:

1. Who decided, and what process was used to decide, who are the intended beneficiaries?

2. How, if at all, were the beneficiaries involved in this decision?

3. What were the challenges or disagreements, if any, with regard to who would benefit and who would not?

These questions bring to the surface information about values, politics, and power—information that will guide what and how to monitor, how to design the evaluation, and how to interpret and value the findings. Here is an example of how engaging with potential beneficiaries influences an understanding of relevance and valuing in an evaluative process. Group R and Group G live in neighboring communities, have similar demographics (the word *demographics* means the characteristics of a group, such as economic status or age), and have received the same intervention. Group R finds the results of the intervention (how they benefitted) to be useful and important (relevant). Group G does not consider the benefits relevant; instead, it views them as nice to have, but not necessary. What can account for these two very different experiences of the intervention? It emerges that before the intervention started, several potential beneficiaries from Group R were asked what they needed or wanted, and a close version of that was provided. Potential beneficiaries from Group G were never consulted. Not being involved in any part of the decision to have an intervention, the shape of it, or its intended results may have resulted in Group G's feeling left out, alienated, or perhaps miffed; hence its members' response. Or maybe a more obvious reason is that because Group G was not consulted, perhaps the intervention did not meet Group G's needs.

Direct and Indirect Beneficiaries: The Barking Dog Example

In the evaluation process, there are typically two categories of beneficiaries: **direct** and **indirect,** sometimes called **primary** and **secondary.** An intervention should have clearly stated direct beneficiaries, and an idea of indirect or secondary ones, which may include persons, animals, places, or things (e.g., children, horses, a forest). Simply put, when a dog is barking nonstop because he is bored (the problem being that the dog is bored), and someone gives him a ball to play with, the dog is the direct beneficiary. The neighbor who has been annoyed by this barking is the secondary beneficiary—meaning that the neighbor does not benefit directly from the ball (the dog does), but they benefit in that the neighborhood is now quiet. Who is the direct beneficiary gets a bit tricky with a slight change to the orientation of the problem. Let's say that the problem is not about the dog's being bored; the problem is that two neighbors have a poor relationship. The dog's barking is just one smaller, pocket problem that has contributed to the poor relationship; the barking dog is not the *only* problem. So when the dog gets the ball and stops barking, the canine-free neighbor is now less annoyed with the dog-owning neighbor, which contributes to a better relationship. The happy, quiet dog is still a beneficiary (he receives the ball), but the neighbors are the primary beneficiaries of the quiet dog. The neighborhood is the indirect beneficiary, as it benefits when neighbors have strong relationships. Problem statements matter. Beneficiaries matter. Perspectives matter.

*Once I worked with an organization that did not like the word **beneficiary**. What then?*

The term *beneficiary* may be a loaded term and should not be used in situations where it brings a negative or uncomfortable meaning. I once had a similar experience where I worked with an organization in which the term *beneficiaries* suggested that a person was passive in receiving something, not an active participant in the process or service. Select a term that is culturally appropriate and acceptable to the organization with which, and the location or context where, you are working.

Eschewing Homogeneity and Examining Heterogeneity

Men are not all the same. Some are married and some are not; some are poor and some are not; and some are well educated and old, and some are young and disabled. Not all young, disabled men are the same; some are sight-impaired, while others have other disabilities. Not even all sight-impaired young men are the same: Some were born blind, some became blind through a degenerative disorder, and some became blind after an accident. A key lesson to remember is that *every difference creates a difference,* and those differences should influence the intervention's design, its implementation, its results, and the ways the results are assessed and valued. In scholastic terms, examining differences is referred to as looking at **heterogeneity** (*hetero-* means "different"); in other words, it is exploring diversity.

The next time you are in a yoga class, a supermarket, a café, or a doctor's office, look around and identify someone who initially seems like you in some basic ways, such as gender, age, height, weight, and race. Then stop and think: In how many ways is it possible that the person is different from you—ways that would make a difference to how they benefitted and valued the same service? What might they value more? Less?

While every difference makes a difference—a way of thinking attributed to Gregory Bateson (1972)—it does not mean that an intervention must necessarily be individualized for each person's circumstances (though it can be). For the evaluator of an intervention, understanding how differences influence people who were assumed to be homogeneous but were not (e.g., school-age girls, forest rangers, athletes, homeless youth) can provide explanations for why an intervention was more effective for certain people, or valued more, or valued less, by different people all assumed to be part of the "same" group. In evaluation, something is valued, and there needs to be an understanding of the source from which these values stem. While Chapter 12 covers values, and Chapters 14 and 15 talk about how different evaluation approaches involve different values, here we focus on how beneficiaries' values and perceptions of the intervention provide one of the more critical places to look for *how* to understand and value a result.

Let's go back to our girls' education intervention. The direct beneficiaries are the school-age girls who currently do not attend school. In how many ways might those girls be different, and how many of these ways would potentially influence the effectiveness of the intervention and how those girls perceive it? Some examples with the potential to make a difference may include girls who have supportive mothers or other supportive males in the family (but not their fathers), girls who want to go to school, or girls who have brothers who go to school.

Who or What Can Be Damaged or Hurt by the Intervention?

A critical, yet often forgotten group consists of those who can be hurt, damaged, or negatively influenced by an intervention, while others (potentially or actually) benefit. To explore who or what (e.g., the rhinos, the environment) might be in this group, consider asking one, if not all three, of the following questions:

- Who or what can be harmed, hurt, upset, or damaged by the intervention?
- Who or what may have diminished power, benefits, or access to resources as a result of the intervention?
- Who thinks the intervention is damaging in some way, regardless of whether or not it is a reality (perceptions)?

Oddly, evaluation theories, models, and frameworks do not provide a specific term to describe persons, places, or things that can be potentially hurt, damaged or intentionally forgotten by the intervention. Not providing a term ignores the importance of understanding one of the more critical aspects in evaluation (and in society). As critical as it is to know who benefits, it is as critical to know who does not, and even more critical to know who is ignored, damaged, or hurt by an intervention. Perhaps we can call them the *un-beneficiaries*. The knowledge of who or what can be harmed, upset, or damaged by an intervention can broaden the insights of a program implementer or designer, which can lead to changing the intervention or mitigating potentially unpleasant situations. For the evaluator, the information regarding who or what may be un-beneficiaries can be obtained from data that explains implementation challenges, unexpected results, or negative findings, such as data on groups or persons who may have either overtly blocked the intervention or subtly sabotaged it. Engaging with the un-beneficiaries also provides a place to explore values that can be used to identify criteria for how to value findings. Perhaps the un-beneficiaries were the group that needed most to benefit and did not, or perhaps the damage done to them by achieving the results outweighs (from their perspective) the intervention's achievements. Consider, for example, the advantage of having a road link between communities. This link may provide access to better medical care, fresher produce, and jobs. At the same time, the road may damage the environment, including local plants or animals and the water supply.

Data provided by the un-beneficiaries can also explain why certain groups or individuals provide critical feedback on the intervention, even when the intervention has achieved all its intended results. Furthermore, asking the question "Who are the un-beneficiaries?" can provide necessary data to explore and understand larger questions of social justice.

Socially Just for Whom?: Some Food for Thought

Thinking about beneficiaries and un-beneficiaries often poses an unspoken challenge for an evaluator who wants to encourage a socially just society through being an evaluator or conducting an evaluation. The evaluator who concerns herself with social justice needs to grapple and come to terms with this question: In any evaluative process, what is considered socially just for whom, and who thinks that? If there are multiple perspectives on what is socially just, how does the evaluator choose to negotiate and engage with those perspectives, and how does that affect the evaluation, its findings, and its recommendations? At the same time, she may need to grapple with the challenge of implementing an evaluation that is *not* focused on social justice— for example, when evaluation users (or clients) are not particularly interested in that issue.

Beneficiaries. Indirect beneficiaries. Un-beneficiaries. Stakeholders. Clients. All these groups are likely to provide useful and varying perspectives (often useful just because they are varying). Yet an evaluator's role goes beyond asking questions and gathering data from multiple perspectives and viewpoints; she also needs to make sense of it all. At times, at least for me, the sense-making role can be a bit (OK, a lot) overwhelming. Yet making sense of data from multiple perspectives is a core reason why evaluators play a critical role in the evaluative process, and in society.

INCLUDING BENEFICIARIES IN THE PROCESS: PLACEBO OR PANACEA?

In a discussion of beneficiaries, the word *participatory*, and the whole notion of *participation*, are often brought into the conversation. Specific evaluation approaches have different meanings and make use of different processes for participation. Some approaches that emphasize participation, yet in different ways, include democratic evaluation, empowerment evaluation, feminist evaluation, developmental evaluation, and, (no surprise) participatory evaluation. See Chapters 14 and 15 if you want to jump ahead to read about evaluation approaches. For now, a very practical discussion wraps up the chapter and takes a down-to-earth perspective on the whole concept of participation.

Irene Guijt (2014) describes participatory approaches as those that in some way involve an intervention's stakeholders (of which beneficiaries are one group, as noted on pages 60–61) at any stage of the evaluation. She notes that the reasons for choosing a participatory approach may be either pragmatic or ethical, or a combination of the two. They may be pragmatic because better evaluations are achieved (e.g., better data, better understandings of the data, more appropriate recommendations, better uptake of findings); they may be ethical because taking such an approach is viewed as the right thing to do. Given these potential benefits, participation in evaluation is often presented as a win–win situation. Nonetheless, such benefits are not a sure thing.

I want to share a stream-of-consciousness reflection on the words *participation* and *beneficiaries*. When someone says, "Oh, I am doing a participatory process," it always makes me wonder: Who is participating? Who chooses whom to participate? What if a group or person does not want to participate (i.e., forced participation or refusal)? How does a person participate, at what level, and at what point in the process? How does it benefit the evaluation? How does it benefit the beneficiary?

When I am asked to implement a participatory process in a community, particularly in an impoverished one, I feel awkward about the fact that I am getting paid and the people participating are probably not. They might get a cup of tea, or have their transportation costs reimbursed, or receive a small honorarium. People often attend meetings, organized for an evaluation process, at a personal or economic cost to themselves; is that OK? It might be; it depends on the context. Using the word *participatory* does not automatically mean that an evaluation is an inherently fair or just process. A participatory process can be quite exclusionary, for example, allowing (or encouraging) some groups to participate and not others. Or the word can be misleading when groups are invited to participate at times when they cannot; when there are other barriers to participation; or when, even if people do participate, their voices in no way influence the evaluation or its related decisions. Then there is the realization that sometimes beneficiaries do not want to participate; should we (the evaluators) badger them until they do, so that we can say the process was participatory?

Sometimes researchers or evaluators think that gathering data from a person through an interview constitutes a participatory process; that makes me shudder. If that were so, then every evaluation that gathers primary data would be participatory. When we label a process participatory, or when we are being asked to conduct a participatory process, we need to be very clear about how the approach will be used in practice, how it is beneficial to the evaluation, and how it is intended to be useful to the people involved.

Consider asking some, if not all, of the following questions:

- How will the process be participatory, and for whom?
- How will participation be compensated, if at all?
- Whose participation is deemed useful and beneficial to the evaluation?
- Who will benefit through participating, and in what ways?
- Who can get hurt if they are, or are not, involved?
- What part of the process is participatory? Is it participatory for different people at different points in the process?
- How does a participatory approach lead to a more credible evaluation? (For a discussion of evaluation credibility, please see Chapter 5.)
- How does participation support a fair and just process?
- And lastly, who is making all of the decisions in regard to these questions, and how are they made?

Phew. It feels good to share.

Let me end this section by stating that participatory approaches, when done well, can be informative, useful, and beneficial to the participants and the evaluation. Here are some examples of how participatory processes are useful: building the capacity of those who participate (when mentoring and training are part of the process); improving the relevance and accuracy of an evaluation report; bringing the local or internal knowledge necessary to interpret findings; increasing process and evaluation use; and contributing to the face validity of an evaluation. *Face validity* means that an ordinary person can understand the evaluation questions, methods, and analysis without special methodological training, and the evaluation makes sense in a straightforward, logical way.

Another concept that is also intertwined in the conversation about beneficiaries and participation is *buy-in*. Obtaining buy-in is a very popular concept when an evaluation brings together multiple stakeholder groups. In these types of evaluative processes, an often-heard expression is "We need to get buy-in . . . through a participatory process." Be careful with the concept and what it implies. If evaluators aim to create buy-in to an assumption or a value, for example, this also likely means that someone or some group is not only dominating, but winning. The aim of an evaluation that has multiple stakeholders is not for one stakeholder to win; the focus is on gathering and understanding those multiple perspectives, and making meaning out of everything that has been heard and gathered. All stakeholders should recognize their voices (e.g., perspectives, needs, insights) in the report, and therefore find the evaluative process, its findings, and the evaluator to be credible and trustworthy.

Engaging Beneficiaries

- *Have a few minutes?* Take a brief look at how Derek Sivers explains that recognizing difference is useful (*www.ted.com/talks/derek_sivers_weird_or_just_different#t-142837*).

- *Have a few hours?* Read Irene Guijt's (2014) report, *Participatory Approaches* (Methodological Briefs—Impact Evaluation 5, published by the UNICEF Office of Research in Florence, Italy). While it focuses on impact evaluation, the document provides a wealth of information on participatory approaches, a useful glossary, and excellent resources in the bibliography.

- *Have a few hours a night?* Consider selecting a few chapters in *Collaborative, Participatory, and Empowerment Evaluation: Stakeholder Involvement Approaches* (Fetterman, Rodriguez-Campos, Zukoski, & Contributors, 2018).

- *Have a few more hours a night?* Sandra Mathison's (2005) *Encyclopedia of Evaluation* provides nice summaries of the approaches mentioned in this chapter, plus a plethora of others. Another place to read about the approaches mentioned is the Better Evaluation website (*www.betterevaluation.org*). Look under the Themes and Approaches tabs.

WRAPPING UP

Writing a nutshell description of an intervention is a useful way to start exploring what to evaluate. This description initiates the discussion of three core concepts: intervention, problem statement, and beneficiary, which are critical to any evaluative process. Identifying the interplay among them demonstrates the necessary interconnected thinking and iterative nature of the evaluation journey. The problem statement, when distinguishing between grand problems and pocket ones, and root causes and symptoms, informs the reason for an intervention, provides guidance in how to design one, and anticipates its results. When a problem statement is well thought out, it provides insight into questions often asked throughout the evaluative process, such as the relevance of the intervention and its results, who aims to benefit, and where results will take place.

Recognizing the role of different stakeholders, one group of whom are the beneficiaries, can generate an awareness of the multiple perspectives that exist; specifically, it can bring to the surface a multitude of values and perceptions that can be used to reflect on the intervention, inform an evaluation design, and influence the criteria for valuing an intervention's results. The discussions in this chapter inform the initial, iterative steps of any evaluative process, and when addressed well, provide a delightful gift to the evaluator. The next chapter delves a bit deeper into the evaluative process and asks you to consider how you know what you know, challenges you to consider how others may think very differently, and explores how to engage with thinking that perhaps does not resonate with your own.

Our Conversation: Between You and Me

The conversation with me is intended to coach you through similar situations you will encounter in the real world.

In the chapter, I shared a stream of consciousness about the concept of participation. I mentioned that sometimes people equate participation with a fair and just process. What was your reaction to that? Pondering about what participation *actually* means helps me to think through what will be my response when a client asks for a participatory process, before they ask me. I use the thought process and questions highlighted in the chapter to do my pondering. What will you do the next time someone says, "I want a participatory process?" How will you respond? What questions will you raise, if any?

CHAPTER 4

How We Know What We Know, and Why We Think That

Asking someone, "How do you know what you know?" can be an infuriating question—yet a fundamental one. In any evaluation process, the question often first materializes during talk about the problem statement. How does someone know that it is actually a problem that is being addressed? Similarly, in an exchange with a colleague or client, sometimes statements will be made that are accepted as facts: "It is just is the way it is." But is it? How do we know? How does someone else know?

This chapter uses the problem statement concept (and segues into a discussion on interventions and results) to begin to explore the topic of how we know what we know. (In academic terms, this type of exploration is called an *epistemological* discussion). The concepts, ideas, discussions, and questions raised in the chapter are relevant to any part of the evaluation process where how *we* know what we know, and how *they* know what they know, can be called into question (which is pretty much the whole process).

THE CONUNDRUM

I have written this book to demystify evaluation. Terms, concepts, and processes are explained to invite people into the conversation, not exclude them. This chapter has brought me my first real struggle in explaining the evaluative process in this way: how to balance an academic discussion with one that will be useful for practitioners. An academic discussion of epistemology (how you know what you know) would teach you about *positivism, postpositivism, constructivism,* and *critical realism,* to name just a few metatheoretical stances. It would also bring in the concept of a **paradigm.** When people talk about different ways of knowing what they know, each way is referred to as a *paradigm.* More specifically, a paradigm is a worldview that presents a way of thinking and making sense of the world (Patton, 2015). An evaluator who knows that different ways of thinking (i.e., paradigms) exist can use that insight to inform her evaluation designs, and/or to better understand why people bring different perspectives and values to an evaluative process. For instance, the evaluator can recognize that disagreements about what are considered credible data or various interpretations of results originate from people's different ways of thinking. This awareness supports the evaluator while she sorts through, and makes sense of, what she is hearing, touching, smelling, or seeing (among other ways of knowing).

As a practitioner, I rarely use the academic terms (e.g., positivism, constructivism, realism) in my day-to-day work, but my understanding of them informs what I do. Do you see the challenge? For example, I never (and I mean *never*) ask my clients or colleagues if they are positivists or postpositivists, or facilitate a conversation by saying, "OK, look, epistemologically, you are taking a postpositivist position and your colleague is thinking like a constructivist. This is why you do not agree on the methods decision, or on what constitutes a fact." However, knowing about these various worldviews or ways of thinking is invaluable for an evaluator; it enables her to think through and understand what happens in the evaluative process, from her own way of thinking and making decisions to those of others. Thus, while the chapter moves forward in a logical progression of demystifying evaluation that purposely avoids academic jargon, there is an unspoken assumption that an evaluator will have the necessary theoretical knowledge to facilitate that practical, evaluative process. Before we get practical, let's get a little academic.

THE ACADEMIC DISCUSSION

This section provides a *glimpse* into the academic discussion of how you know what you know by highlighting three competing social sciences paradigms: positivism, constructivism, and critical theory. Postpositivism is a fourth paradigm closely related to positivism. Although each of these four is briefly covered, note that other paradigms exist, such as transformative realism and pragmatism.

- *Positivists* believe that there is a truth, and that this truth can be identified through objective research. Some key aspects of positivism include a strong belief in quantitative data inquiry, testing hypotheses, having representative data, and minimizing sources of bias. According to positivists, in other words, the research shows that a chair is a chair.

- *Postpositivists* are similar to positivists. The main difference between the two groups is that postpositivists acknowledge that various factors, such as researchers' prior knowledge and values, can influence what is observed. Thus postpositivists acknowledge the reality of bias while they aim to minimize it.

- *Constructivists* argue that human beings construct their own social realities, and thus that realities are subjective and experiential. Some key aspects of constructivism include a strong belief in qualitative data inquiry, exploration, in-depth understanding, and recognizing different perspectives and lived realities. Different religious beliefs constitute an example of competing explanations of similar realities. To give another example, for a constructivist, the research shows that, for the child, the thing over there that looks like a chair is actually being used to hang clothes, and therefore is a clothes hanger.

- *Critical theorists* examine the world with attention to power and politics. Critical theory acknowledges and seeks to understand power relations and patterns of dominance. Critical theorists value exploring social change in relation to social struggles. For example, as they see it, that thing over there is a chair for the mother and a clothes hanger for her child, even if the mother tries to convince her child to use it as a chair.

Having a firm grasp of various paradigms is likely to influence the evaluation design and approach; help make decisions transparent; support an evaluator to sort out, explain, and understand others' experiences and perceptions of the evaluative process; and assist the evaluator in valuing its findings. Most likely (though not necessarily), an evaluator will bounce around among the different paradigms, as different evaluation questions and contexts often require different evaluation approaches (and ways of thinking).

SOCIAL RESEARCH PARADIGMS

There are numerous resources on social research paradigms. Here are a few to consider.

- **Have a few hours?** Read *Research Terminology Simplified: Paradigms, Axiology, Ontology, Epistemology and Methodology* by Laura Killam (2013). This short (55-page) book, while aimed at nurses, provides a solid, basic understanding of numerous research concepts discussed here, among others, for any evaluation practitioner.

- **Have a few hours a week?** Read *Social Research: Paradigms in Action* by Norman Blaikie and Jan Priest (2017). The book carefully explains how research paradigms influence practice.

- **Have some more time?** Consider taking a course, either online or at your local university. Look for a course on research epistemology or an introductory course to social science research. Or, look for short introductory courses in research psychology, education, sociology, and anthropology. Ask for the syllabus to confirm that these topics are covered.

Searching for and reading online definitions of the terms covered in this section are *not* recommended. Various interpretations are out there, and a web search is likely to result in more confusion than clarity.

THE PRACTITIONER CONVERSATION
The Facts about Facts

The practitioner conversation on how you know what you know (which includes how we-the-evaluators know what we know) can be grounded in a discussion centering around facts. The conversation starts with a general chat about facts, and then distinguishes them from assumptions. Let's first consider the term *fact*. Organizations often have "Fact Sheets." I grew up where a common expression after someone said something interesting was to respond casually, "Is that a fact?" I often hear people say, "As a matter of fact . . ." So the word *fact* is one that most people hear in everyday conversation. In evaluation, when we talk about a fact, we are almost always talking about something that can be backed up with evidence. Evidence comes from one of our five senses—we can hear it, touch it, smell it, taste it, or see it (for more discussion of evidence, go to Chapter 5). And other people can, too. Why do I say "almost always"? There are other ways to consider what is a fact, and therefore what is evidence (for more on other ways of knowing, see discussions in Chapter 13). One example is a tacit way of knowing. *Tacit* means something that is understood without being directly stated or written down. An example of tacit knowledge is intuition; some people use this kind of knowledge to make important decisions, such as whom to trust or to marry. There may be other ways of knowing in the context in which you work; it is important to be aware of what is accepted as a fact, and what is not, early in the evaluation process. Put bluntly, if an evaluator answers evaluation questions with what he considers to be facts, and not what his evaluation users do, the evaluation findings are likely to be rejected.

> ### BOX 4.1. Recognizing Other Ways of Knowing
>
> Being clear about what you accept as a fact or as knowledge, and seeking out, understanding, and accepting how others view what is a fact and what is knowledge, are core elements of being an evaluator. An evaluator honors that there are multiple ways of knowing by exploring what is a fact, how facts are valued, and what is considered knowledge, and by accepting ways of thinking that are potentially different from her own. These conversations then influence decisions, such as what methods of inquiry to choose, how to analyze and interpret the data, how to value them, and how to discuss and present findings.

In mainstream evaluation, there are two different kinds of facts: a *scientific* fact and a *socially constructed* fact. It is highly likely (though not necessary) that both types of facts will be used in most evaluative processes. The discussions below lay the foundation for the conversation in Chapter 5 that introduces different methods of inquiry for answering evaluation questions, a conversation that is then carried into Chapters 14 and 15, which focuses on evaluation approaches. *Inquiry* is a general term for the gathering of data and evidence.

Scientific Facts and Socially Constructed Facts

Let's look at the two different kinds of facts: a scientific fact and a socially constructed fact. It is a fact that the human body needs water to survive. This is a scientific fact. All human beings, everywhere in the world, need water to live. There are also socially constructed facts. Guba and Lincoln (1989) write about socially constructed knowledge. They suggest that knowledge emerges in an evaluative process, and that what is known (knowledge) is created by humans (p. 67). Here is an example: At one time, some societies valued the salt we use for flavoring so much that they could use it to purchase other items, such as food, a boat, or land. Contrarily, today we find salt at restaurants where we can take all that we need to flavor our food or easily buy it in a grocery store; today's society does not place a purchasing value on salt, though we often need money to purchase it. The value of salt is socially constructed; it has changed with time. The compound we know as table salt is made of sodium and chlorine. That is a scientific fact. It is a fact today, and it was fact when salt could be used to buy a ship.

Thus the question of what constitutes a fact, and what does not, is a demanding one that needs to be answered to ensure that an evaluation is accepted and used. It can become somewhat complicated when different users have different ways of thinking (i.e., paradigms), and therefore different value systems, about what constitutes a fact. Some advice is provided below.

Few evaluation audiences, clients, stakeholders, beneficiaries, or others want to have an in-depth theoretical conversation about what constitutes a fact (though some do). Thus I recommend keeping two words in mind when addressing the "what is a fact" question: brevity and levity. Here are three ideas that will support a nonphilosophical approach to identifying what an evaluation user considers a fact.

Do Some Research

Ask for a previous evaluation report, project report, or other document that contains data—a document that the stakeholders (e.g., beneficiaries, clients) considered to be a good piece of work or that they used to inform decisions. Reviewing the reports will provide a hint or an idea of what is accepted as a fact. Keep in mind, however, that there may be other reasons why people thought the report was useful (see Chapter 13, specifically about the fabulous five, for other reasons).

Have a Practical Discussion

Think up different kinds of potential "facts" about the intervention, and ask, "If I were to provide [these data] to you, would you believe them? What about if I provided [these other data]?" Ensure that the examples are straightforward and realistic. Or, if you have done a similar evaluation previously, show them the relevant parts of that evaluation's report (highlight a few paragraphs or sections; do not just hand them the report) and talk them through these excerpts, asking if they would consider that kind of data and information useful.

Present Some Different Ideas for Collecting Data

On the basis of the evaluation questions, identify what kinds of ways the data can be addressed, and present these data inquiries and potential responses to the clients. Discuss whether they would find data addressed in those ways believable. If not, why not? What would they consider believable? You may want to skip ahead to Chapter 5 for a more in-depth look at the kinds of options that exist.

What do I do when evaluation users and beneficiaries have different ways of seeing the world—in other words, when they have different ideas about what constitutes a fact?

When different evaluation users believe in different kinds of facts, consider more than one way to answer the same evaluation question; only collecting data that supports one viewpoint privileges one group over another. While providing multiple kinds of facts is often a good solution, this recommendation has two common drawbacks. First, more resources are likely to be needed (though not always). Second, sometimes different ways of gathering evidence may also produce different findings, simply because these are different ways of seeing something. The evaluator then needs to engage with those different findings. (Chapter 2 addresses this through the Listen–Speak–Listen activity; also see Chapter 5.)

THE DIFFERENCE BETWEEN FACTS AND ASSUMPTIONS

After clarifying the term *fact*, move to the term *assumption*. A common definition of an assumption is something that is not a fact. This is not exactly helpful. The *Cambridge English Dictionary* describes an *assumption* as "something that you accept as true without question or proof" (*https://dictionary.cambridge.org/dictionary/english/assumption*). That is better: An assumption is something that is thought to be true, with no proof. Assumptions may be grounded in facts, informed by values, based on personal experiences, or a mix of all three.

> **BOX 4.2. The Use of Assumptions**
>
> Assumptions guide our everyday behavior, both consciously and tacitly. While an evaluator aims to identify facts, she also needs to uncover core assumptions that influence decisions and how results are valued. Knowing what are the facts, and what are the assumptions, is critical in any evaluative process. A problem statement is (or should be) a fact or set of facts. An intervention is an assumption (which sometimes mixes in a few facts) of what might work to fix or otherwise address that problem. That is why we monitor and evaluate an intervention—because it is not a fact that it will produce the desired results in that time, in that place, for those beneficiaries.

The Bus Example: Take 1

Let's look at an example of how assumptions are used in everyday life to inform decisions.

In the morning I get up and have a cup of tea. What I drink is tea, and it is in a cup. These are facts. I then walk, in the pouring rain, to the bus station to take the 6:45 A.M. bus to work. That I walk, and that it is raining, are facts. The bus never arrives. That is also a fact, and it is a problem because I am now late to work. Everyone at the bus stop agrees that the bus is late because it is raining. That everyone agrees is a fact, but that everyone agrees that the bus is late because it is raining does not make *that* (i.e., the agreed-upon reason for the lateness of the bus) a fact. Maybe the bus has mechanical challenges, or perhaps the bus drivers are on strike. Based on prior experience, the given facts, and my values, I need to decide whether to wait for a bus and be late for work, or to start thinking about other ways to get to work.

Facilitating Conversations

In having discussions with colleagues or others to explain the difference between facts and assumptions—or, indeed, in having any conversation described in this book—try to use an example *very far away* from the context in which they are working, yet one in which they can engage. Why is that? When people are familiar with a sector (say, education, health, or environment), and an example is drawn from that sector, sometimes people find a flaw in the example—and that flaw then becomes the discussion focus. Sometimes people add more details about context, which turn the simple example into a tricky one that draws away from the point of the activity. Furthermore, the person providing the details, or picking apart the example, is not focusing on the point of the learning exercise or discussion. So select something that most people can relate to, as I have done in the previous paragraph with the late bus and rainy weather (food is also often a good theme), to explain a key point, term, or concept.

As demonstrated with the rain-and-bus example, a common challenge faced in an evaluation process is that people often mix facts and assumptions into one sentence or paragraph, making it difficult to discern which is what. The example given on the previous page is that everyone agrees that the bus is late (fact) *because it is raining* (assumption). (For a similar example, read the following question and answer on facts and opinions.) In any evaluative process, an evaluator needs to sift through whatever she gathers and identify which are facts and which are assumptions, as they are (or should be) used differently in the evaluation process. Facts are used to establish that a problem exists, to show that a result has happened, and to answer or inform evaluation questions; by contrast, an evaluator continually asks questions about assumptions, which can be used to identify the desired results and interpret the data. Facts and assumptions often combine to inform an intervention and the evaluative process.

What is the difference between an assumption and an opinion?

They are very similar, though the two words tend to be used in different ways. An opinion is based on a belief. Here is an example. I think a Boerboel, a South African mastiff (fact), is the best breed for a family dog because families need dogs to protect the home (opinion) and yet to be gentle with small children (opinion). Others may disagree and think that German Shepherds, which are also called Alsatians (facts), are the best dogs for that purpose (opinion). These are statements that mix facts and opinions. A challenge in evaluation is that when statements are mixed, people do not often stop to separate facts from opinions before they disagree with the whole statement (or accept the whole statement as a fact or set of facts). However, with what are they disagreeing (or accepting)? The facts, the opinions, or both? Here is where the evaluator needs to take apart statements and determine what are the opinions and what are the facts, which in many circumstances can be challenging. For example, some opinions are so common that they appear to be facts. Here is one: Going outside in cold weather, with wet hair, will make you sick. Although my grandmother believed this (and many people I interact with today still believe it) to be a fact, it is, in fact, an opinion.

In any part of an evaluative process, separating out facts, assumptions, and opinions will help to facilitate useful conversations. Keep in mind, too, that providing different kinds of facts (e.g., "It is a chair" vs. "It is a clothes hanger") is an extremely different type of conversation from providing facts that contradict popular opinions or common assumptions.

ENGAGING WITH FACTS: BEFORE AND AFTER THE FACT

Throughout the entire evaluative process, an evaluator continually engages with the use of facts from at least two different perspectives: (1) "How do *we* know what we know?" (the evaluator's perspective), and (2) "How do *they* know what they know?" (the implementer's perspective). Other common perspectives are that of beneficiaries and other key stakeholders.

While an evaluator can be part of identifying the problem that the intervention will address, and then an integral member of the team who develops the intervention, the evaluator *most likely* enters the scene once an intervention has been designed, often after it is implemented, and sometimes after it has ended. Since she is thus not likely to have been the person who collected the data to determine that there was a problem to begin with, she is often in the position of establishing how someone knew that there was a problem, and for whom, and asking what facts were used to establish that problem. This is a very different situation from when an evaluator is invited to be involved in determining the problem that needs to be addressed, and thus inform the intervention's design and intended results (see Chapters 6–8). The evaluator's role in how she engages with facts (identifying them or questioning them) will shift depending on when she enters the process and what role she is asked to play (see Chapters 2 and 11 for more on evaluator roles).

Establishing that a problem statement is indeed a fact or set of facts is an essential part of the evaluation process. A problem statement needs to be based on facts, not assumptions of facts. The differences between facts and assumptions is highlighted for good reason: If someone is going to spend time, money, and other resources on a problem, only to realize months or years later that what they thought was a problem was just an assumption of a problem, the intervention was probably (though not always) a waste of resources. Why do I say that? The intervention aimed to address something that was not ever a problem, and did not need to be fixed or otherwise improved. Imagine that 10 million U.S. dollars (or euros or British pounds or South African rands) are invested to solve a problem that turns out not to be a problem after all, just an assumption of one—and that this assumption was wrong. This would mean that the intervention was not needed, and that barring potential unintended positive effects, millions were spent that could have been used to address an *actual* problem. And let's not forget the evaluator who is brought in to implement an evaluation to understand why the intervention did not have the intended effects it was meant to have. Was the reason poor implementation or lack of resources? No; he finds out that there was just no problem to fix in the first place. Most would consider that a waste of evaluation resources.

Psst. Come a bit closer. The other reason a fact-based problem statement is needed is an open trade secret: The evidence to show that there is a problem is the same evidence used for determining a baseline. To read more about a baseline, a retrospective baseline, or the lack of a baseline, skip to the "Baseline Study" section of Chapter 5. For a recap of what is evidence, go to pages 106–109. Fact-based problem statements inform interventions, their intended results, and the ways to assess them.

A challenge often encountered with a problem statement is that people make assumptions about a situation and declare it to be true. Now, while an intervention is full of assumptions (further described in Chapters 6 and 7), a problem statement needs to be supported with facts. To explore how we know that the problem statement is a fact-based problem, we need to ask two questions:

- How do you know that there is a problem, or that something needs to be improved, fixed, changed, or influenced in some way, and for whom?
- What makes you think that?

In other words, how do they know that the problem statement is based on facts and not on assumptions? These two questions can be used to guide document reviews or interviews. Asking for data to answer the two questions can lead to an enlightening conversation. Here are three proactive strategies to consider using to gather information about the problem statement.

Strategy 1

If you are working closely with the people involved, and there is time (i.e., 4–6 hours),

- Have a hands-on session that thoughtfully explains the purpose of a problem statement (draw on key messages and ideas provided in Chapter 3) and the ways it is used in the evaluation process.
- *Ask the two questions.*
- Identify who is likely to have the data (e.g., a person's name or a position, such as "the education officer" or "Mr. Banihashemi"), and/or where the data are likely to be found (e.g., "the county health department"). Do not ask for the data in the meeting, as the interaction is intended to encourage engagement rather than put people "on the spot."
- Through a facilitated discussion, determine who will follow up to identify what data exist. It helps to divide up the responsibilities; it is less overwhelming. Finally, determine how that information will be shared (e.g., a meeting, an email, Dropbox).

Strategy 2

If you are planning to visit the intervention to hold a meeting (1–2 hours),

- Give the personnel a "heads-up" before you arrive. Describe what kind of information you will be asking for during the initial visit, or what you would like to observe.
- Explain why the information is needed and how it will be used.
- *Ask the two questions.*
- When you arrive at the site, take the time to (re)explain the need for clarity on the problem that is being addressed, and ask for the information.

Strategy 3

If time is extremely short, or you are not physically near the group,

- Consider sending an email that specifically explains what is needed, provides examples if possible, and gives a short explanation of why these data are needed.
- *In the email, ask the two questions.*
- Follow up with a phone call, Skype, Zoom, or similar medium of communication, to provide further explanation if needed, and to ask for the information.

It is important to note that someone cannot just randomly provide figures or statements; these need to be supported by evidence. For example, if someone says, "90% of the people needed the intervention," ask to see the research that supports this statistic (i.e., that supports how they know what they know). Sometimes people provide statistics that sound factual, but are assumptions. Although this can also happen when someone just describes a situation (e.g., using words), for some reason people are less likely to question a statistic.

For a bit of fun, next time you are in a conversation with a friend, notice if they throw in a percentage as if it is a fact, and ask them, "How do you know that?" What may not be as much fun is questioning a program manager or implementer about their problem statement (or their identified results). Table 4.1 presents some common challenges that can occur when you are asking implementers (or other relevant persons) how they know that what is being addressed is indeed a problem.

The Girls' Education Intervention: Example of a Practical Discussion

Let's apply the two questions from page 79 to our example of a girls' education intervention.

- How do you know that there is a problem, or that something needs to be improved, fixed, changed, or influenced in some way, and for whom?
- What makes you think that?

The answers are likely to include several responses, each of which will need to be a fact and not an assumption. At the end of the discussion, there should be clear information. The responses are first described in Table 4.2.

In the real world, things are likely to be more complicated, and the process may take more time than the sample provided in Table 4.2 suggests. The girls' education problem has three possible pocket problems, and only two are facts. So we have two pocket problem statements, and the intervention needs to address those problems, not the one identified as a perception. The narrative on the next page describes the problem statement for the girls' education intervention in a bit more depth. (You might compare this with the nutshell description for this intervention in Chapter 3.)

TABLE 4.1. Challenges and How to Address Them

Challenges with asking for facts (How do you know what you know?)	Strategies to address the challenges
Requesting data essentially to prove the problem statement can be perceived as a confrontational question. The question challenges the need for the intervention, and thus it questions whoever made the decision to have the intervention. It also probably confronts other commonly held assumptions, such as "What do you mean you doubt why we are doing what we are doing?" Or, for a more personal spin, "Why do you doubt me?"	Explain that how we know that there is a need for an intervention is critical to knowing how to evaluate, and therefore to understand, whether the intervention is making a difference. As such, it is a question that we evaluators ask in all evaluative processes. In other words, we are not doubting the value or need for the intervention; we are just trying to understand it.
Data may not exist, may not be accessible, or may be of poor quality. If one or more of these is the case, the respondents may be defensive, feel inadequate, or consider themselves helpless when asked to produce data related to the problem statement.	Explain that many interventions lack data on the problem statement; such a lack is not a disaster. As the evaluator, it may be useful for you to explore why this is the case (if it is), and to explain in any case that even without these data, a credible evaluation can be implemented. (For what to do in the case of a lack of baseline, see Chapter 5.)
Asking for facts may not result in getting the facts anticipated; it may be facts that are politically sensitive and not often mentioned—especially to an evaluator.	A political reason to have an intervention can be a fact, just not the kind anticipated. Maybe the reason was to spend down a budget, which is a fact. Explain that lots of reasons often exist for implementing a program, and that even when these reasons do not provide facts to support the problem statement, each answer is useful to provide insight and explanations for understanding the context, the intervention, and ways to value the results (or lack thereof).

Girls' Education Intervention: Problem Statement

Several years before the intervention was designed, a study identified that the community's school-age girl population is double the school-age boy population for the same age brackets. However, few girls attend school, while all school-age boys attend. The exact numbers are provided in the appendix [note that here in this book there is no appendix, but in real life there would be]. A mixed methods inquiry [see Chapter 5 for further explanation] has established two reasons why girls do not attend school, which have been triangulated: Girls do not attend due to (1) concerns about their safety, and (2) the belief held by their fathers or father figures that girls do not need to attend school. Teachers, community leaders, and school-age girls in neighboring communities think that few girls attending school is a problem, for many reasons. In the community where the intervention will take place, the implementing organization, a nonprofit organization (NPO), identified that girls' not attending schools is a societal problem through a review of multiple published and peer-reviewed articles. The NPO's research (based in literature from the fields of gender studies, education, and development studies) has found that girls' not accessing formal education often leads to their having fewer choices in life, as well as higher incidences of abusive relationships, unwanted pregnancies, and higher poverty levels, compared to girls who receive education until the age of 18.

TABLE 4.2. Facts versus Assumptions in the Girls' Education Intervention Example

Grand problem	Is it a fact or an assumption?
In the community, there are high rates of unwanted pregnancy for teenage girls, as well as high rates of spousal abuse.	A document review of government statistics has determined that these are facts, and other studies show that the lack of education leads to these problems. FACT.
Grand problem (though at a lower level)[a]	**Is it a fact or an assumption?**
Most girls do not attend school.	A document review has identified that the community's school-age girl population is double the school-age boy population for the same age brackets. However, few girls attend school, while all school-age boys attend. FACT.
Pocket problems	**Is it a fact or an assumption?**
The road to the school is not safe for girls, due to several attacks in the past few years on women in the area between the school and the community.	Primary research has been conducted and determined that this is a fact. FACT.
Fathers or father figures do not permit their daughters to go to school. They think girls do not need a formal education.	Primary research has been conducted and determined that this is a fact. FACT.
Girls do not attend school because they do not have uniforms.	Primary research has been conducted and determined that this is not a fact. It is an assumption. Therefore, no intervention has been designed to address it, and there are no results linked to it. ASSUMPTION.

[a]The label is not important; the flow of the logic is. See Chapter 3.

Ta-da! The facts demonstrate that there is a problem that needs to be addressed. Therefore, the problem statement has established that an intervention is relevant, has clarified for whom the intervention is intended, and hints at the results that are likely desired. Now let's move on to looking at how facts and assumptions are often lumped together to design an intervention.

HOW MIXING FACTS AND ASSUMPTIONS CAN INFLUENCE AN INTERVENTION

The Bus Example: Take 2

Earlier in the chapter, I described a scenario about my standing in the rain and waiting for a bus that never arrives. The mix of facts and assumptions will influence my decisions about what to do. For example, based on the mix of fact and assumption described on page 76—the bus is late (fact) because it is raining (assumption), and as it turns out, I am late to work (fact)—the intervention (solution) may be to buy a car. Now when it rains, I can drive to work. This is an expensive intervention, however, and has all sorts of other costs (e.g., gas, parking, car insurance) and other assumptions (e.g., I know how to drive) associated with it. It solves my problem; I have more control about arriving to work on time when driving my own car. But it does not solve the problem that the bus does not arrive, or help the other people at the bus station (the larger social issue). Identifying the cause, such as the bus drivers' poor working conditions and low pay (root cause) that have led to a strike (symptom) and the lateness of the bus (symptom), may lead to an entirely different solution, intervention, and potential result that might also solve the issue of my being late to work and address the larger social issues.

The actual intervention, perhaps, may be working with unions to provide better working conditions for drivers and meet the bus drivers' demands for higher pay, which could end the strike. The end of the strike will mean, barring any other external causes (like a flat tire or traffic), that the bus will run on time in the future. It will also solve the larger social issue for everyone who has to rely on the bus and cannot afford to buy a car, or cannot drive a car. The example demonstrates that in most interventions a mix of facts and assumptions (and values) influences the possible choices, and that what the intervention does, where it intercedes, and for whom all influence what results are expected. An evaluator needs to distinguish which facts (including root causes and symptoms; see Chapter 3) and which assumptions have informed the intervention's shape, as well as where the intervention has chosen to intervene, for whom, and with what expected results. Knowing these details provides clearer guidance on what to evaluate.

The program that I monitor has facts in the intervention, not just assumptions. Can you explain a bit more about facts and assumptions in the intervention, and how that influences what you monitor or potentially evaluate?

A common challenge in practicing evaluation is discerning facts from assumptions. Sometimes parts of an intervention are facts. Let's look at an example. It is a fact that immunizing infants against polio will prevent the infants from contracting polio. Infants who get the right dosages of an effective vaccine, at the right times, will not get polio. That polio vaccines work is a fact and does not need to be monitored. Then why monitor or evaluate any vaccination campaign, or any intervention that has embedded facts in its design? Basically, interventions are implemented in the real world with real human beings; this means that many things can go wrong, or may not go as expected. For instance, people may not bring infants to be vaccinated because they think the vaccine will damage their infants. Or maybe infants do not get vaccinated because the cost of the visits is too much, it is too far to travel to the clinic, or people do not know that the vaccinations are being offered. Another example is that maybe all infants in the community are vaccinated, but some contract polio. This last example would suggest evaluation questions such as whether the vaccine was tainted or wrongly administered (e.g., the wrong dosage). Thus, even when an intervention contains facts, aspects of the real world (people, policies, environment, economy, and/or culture) may influence whether the intervention was implemented as intended, and whether it achieves its intended results.

VALUES, VALUES EVERYWHERE

In evaluation, a myriad of perspectives and interests, as well as social, cultural, and political norms, influence how an intervention and its results are valued. Those are a lot of influences, and thus a lot of values. While Chapter 12 is dedicated to values, the topic is so complex that an evaluator should be constantly identifying from where and from whom which values stem, at every stage of the evaluative process. If possible, the evaluator should not wait to identify values in one sitting (e.g., right when it is time to value the findings); doing so often results in a process that is too rushed and too late.

In the quest to understand what is accepted as a fact, values are unearthed. My colleague and fellow evaluator Susan Tucker contributes this interesting insight:

> "The use of the scientific method, the adherence to empirical evidence, the willingness to believe the evidence even when it conflicts with religious or cultural assumptions—these are all characteristics of a value system that puts a high priority on logical and scientific thinking. . . . Many people around the world subscribe to different values, which places much more importance on religious or cultural traditions, and see the work of science as worthless when it conflicts with those traditions."

The assumptions someone makes are based on values. Deciding to have an intervention to address a problem exposes values. Values are apparent again when the intervention is designed, and yet again when it is decided who are the beneficiaries (and often by default, the un-beneficiaries). In other words, there are millions (and likely billions) of problems in the world; why address this one, in this place? Why use that intervention? For these people or those animals? The answers to those questions reveal values that can be used to inform evaluation decisions (e.g., what to evaluate, whom to involve in the process) and how to value the results. Therefore, exploring the problem statement and intervention decisions, clarifying who aims to benefit from the intervention, determining what is regarded as a fact, and discovering which assumptions are used, all provide a multitude of clues with regard to how to determine criteria to value the intervention results.

Sometimes, however, people (e.g., evaluators, program implementers, managers, and donors, just to name a few) make a drastic leap from looking at some facts and assumptions to valuing an intervention. Activity 4.1 explores that leap, and how to address it.

ACTIVITY 4.1. Facts, Assumptions, and the Leap to Valuing

Purpose of the discussion: The facilitated discussion encourages people to discern the differences among a fact, an assumption, and a value judgment.

Time needed: Allow 2 minutes to prepare and introduce the activity, and 3 minutes for small-group discussion. The focus is on the large-group discussion, which needs about 20 minutes. Total approximate time: 25 minutes.

Materials: You will need a bottle of drinking water (if you can, tap water in a reusable plastic or glass bottle), a well-marked measuring cup, a clear glass that is big enough to hold the water from the measuring cup, and the following statements, each written on a separate piece of paper:

1. There is one person who is thirsty, but does not like water.
2. There is one person who is not thirsty; she just drank a glass of water.
3. There are three kids drenched in sweat after having a fun game of football.
4. There is one person who is not thirsty, but who would like to sip a tiny bit of water as he thinks about his day.

If there are additional groups, you can duplicate the statements.

The exercise: Place the bottle of water on the table. Tell the participants that there is clean drinking water in the bottle. Point out that this is a fact, not an assumption. Then fill the measuring cup with the water from the bottle. Have participants confirm that it is a fact that there are 500 milliliters (ml) of drinking water in the measuring cup (or whatever the measurement is). Then pour the water into a large glass, with no spillage, so that the glass now holds the water. Have the participants agree that there is 500 ml of potable water (or the amount measured) in the glass (facts).

Divide the room into groups of three to five participants. Give each group one prepared statement. Then say, "In your small groups, share the statement that I just provided, and then discuss and make a judgment on whether this glass of water is adequate." Allow a few minutes for group discussion, and then ask each group to respond with one of the following responses: "Yes, it is adequate," "We are not sure," or "It is not adequate." Puzzled looks or (ideally) some heated discussion will ensue. Although each group has been provided with different facts (the statements that you gave out), the participants do not realize that. Then ask a member of each group to read the statement the group was given. Then ask some or all of the facilitation questions that follow.

The facilitation questions: You do not need to ask all the questions.

- *Questions on facts:* What were the facts? Why did I [the facilitator] ask you [the participants] to confirm that these were the facts? What if someone did not agree? How would disagreeing on facts influence an intervention? An evaluation?
- *Questions on values and judgments:* What was your immediate reaction when other participants provided judgments that differed from your own (e.g., perhaps that the persons were wrong)? When you relate this exercise to evaluation, what roles do description and context play in making a judgment? How does making decisions explicit encourage evaluation use?

Optional step: If you have time, consider adding this step. Empty the glass, and refill it halfway. Do not measure the water first. Ask whether the glass is half full or half empty. How does this make the conversation challenging? (Hint: What's the fact, and what are the opinions?)

Optional step: If you have more time, ask how a type of participatory approach might have influenced the value judgment (i.e., asking the intended beneficiary if the water was adequate).

Critical learning points: There should never be any doubt about the facts. Who benefits, and their circumstances and needs, should influence how something is valued. Making an evaluative judgment is based on facts, assumptions, and values, all of which need to be explicit.

WRAPPING UP

Exploring how we know what we know is a conversation that should be informed by the academic discussion described in this chapter and practiced with the practitioner discussion. There are three key messages in the chapter. First, distinguishing between facts and assumptions, and determining what people consider facts, are relevant to the entire evaluative process and it brings values to the surface. Second, an evaluator is often in one of two positions: She is either questioning facts (identified before her arrival), or determining them herself (or with a team).

Questioning facts often first emerges during the exploration of the problem statement. It is difficult to discuss a problem statement without discussing the need for a fact. And to discuss the need for a fact, an evaluator probably needs to know what is an assumption. And in this conversation about facts and assumptions, an evaluator needs to understand that different people may have different viewpoints about what constitutes a fact, and different thought processes for how to make assumptions.

The chapter ends with a discussion of values. Values are a topic often brought in toward the end of the evaluation journey to determine what criteria should be used to weigh an intervention's results, but near the end is much too late in the evaluative process to begin a discussion on values. Values need to be identified throughout the entire journey. This chapter is titled "How We Know What We Know, and Why We Think That." If I could have had a longer title, I would have added, "How Do *They* Know What They Know, and Why Do They Think That?", to emphasize that what an evaluator "knows" and what a client, colleague, or beneficiary "knows" may be very different indeed. Combined, both titles accurately describe the inquisitive thought process that an evaluator needs to engage in while conducting any evaluative process. Before you leave this chapter, I invite you to have a conversation with me.

Our Conversation: Between You and Me

We have covered a lot of information in this chapter. As in other chapters, the conversation with me is intended to coach you through similar situations you will encounter in the real world.

A situation arises where different stakeholders are arguing over a finding in an evaluation report. One key stakeholder agrees with the judgment, and the other key stakeholder does not. They ask you to facilitate the conversation so that they can come to some sort of agreement. Where do you start? First, I would move the conversation to neutral space—in other words, a place that does not belong to one stakeholder or the other (e.g., not one stakeholder's office). In the neutral space, I would ask each to explain the finding (not his opinion of it, just the finding). If there are multiple findings under discussion, choose one to start. I would then untangle what is it about the finding that they disagree with, and break that down as follows:

1. The evaluation report answered Question X. Did you find that question an important one to answer?

2. The method of inquiry was Method Y. Did you find that appropriate?

3. The evaluation team collected the data in these ways, from these people, in this time frame, with this sample. Were there any challenges with how the data were collected, or from whom?

4. Did you find the facts credible?

5. How would you interpret those facts differently, and why?

In other words, I would break down the process to identify what was causing the argument to happen, and explore any differences identified at each step. What would *you* do? What would *you* say?

POSTSCRIPT: FACTS AND ASSUMPTIONS IN DICKENS'S "A CHRISTMAS CAROL"

In 1843, Charles Dickens wrote "A Christmas Carol"; many of us know that this is a story about Ebenezer Scrooge, a mean, stingy old man. On Christmas Eve, Scrooge is visited in dreams by the Ghost of Christmas Past, the Ghost of Christmas Present, and the Ghost of Christmas Yet to Come. Each ghost takes Scrooge on a journey. Christmas Past shows him his Christmases as a child. Christmas Present shows how people he knows are celebrating Christmas on that very day, and how his miserly ways have negatively affected those around him. The present-day scenes are awful and greatly upset Scrooge. Yet the past and present are facts he cannot change. The Ghost of Christmas Yet to Come shows him what future Christmas days will look like, and they are even more dismal. Scrooge realizes that there is still time for him to change, however, and he becomes a generous and kind-hearted man when he awakens from his dreams. The Ghost of Christmas Yet to Come shows Scrooge assumptions, and by changing his behavior, Scrooge proves the assumptions to be wrong.

CHAPTER 5

Data and Credibility

What Inquiring Evaluator Minds Need to Know

Packed inside my assessment suitcase are the methods of inquiry used to answer evaluation questions credibly. The chapter discusses how to choose from among different methods of inquiry: qualitative (words), quantitative (numbers), and mixed methods (a combination of both), with a particular focus on credible data, credible evidence, and a credible evaluation. Establishing baseline data to monitor change over time warrants its own section at the end of the chapter.

QUALITATIVE INQUIRY

Essentially, **qualitative inquiry** (1) explores something to understand its meaning (2) from the perspective of those experiencing it, and (3) provides an in-depth description of that something (also called a *thick description*), which (4) enables readers to immerse themselves in the experience (Patton, 2015; Stake, 2010).

According to Patton (2015, p. 13), there are seven reasons to use qualitative inquiry: (1) to illuminate meaning, (2) to study how things work, (3) to capture stories to understand people's perspectives and experiences, (4) to elucidate the ways systems function and their consequences for people's lives, (5) to understand context, (6) to understand how and why identifying unanticipated consequences matters, and (7) to make case comparisons to discover important patterns and themes across cases. *If an evaluation question fits into one of these themes, qualitative inquiry is likely an appropriate match.*

Data Collection Methods

Qualitative research aims to provide insights for one or more of these seven purposes through collecting words and pictures (data). These data are collected by using one of three methods (Patton, 2015, p. 14):

- In-depth, open-ended individual and group interviews
- Direct observation
- Written communications

A *focus group* is a type of group interview often used in evaluation. Here, a few primary questions are asked (often one or two), and the facilitator probes participants for deeper responses as needed, with the hope that the group interaction will encourage richer reflection and insight (Krueger & Casey, 2009). Note that a group interview is different from a focus group: Although the facilitator is again trying to gather information from the group, there is no encouraged group interaction; the evaluator is simply collecting data from several people at the same time.

In qualitative inquiry, the evaluator is considered the tool. She is immersed in the inquiry through not only data collection (obtaining the data), but data analysis (i.e., taking apart what she has collected so that she can re-sort it) and data re-sorting (i.e., making sense of meaning, interpreting). This type of inquiry is an iterative process.

Data Analysis

Three types of data analysis are common in qualitative research: *content*, *pattern*, and *thematic* analysis. In a content analysis, words and phrases (also called *search terms*) relevant to any of the evaluation questions are identified. The evaluator can use these terms to explore her data set to identify any patterns. A pattern analysis identifies words (or meanings of words) that suggest a pattern, such as similar actions, perceptions, experiences, relationships, and behaviors in the group being studied. The process of identifying patterns from the data is not formulaic. Rather, it is based on the exercise of reasonable judgment and an understanding of the contexts in which the intervention took place. The third analytic approach is to develop conceptual categories, or *themes*. These themes represent the patterns at a higher level of abstraction and allow for findings that are more analytically generalizable (Maxwell, 2013; Patton, 2015).

Presenting Qualitative Data

Qualitative data are words and pictures. Having the skills to construct a logical and engaging story, and to present evaluation findings so that they convey meaning and insight, is an important part of qualitative inquiry. There are some common approaches to visual data presentation in qualitative research. Photographs (used with the permission of the people portrayed in them), drawings, or animated pictures can help the readers immerse themselves in the story being told. Other approaches include quotes taken from interviews (again used with permission, or with the interviewees' identities disguised) that provide deeper insights into a finding or represent unique voices. Sometimes the visual presentation can show part of an actual interview. For example, a video excerpt from an interview or a section from a transcript can be used:

> DONNA, THE EVALUATOR: So tell me about your experience with qualitative research.
>
> RESPONDENT: I love it! I use it all the time.

Other innovative ways of visually presenting qualitative data exist, such as the use of pictographs, which are drawings that represent something or someone. For more ideas, refer to the section on quantitative inquiry for data visualization resources.

Sometimes—even after my client agrees that qualitative inquiry is the best method for the questions being asked, after I finish the evaluation, and after I answer the evaluation questions with technically credible data—the client says, "Where are the numbers? Can you quantify the data?" What do I do?

When people ask questions like these, try to find out what is it about numbers that would be helpful to them. For instance, ask them to explain how quantifying the data would help them to learn, or how not having numbers affects their ability to use the findings. For example, what do they *not* know because of the lack of numbers? A second, slightly different approach is to ask a specific question, such as "How many interviews would produce a credible response to the evaluation question for you?" Finally, if time, budget, and other resources permit, you might consider supplementing the evaluation by providing the types of numbers that the user finds credible. Of course, if the qualitative data are of good quality, the number of interviews has no bearing on the actual technical credibility of the evaluation data; the perception of the data as credible can be just as important. This is not to be confused with having poor-quality data that the client thinks are credible; such data are not acceptable.

My government department accepts different methods of inquiry as producing credible evidence. However, I recently presented a qualitative evaluation to my management team, and they criticized the evaluation, saying that it was biased and subjective. Can you help me?

There are a few ways to approach this situation. First, let's clarify some language. According to the *Oxford Living Dictionaries: English* (2018), *objective* means "not influenced by personal feelings or opinions in considering and representing facts." *Subjective* is the opposite, and is defined as "based on or influenced by personal feelings, tastes, or opinions." *Biased* is defined as "unfairly prejudiced for or against someone or something." So the comment that the research is biased and subjective is some pretty harsh criticism. Let's dig down and figure out some of the reasons why the management team may have said that the evaluation is biased or subjective, and then systematically address each one.

The criticism may have been focused on the evaluator. If so, ouch! A qualitative evaluator (just like a quantitative one) does not set out to prove a particular perspective. Ever. The researcher is neutral. However, she is likely to be empathetic to the situation she is studying (e.g., she does not have neutral feelings about HIV/AIDS orphans, or ice caps melting and polar bears starving). Being empathetic does not make the evaluator biased; it makes her human. *An evaluator's caring that people or animals are suffering because of a situation shows that the evaluator has empathy and makes the evaluation more credible.* In fact, empathy is a built-in strategy that strengthens the quality of the data; it does not weaken it. Because an evaluator is empathetic, she knows that *only* credible data (and, in some cases, *only* her evaluation) has the capability to inform decisions that will positively affect the social problem.

Perhaps the criticism was aimed at the evaluation findings. That's still an ouch, but perhaps a little less so, as it is not so personal. In this instance, I would describe in detail the strategies used to address bias and strengthen data credibility. These include **data triangulation** (in which data are gathered from different participants, sources, or methods, as further explained on pages 92–93); **data saturation** (in which the same question receives the same response from different people and different groups); **member checks** (in which the persons interviewed review the data transcripts or summarized information about them or their surroundings, and makes any necessary corrections); and a review of the data against set criteria to ensure their quality. Other strategies include prolonged engagement, persistent observations, and peer debriefing (Guba & Lincoln, 1989; Maxwell, 2013; Patton, 2015).

I thought that in qualitative inquiry, the whole idea was to seek people's perceptions and to make meaning of those data (with an emphasis on meaning) to address the evaluation questions. Yet my client is telling me that the findings are not credible because I am only reporting people's biases and perceptions.

This third type of bias labeling calls for a completely different discussion from that needed for the two types already mentioned. In interviews, the very core of what the evaluator wants to hear and understand *consists of* the interviewees' biases, perspectives, and subjective opinions. What moves these from "A person randomly said that" to data is the use of a transparent, logical, and consistent approach to obtaining the data.

I have a colleague who says that she is going to use qualitative research because it is easier than quantitative.

I am not sure why that damaging myth continues to float around; it is simply not true. Using qualitative methods in monitoring and evaluation takes training, and often years of practical fieldwork. Qualitative inquiry is not easier than quantitative inquiry; rather, each type requires a different skill set.

*I hear a lot about **triangulation** in qualitative research. Can you talk specifically about what that is and why it is used?*

Triangulation is a strategy that addresses data credibility. It is an evaluator's avoidance of being dependent on any one source of data, or any one understanding of it (Denzin & Lincoln, 1998; Guin, 2002; Patton, 2015; Schwandt, 1997). There are five types of triangulation.

- *Data triangulation* is the use of different sources, such as interviews with program implementers and beneficiaries.
- *Evaluator triangulation* occurs when different evaluators review the same data and provide their interpretations (Denzin & Lincoln, 1998; Guin, 2002; Patton, 2015; Schwandt, 1997).
- *Methodological triangulation* is the use of two or more qualitative and/or quantitative methods, such as surveys and interviews (Greene, 2007; Patton, 2015).
- *Theory triangulation* occurs when individuals from different disciplines employ their own theories of how the world works, and therefore interpret the data in different ways—reaching either the same conclusion, or different ones (Donaldson, 2007; Funnell & Rogers, 2011; Patton, 2008).
- *Environmental triangulation* explores different settings or other different factors (such as time, day, or season) that may influence the information (Guin, 2002).

The first four strategies enable the evaluator to gather data that engages with and honors diversity in people's ways of thinking, ways of seeing the world, and ways of knowing (e.g., nontraditional ways of gathering or accepting what are data). Those different viewpoints can be sought both among the people who are being studied (data triangulation) and among those who are studying them (evaluator triangulation). Methodological triangulation and theory triangulation bring in different ways of knowing (what is a fact and how to interpret that fact), although how these bring in that diverse thinking is often more obscured in an evaluation, as it is usually buried more deeply in the methodology section of an evaluation report.

Can you provide an example of how you use data triangulation for data analysis?

Here is one of my "go-to" strategies when I am working with a team of evaluators. Data are gathered, cleaned, and shared with each team member, and then the team is brought together for a data analysis workshop. At the workshop, the evaluation questions are posted on a flip chart, and each team member is asked to use the data to explain how they would answer each question. There is often divergence among team members, though not always, and the areas of divergence usually produce rich discussions that strengthen the findings. Even when there is no divergence, sometimes how an evaluator arrived at that answer results in a rich discussion that also strengthens the findings. These workshops can be expanded to include, for instance, implementers or technical experts in the area under study (e.g., education experts, nurses, environmentalists). This is just one example of how to use triangulation of these methods.

The example provided shows how different interpretations of the data strengthen findings. In addition, the data from different sources (e.g., a survey and in-depth interviews) may produce different or even conflicting findings. Do not be concerned; rather, be thrilled. The inconsistencies among the data are useful for learning why these inconsistencies exists, and bring higher-level insights to an evaluative process.

SOME FURTHER READING ON QUALITATIVE INQUIRY

- *Have a few minutes?* Watch John Creswell's video, which uses a case study to show the value of qualitative and mixed methods research (*www.youtube.com/watch?v=l5e7kVzMIfs*). Or check out a conversation between Albert Einstein and Queen Elizabeth II (*www.youtube.com/watch?v=MlU22hTyIs4#funny*).

- *Have an hour?* Check out some articles in Sage Publications's *International Journal of Qualitative Methods*. Specifically, look at an editorial by Paul Galdas (2017), titled "Revisiting Bias in Qualitative Research: Reflections on Its Relationship with Funding and Impact."

- *Have a few hours?* In the fourth edition of the *Handbook of Practical Program Evaluation* (Newcomer, Hatry, & Wholey, 2015), read Krueger and Casey's chapter on focus group interviewing or the chapter by Goodrick and Rogers on qualitative data analysis. If you are interested in engaging in qualitative research that involves using the internet and digital applications, or videos, photographs, and the arts, check out Chapter 7 in Marshall and Rossman's *Designing Qualitative Research* (2016). That book provides numerous other suggested readings and resources, so if you have time, take a quick skim through the rest of the book for further resource guidance.

- *Have an hour a few nights a week for the next several months?* Then there are several options. For a very practical exploration of qualitative research, and one filled with numerous examples and stories, read Michael Quinn Patton's *Qualitative Research and Evaluation Methods* (2015), spreading one chapter over several nights. It is a book well worth having on your shelf. For a more academic yet accessible book, try reading Robert E. Stake's *Qualitative Research: Studying How Things Work* (2010).

QUANTITATIVE INQUIRY

Let's now turn to quantitative inquiry. Quantitative inquiry can be used to measure attitudes, opinions, behaviors, and other defined variables by collecting numerical data that are then statistically analyzed. Quantitative research analyzes numbers, uncovers patterns in those numbers, and then generates conclusions (Creswell & Creswell, 2018; Johnson & Christensen, 2012).

Quantitative inquiry is best suited to an evaluation that seeks (1) to answer causal or predictive questions, and/or (2) to generalize findings from a sample to the larger population.

- *Descriptive* questions ask "how often" or "how much" in terms of numbers. An example would be "How often do teenagers visit the tutoring program during the school week?"

- *Causal* or *relationship* questions (which are elaborated on, as they are common in evaluative practice) compare variables to try to determine a relationship: Did one variable cause another, or is one related to another? An example of a causal question would be "Did the improved recruitment activities targeting women for the personal finance training program increase female attendance at the training?" An example of a relationship question would be "Does implementing free breakfast at the primary school relate to attendance of primary school children?" (Johnson & Christensen, 2012; Salkind, 2000).

- *Inferential* questions try to figure out what actions (dependent variables) will cause a desired (or undesired) outcome (independent variable). An example of a predictive question would be "Does playing an after-school sport lead to higher rates of anorexia nervosa in girls?"

Data Collection Methods

Quantitative inquiry relies heavily on validated data collection tools (e.g., surveys, assessments, measures). In a quantitative evaluation, a common method of inquiry is a survey (also called a structured questionnaire). These questionnaires can be administered in several ways: in face-to-face interviews, via some type of telephonic interview (e.g., mobile phone, Skype, Zoom), on paper, or via an internet survey. Structured questionnaires are just that—sets of structured, closed-ended questions, in which the answer choices are already provided, and the order of questions stays the same. In addition, quantitative inquiry uses statistical modeling with "big data," observations that score behavior, and (of course) all kinds of tests. And let's not forget quantitative indicator data (see Chapter 9) and management information systems. At its core, quantitative data are numbers that can be subjected to statistical analysis.

Data Analysis

Quantitative data are analyzed through some form of statistical analysis, and in evaluation, most of that analysis is informed by the *general linear model* (GLM; see Trochim, 2006). There are two kinds of statistical analysis: *descriptive statistics* and *inferential statistics*. Trochim (2006) offers a succinct description on his website of what these are, and their differences:

> Descriptive statistics are typically distinguished from inferential statistics. With descriptive statistics you are simply describing what is or what the data shows. With inferential statistics, you are trying to reach conclusions that extend beyond the immediate data alone. For instance, we use inferential statistics to try to infer from the sample data what the population might think. Or, we use inferential statistics to make judgments of the probability that an observed difference between groups is a dependable one or one that might have happened by chance in this study. Thus, we use inferential statistics to make inferences from our data to more general conditions; we use descriptive statistics simply to describe what's going on in our data.

For most evaluators, it is useful to know descriptive statistics, such as how to calculate a *mean, mode,* and *median,* and how to interpret a *standard deviation.* Descriptive statistics are the simplest ways of combing through data to understand the story behind the numbers. My colleague Benita Williams, an evaluator who specializes in evaluating education interventions in South Africa and someone with whom I often work, has provided an example of how she uses descriptive statistics in her daily work. She explains:

> "Here is an example of how I use descriptive statistics, and I think most evaluators would find knowing these kinds of analysis useful. Say that children take a test at the beginning of the school year so the teacher knows the class's level of math knowledge. Then, 6 months later, the teacher gives the class the same exact math test. How would you know if the class improved? You would simply calculate means (averages) for the baseline and endline, and look at the standard deviations to make sure you have some idea of how your data are distributed around the means. And if someone tells you that there is a correlation of $r = .60, n = 55, p < .000$, you could either run away scared, or spend 20 minutes to read this and understand what are a correlation coefficient and a *p* value: *www.socialresearchmethods.net/kb/statcorr.php.*" (Note that the link Benita provides is to the "Correlation" page of Trochim's [2006] website. Other pages on this site are worth studying as well.)

Thanks, Benita, that was helpful. Can you provide a table that shows how to calculate the mean, median, and mode? Since it is something I should know, it would be helpful to see an example.

Having examples is helpful. Table 5.1 demonstrates how to calculate a mean, median, and mode, and provides an explanation of the differences among the three.

TABLE 5.1. Calculating a Mean, Median, and Mode

The data: Five children take a math test. One child scores 50%. One child scores 75%. One child scores 60%. Two children score 100%. What is the average score? There could be three answers.

Mean	Median	Mode
A type of average where scores are added (summed) and divided by the number of observations.	The point where 50% of the cases in the distribution fall below, and 50% fall above. If there are an even number of observations, the two middle scores are averaged (the same math used to get a mean).	The most frequently occurring score in a distribution. It is the least precise (Salkind, 2000).
50 + 60 + 75 + 100 + 100 = 77. The mean score is 77%.	50, 60, 75, 100, 100. The median is 75 (it is two scores from the bottom and two scores from the top).	100% is the most frequently occurring score, as it occurs twice and other scores only appear once.

Before we move along, Benita mentioned standard deviation. Can you talk a bit more about that?

A standard deviation is a measure of the dispersion of a set of data from its mean. In other words, a standard deviation shows how spread out the numbers are from the average. To understand this concept, consider what statisticians call a *normal distribution* of data. Such a distribution means that most of the examples in a data set are close to the *average*, while relatively few examples tend to one extreme or the other. So the standard deviation is a statistic that tells you how closely each case (in the example in Table 5.1, how many students) are clustered around the mean in their class (also known as the *data set*). When the cases are tightly bunched together, the standard deviation is small. When the cases are spread relatively far apart, the standard deviation is large.

I was running away pretty fast when Benita talked about correlations. I know she's provided a link to a page of Trochim's website to learn more; can you explain what it means if a correlation coefficient is reported as r = −.68, p < .000?

A correlation coefficient is represented as *r*. So in the statement you give, the correlation coefficient is the −.68, and the probability (*p*) is 0. Correlation is a statistical measure that indicates whether two variables are associated, and in which direction they are associated.

Let's take a question. An evaluator wants to find out if older people visit health clinics more than younger people. So, she asks, is the average age related to the average number of visits?

A correlation coefficient can range from −1 all the way through 0 and then to +1. You should pay attention to the size of the correlation coefficient and to whether it is a positive or negative number. In addition to the correlation coefficient, you need to take note of *p*.

If there is an association between the two variables—in this example, average age and average number of clinic visits—you will have a correlation coefficient closer to 1 than 0, or a correlation coefficient closer to −1 than 0. Basically, if the correlation coefficient is close to 0, it means that there is no relationship.

- If the correlation coefficient has a negative sign, it means that there is an inverse relationship: The *higher* the average age, the *lower* the average number of clinic visits. The one variable is high, and the other is low. The fact that it is an inverse relationship is indicated by a negative sign.
- If the correlation coefficient has a positive sign, it means that there is a direct relationship: The *higher* the average age, the *higher* the average number of clinic visits. Or the *lower* the average age, the *lower* the average number of clinic visits.

Where the p value comes in is to tell you whether these two variables are related (the hypothesis) or not related (the null hypothesis). If p is smaller than .05, it means that there is *no* evidence that the two variables are *not* related; in other words, they are probabilistically (yes, this is the real word!) or statistically significantly related.

So, an evaluator would then ask, what is considered a strong correlation and what is considered a weak correlation?

- First, look at p. If p is higher than .05, it means that there is probabilistically no statistically significant relationship. If it is lower than .05, then look at the sign (positive or negative) and size of the correlation coefficient, r.
- If r is positive, a value of 0 to .3 is considered a small or weak correlation; a value of .3 to .6 is considered a moderately strong correlation; and a value of .6 to 1 is considered a strong correlation.
- If r is negative, a value of 0 to −.3 is considered a small or weak correlation; a value of −.3 to −.6 is considered a moderately strong correlation; and a value of −.6 to −1 is considered a strong correlation—again, only if p is smaller than .05.

Presenting Quantitative Data

How quantitative data are presented is an important part of using statistical analysis. Tables with means (averages), frequencies (how often something happens), and cross-tabulations (comparisons of the relationship between two variables) are extremely useful for an evaluator to understand her quantitative data, and to share it with her client. If you want to ensure that your quantitative data (e.g., tables, graphs) are useful to the people who will read your report, pay attention to the growing body of work on data visualization. One important tip from the data visualization field is never, ever, ever to use a pie chart with more than three categories. Some evaluators do not like pie charts at all, and prefer to use only bar graphs. Some data visualization references can be found on page 99.

A more advanced level of statistical analysis is inferential statistics. Examples of inferential statistics are *t*-tests or analyses of variance (often abbreviated as ANOVAs). These kinds of analyses look to see if the means of various comparison groups are statistically significantly different from one another. A good place to use this level of analysis would be a situation when the baseline and endline mean scores for a math class are very close to each other, but the standard deviations look very different. You may need a statistical package such as IBM SPSS or STATA or R for this kind of analysis, although you can load something called the Data Analysis Toolpak onto Microsoft Excel (*www.statisticshowto.com/how-to-do-a-t-test-in-excel*).

I just did the most amazing quantitative evaluation. I answered the evaluation questions by using all kinds of sophisticated statistical software and analysis, and I provided detailed information to my client. The client wanted to see the data that supported the findings, and he wanted graphs and charts in the report. But then when he read the report, he seemed uninterested in all the data.

Although other reasons might exist, perhaps the evaluation user did not fully comprehend the statistical analysis and/or the resulting graphs and charts. While quantitative data and high-level statistical analysis may be necessary to provide credible data to answer evaluation questions, they may at the same time be the reasons an evaluation is underused or not used. When an evaluation report is laden with necessary statistics, charts, and graphs, it is helpful to provide an interactive session in which the data can be verbally presented, and to ensure that the visualization of those data is well done (see the Resources feature that follows). If the client does already understand the data, he may welcome the time to engage with the evaluator at a more intensive level; if he finds some of the statistics challenging to interpret or engage with, he will welcome the additional understanding that the meeting can provide.

SOME FURTHER READING ON QUANTITATIVE INQUIRY

- **Have a few minutes?** William Trochim's (2006) website provides clear and succinct explanations on quantitative analysis, along with many other social research methods. (Trochim is a professor at Cornell University.) Check out the table of contents on his website (*www.socialresearchmethods.net/kb/contents.php*).

- **Have a few more minutes?** For specific help from Trochim's site on how to select the right statistical analysis for your data, look at this webpage (*www.socialresearchmethods. net/selstat/ssstart.htm*). The page will ask a series of questions about your data, and based on what you choose, it will select the correct statistical test. If you want to understand *why* a specific test is the right choice, look at a page of Graphpad's website (*www. graphpad.com/support/faqid/1790/an*).

- *Have an hour?* Choose some statistical topics that are of interest to you from David M. Lane's HyperStat Online website (*http://davidmlane.com/hyperstat*). The website provides 18 different topics on statistics, from an introduction to stats to measuring effect size. It also provides numerous other links on statistical analysis.

- *Have some more time?* Consider reading Shadish, Cook, and Campbell's (2001) *Experimental and Quasi-Experimental Designs for Generalized Causal Inference.* Another text worth having on your shelf is the fifth edition of Creswell and Creswell's (2018) *Research Design: Qualitative, Quantitative and Mixed Methods Approaches.* The book discusses the terms used in all three approaches, shows how to apply these approaches, and describes how to engage in the data quality discussion for all types of inquiry.

- *Want to learn more about data visualization?* Check out the websites by Stephanie Evergreen (*http://stephanieevergreen.com*), Ann K. Emery (*http://annkemery.com*), and Edward Tufte (*www.edwardtufte.com/tufte*).

MIXED METHODS

Now we turn to the third type of design, **mixed methods research,** which is exactly what its name suggests—a mix of qualitative and quantitative research. Johnson and Onwuegbuzie (2004) provide a description of mixed methods research. These authors note that because quantitative and qualitative inquiry bring different assumptions and worldviews into methods of inquiry, combining the approaches can be very useful. Mixed methods approaches are often explained in this manner, with a focus on how to combine qualitative and quantitative methods.

Consider this example. An exploratory open-ended qualitative interview is used to gain an understanding from select groups about what people appreciate most about the local community watch, and what they want to change. Based on information from those interviews, a focused, closed-ended survey is designed and sent to the larger community (e.g., 5,000 people). The evaluator now knows that 82% of women in the community think an evening patrol is necessary or very necessary; however, only 21% of men report that it is necessary, and none report that it is very necessary. While it is clear what women and men think with regard to the evening patrol, it is not clear what accounts for the difference. An evaluator could then, using a purposeful sampling strategy, select participants to take part in focus groups (a qualitative method) with women and men in the community. The data from the focus groups are then used to further understand these quantitative results.

In Jennifer Greene's (2007) explanation of mixed methods, she suggests that mixed methods inquiry involves "considered and thoughtful attention to various ways of knowing and various ways of conducting social inquiry. . . . [Such attention is] a central and defining characteristic of mixed methods inquiry . . . for better understanding social phenomena" (p. 14). She goes on to discuss mixed methods research as requiring more than a series of choices between qualitative or quantitative methods. Rather, it is about respecting and including what she calls people's different "mental models"—how they think about how the world works, and therefore how they go about collecting information to answer questions, and what they consider to be credible data. Greene thus provides a working and practical definition of mixed methods inquiry in the real world, where different people, perhaps influenced by politics, culture, religion, education, or other factors, have different ways of engaging with, seeing, and valuing an intervention and its results. (See Chapter 4 for more on different ways of thinking and knowing what is a fact.)

Mixed methods are useful for two reasons:

1. *Evaluations may be strengthened through having the perspectives brought by qualitative and quantitative data.* As noted by Palinkas and colleagues (2015), "the challenges of implementing evidence-based and other innovative practices, treatments, interventions and programs are sufficiently complex that a single methodological approach is often inadequate."

2. *Clients or colleagues may simply prefer having both kinds of data, even though one type of data may technically answer the evaluation question.* For instance, evaluation users, or commissioners of evaluation, may like to see numbers in an evaluation report, such as 80% of the beneficiaries liked the services provided, along with stories and pictures that depict some of the beneficiaries, and often bring a more "organic" feel to the evaluation.

SOME FURTHER READING ON MIXED METHODS INQUIRY

- *Have about 7 minutes?* Watch John Creswell's video, recommended above in the Resources for qualitative inquiry, which uses a case study to show the value of qualitative and mixed methods (*www.youtube.com/watch?v=l5e7kVzMIfs*).

- *Have an hour?* Read Jennifer C. Greene's (2008) article, "Is Mixed Methods Social Inquiry a Distinctive Methodology?" *Journal of Mixed Methods Research, 2*(1), 7–21.

- *Have some more time and a serious interest in mixed methods approaches?* Read Jennifer C. Greene's *Mixed Methods in Social Inquiry* (2007), which is an informative text on these approaches, or John W. Creswell and Vicki L. Plano Clark's third edition of *Designing and Conducting Mixed Methods Research* (2018).

SAMPLING

Although a researcher or evaluator could study an entire population, it is often not feasible, cost-effective, or even necessary to do so. Thus evaluators select a sample (with each person, place, or thing selected called a *case*) from the identified population, in order to provide data that answer the evaluation question. An evaluator using sampling needs to provide a transparent strategy that clarifies the criteria used to select the sample, and recognizes the limitations. Qualitative sampling is fundamentally different from quantitative sampling.

Qualitative Research: Purposeful Sampling

In qualitative inquiry, evaluators select specific people, places, or things within the larger population because of the unique insight and rich information they bring to bear on a particular evaluation question. In an evaluation, it is *not* enough to say that purposeful sampling will be used (or was used); the evaluator needs to specify which type of purposeful sampling, and why that strategy was chosen. Here are four of several kinds of qualitative sampling that exist.

Criterion sampling involves identifying specific criteria, and then exploring all cases that meet those criteria. In *extreme* or *deviant case sampling*, the evaluator selects cases where the intervention was notably perceived as a success or a failure. Realist evaluation (see Chapter 15) is an evaluation method that is likely to draw on this approach, as this type of evaluation (Pawson, 2006) is interested in understanding what works under particular circumstances. Extreme or deviant case sampling identifies cases that are likely to provide rich data for examining successful as well as unsuccessful implementations of the intervention. Another type of qualitiative sampling is *homogeneous sampling*. Here an evaluator selects a small, homogeneous group (i.e., a group whose members are all the same or very similar) in order to better understand a particular group in depth; the homogeneous group could even consist of one person. A final example is *snowball* or *chain sampling*. Here the evaluator identifies initial key informants (people who are likely to have or provide information needed to address the evaluation question) and then, from these key informants, seeks details of other "information-rich cases" in the field (Patton, 2002, 2008, 2015).

Quantitative Research: Probability or Random Sampling

Quantitative researchers and evaluators use *probability* and *nonprobability* strategies to select samples to study. A probability sample utilizes some form of random selection. In probability sampling (also known as *random sampling*), any case (i.e., person, place, or thing) has the same chance of being selected, thus eliminating the possibility of bias. In other words, a sample chosen randomly is meant to be an unbiased representation of the total population (Bickman, 2000). Aimee White, a methodologist and empowerment and collaborative evaluator, explains the thinking behind probability sampling:

> In the quantitative world, there is this concept that across large numbers of persons there is a "normal curve" that implies odd experiences or "outlying" responses can be **normalized** if enough persons are selected to collect data from, and those persons are all selected **at random.**

If you're ever at a party and want to sound smart, drop the term that describes this, the Central Limit Theorem. People will think you are brilliant. (personal email, January 15, 2018)

White goes on to explain that the aim of normalization is to have as "representative" a sample of the full population of interest as is possible, and that in doing so, the researcher works toward "generalizability" (being able to take the answers from a few in order to generalize those answers to the larger group affected) of the findings.

BOX 5.1. Random Assignment or Random Sampling: There Is a Difference

White, Sabarwal, and de Hoop (2014, p. 1) explain:

> Random assignment should not be confused with random sampling. Random sampling refers to how a sample is drawn from one or more populations. Random assignment refers to how individuals or groups are assigned to either a treatment group or a control group. RCTs [randomized controlled trials] typically use both random sampling (since they are usually aiming to make inferences about a larger population) and random assignment (an essential characteristic of an RCT).

PRACTICAL GUIDANCE IN CHOOSING AN INQUIRY METHOD

1. *Match the method to the question.* The advice commonly given when evaluators ask which method of inquiry to choose is to match the inquiry to the evaluation question. For example, if the question is how well a student reads, a reading test will be needed. If the question is how students feel about reading, students should be interviewed.

2. *Take users' preferences into account.* If a client, colleague, or boss states a preference for a particular method, listen closely, for this preference provides insight into what type of evidence the user considers to be credible (i.e., believable). Thus the second consideration in choosing methods is to consider the user's beliefs, assumptions, and perceptions.

3. *Match the inquiry to the resources available.* Consider the resources allotted for the evaluation, such as finances or time (e.g., when decisions based on the evaluation findings need to be made, or whether there are enough funds to visit 10 sites).

4. *Assess contextual and logistical factors.* Context means the characteristics and features of the setting in which the evaluation takes place. For example, is it feasible to do mail surveys, or is it safe for an external evaluator to conduct inquiry in a community? Consider the appropriateness of the inquiry to the cultural, political, and social context.

Toss all four considerations into a pot (the evaluation question, user's preference, resources, and context), mix well, and the type of inquiry to use will bubble to the top.

CREDIBLE DATA

No matter what kind of inquiry design is chosen, there needs to be an explicitly described inquiry approach that leads to credible data, led by an evaluator who is neutral. Having good-quality, and therefore credible (believable), data is always critical. Qualitative data (words and pictures) and quantitative data (numbers) require different criteria for judging the quality of the data because they involve different ways of knowing what is a fact. (See Chapter 4 for discussions of ways of thinking and ways of knowing what is a fact.) The present section briefly identifies the different criteria used to judge data quality, which then feed into the conversation on credible evidence.

Listen closely; I have another trade secret to share. Having good-quality data is essential to having credible evidence, and credible evidence is an essential part of having a credible evaluation. The three—credible data, credible evidence, and credible evaluation—are connected but different, as we will soon find out.

Good-quality data are critical for any study. Qualitative and quantitative approaches bring different ways of thinking about data, and therefore require their own criteria for whether the data are credible or not. An evaluator who uses qualitative data needs to use criteria identified in qualitative inquiry—namely, their credibility, transferability, dependability, and confirmability. An evaluator who draws on quantitative data needs to employ quantitative criteria, which are internal validity, external validity, reliability, and objectivity. Different methods of inquiry; different kinds of data; different criteria. Qualitative criteria should be used to judge qualitative data, and quantitative criteria should be used to judge quantitative data. Just as a person does not judge a quantitative study with qualitative criteria, a qualitative study is not judged with quantitative ones.

At the same time, regardless of the method of inquiry, an evaluator needs data that are precise and accurate. The more precise information is, the more useful it is. For instance, when the question is "How old is your daughter?", it is more useful to know the daughter's birth date than her age, as her age will change tomorrow. Even so, the amount of precision will be determined by the research question, as perhaps the research only requires that the person's daughter be under 18. Her response that her daughter is 11 is adequate precision in this instance. Whereas in quantitative inquiry *precision* often means precision with regard to a number, in qualitative inquiry it means a thick, rich description that enables the researcher (and the reader of the data) to know what a person is talking about, with enough exactitude to answer the research question. Precise data are not necessarily accurate data, and this holds true for qualitative or quantitative data. For example, stating that someone is a second-year anthropology student at the local university is more precise than saying that she attends the university, but she may actually be a graduate student in sociology (Babbie & Mouton, 2001).

Now that we have looked at what are considered good-quality data, let's look at what is considered credible evidence.

CREDIBLE EVIDENCE

An evaluator needs not only to gather credible data, but to present evidence (for a discussion on data vs. evidence, see Chapter 1) that is viewed as credible (believable) by those whom an evaluation is trying to support, help, inform, or otherwise persuade. Evidence that is not perceived as credible can contribute to an evaluation's crashing at the end or stumbling along the way. While having good-quality data are an integral part of having credible evidence, such data form only one part of the discussion.

What is considered credible evidence is a topic fraught with diverse perspectives informed by values, culture, the evaluation literature, and academic training, to name a few of the weightier influences (Schwandt, 2009). When evaluation users have different understandings of what counts as credible evidence, it is the evaluator's role to facilitate discussions that bring clarity and agreement. To provide a useful way to discuss credible evidence, Donaldson's (2009) five characteristics of credible evidence have been expanded, adapted, and molded into a framework that can help an evaluator facilitate a discussion that identifies what is considered credible evidence, and by whom (see Table 5.2, left column). This adaptation of Donaldson's work was heavily influenced by Greene (2000, 2009), House and Howe (1999), Patton (2008, 2015), Schwandt (2009), and my own research (Podems, 2007, 2010, 2017). Table 5.2 also provides a simplified set of questions and practical points to consider (middle and right columns) that can be combined with the framework, or used as a stand-alone option.

While the framework presented in Table 5.2 is intended to provide concrete guidance, questions like the following provide a less structured way to engage in a credibility discussion, which can be used either on its own or as a supplement to the Table 5.2 framework. Engage people in a conversation by asking questions like these:

- What do you consider credible evidence?
- If I provided X and Y, through doing A and B, which resulted in good-quality data, would you find the evidence that resulted credible?
- Please show me a few evaluations or other evaluative reports that you consider not to be credible. Can you explain to me what makes you think that?

TABLE 5.2. Facilitating a Dialogue on Credible Evidence

Influencer of credibility of the evidence	Questions to answer	Practical points to consider
Multiple voices: How does the evidence address questions from multiple viewpoints?	Whose viewpoints need to be considered? Are there different viewpoints for different questions?	Identify the multiple voices (meaning people) that need to be heard. For all questions in the framework, consider these perspectives. Then consider: What if the viewpoints conflict? Who makes the decision to value one voice over another? How will that be managed? Does one voice have more power than others, or power over others? Is the research budget large enough to address different viewpoints? If not, what then? Consider multiple views. Confirm what multiple users consider acceptable.
Practicalities	What are the practical and logistical constraints that may influence the evaluation process and the evidence provided?	These questions are likely to be discussed between the evaluators (who identify and explain the constraints) and whoever is funding the evaluation. Once the constraints are clear, it may be possible to make needed adjustments (e.g., to increase the budget or make other accommodations). If there are no options, be explicit in describing to all evaluation users how these practical and logistical constraints can influence the credibility of the evidence *before* the evaluation commences (or as they become evident in the process). If these constraints are only mentioned after the evaluation is completed, or as a response to an attack on the credibility of the evidence, the constraints are likely to be perceived as excuses. Consider multiple views. Confirm what multiple users consider acceptable.
Research approach	How well do the methods answer the evaluation questions? What are the strengths? What are the weaknesses?	It may be necessary to explain the research approach, and its strengths and weaknesses, to the evaluation users. Provide concrete examples that demonstrate the strengths and the weaknesses (not theoretical explanations). Then ask, "Do you find this acceptable? If not, why not?" If users say that the weaknesses in the approach will lead to their not using the evaluation, consider alternatives, one of which is not conducting the evaluation. Implementing an evaluation when the evidence will not be found credible, and the evaluation will then not be used, is a waste of resources. Consider multiple views. Confirm what multiple users consider acceptable.
Evaluation and the evaluation approach	What are the users' assumptions about the evaluation in terms of what it will, and will not, do? Do users find the evaluation approach credible?	Describe the advantages and limitations of any evaluation (e.g., its time-bound nature, the role of values). Explain the evaluation approach, its strengths, and its weaknesses to the evaluation users. For example, if using a participatory approach, what will that involve? If there are options or tradeoffs, present those in a straightforward manner. Consider multiple views. Confirm what multiple users consider acceptable.
The social, cultural, and economic context of the intervention	How do social, cultural, and economic factors influence the choices of data to be gathered? Data-gathering methods? Interpretation of the data?	Consider these questions in developing the nutshell description (see Chapter 3). Different users may have very different insights. Identify specific social, cultural, and economic influences (do not use labels only) and then ask evaluation users if they have other ones to add. Consider how all these influences may affect the evaluation. Consider multiple views. Confirm what multiple users consider acceptable.

An evaluator needs to know which stakeholders consider what to be credible evidence because an evaluation that is regarded as lacking such evidence will not be used (Donaldson, 2009; Patton, 2015; Schwandt, 2015). Credible evidence is in the eyes of the beholder, so to speak. Providing credible evidence, however, does not mean that an *evaluation* will be credible or even be used, as an evaluation is more than its evidence. Factors such as the credibility of the conclusions, interpretations, and recommendations; timing; and the readability of the report will all affect its credibility, and therefore its use (Calhoun & Risendal, 2018; Patton, 2015; Schwandt, 2015).

BOX 5.2. An Evaluator's Role in Producing a Credible Evaluation

An evaluator needs to know when to use which inquiry method in an evaluation to answer what evaluation question. An effective evaluator does not need to be an expert in all three methods of inquiry, but she needs to be an expert in at least one, and to understand enough to be at ease with the others. Throughout, the evaluator needs to pay close attention to, and actively engage in, making decisions and employing strategies to produce credible data, credible evidence, and a credible evaluation. Sometimes making these decisions is not within the evaluator's power; see Chapter 17 for what to do when that happens.

BASELINE STUDY

A **baseline study** is a form of assessment; however, a baseline study has its own suitcase because of the unique role that its data play in the evaluative process. A *baseline* shows what was in place, or what existed, when the intervention started, and is directly related to what the intervention aims to fix, change, or otherwise improve. A baseline study, then, provides information with which to monitor an intervention's progress during implementation, and to assess its effectiveness along the way, and after the activity is completed. Some interventions have baseline data; sometimes the data are incomplete or of poor quality; and often they are nowhere to be found. Baseline data are needed for each problem addressed by the intervention (see Chapters 3–4 and 10). When planning a baseline study, an evaluator (or researcher or program manager) needs to determine what change needs to be assessed, and what sort of data are needed for that comparison (see Chapters 3–4 for more on problem statements).

Here is an example. A person weighs 150 pounds at the start of her exercise program; that is the baseline for her weight. The person wants to lose weight (i.e., the intended result is weight loss), and she wants to weigh 130 pounds (target). After 3 months of running, she weighs 130 pounds. As the evaluator, you know the baseline (where the person started—150 pounds) and where she ended (130 pounds). You can confidently state that she lost 20 pounds because you know from where the person started (baseline) and where they ended. A qualitative baseline uses words rather than numbers. Here is an example. Most people who live within a 2-kilometer radius of a certain lake describe the level of garbage in and around the lake as unacceptable. While this description is in words, it is evaluable; after an intervention is implemented, it provides a place to compare what is with what was.

Sometimes, an implementer will decide months or even years into implementation to identify the baseline. The data gathered after an intervention has started are not baseline data (unless these are historical data taken from records that reflect the context at the start of the intervention). They are not baseline data because they were not collected prior to the intervention's implementation (the base). Collecting data after the intervention has started may be a useful figure to gauge progress from the point in time data are gathered; however, these data ignore the progress that was made in getting to that point, which may be where the most significant changes took place.

Let's go back to the weight loss example. Imagine that the same person does *not* weigh herself. A few weeks after her intervention (the running program) is implemented, her running coach contacts you to see how successful the person has been in losing weight, and asks you to collect baseline data. At this point, after the person has started the running program, you meet the person and (as requested by the running coach) weigh her. The person's weight is 143 pounds. A month later you return and weigh the person again, and she weighs 140 pounds. Since you wrote down 143 as your baseline (as requested), it looks as if the running intervention resulted in the person's losing 3 pounds. However, if the person's weight has been measured from the first day of the running program (which, for this example, we know to be 150 pounds), before the running program started, then the intervention will demonstrate a bigger weight loss and is likely to be perceived as more successful by the running coach (since he is judging the person's success on weight loss). When an intervention is assessed, most people want to show *all* their achievement, not part of it. Thus collecting data after an intervention has started, and labeling these as "baseline" data, should not be done.

Let's keep twisting the example, though. The person losing the weight may not need a scale as her baseline; for her, perhaps reporting feeling overweight and not fitting into her favorite jeans before the running program starts, and now fitting into her favorite jeans, is enough for her to be happy with the running program. How the problem is perceived, and how success is determined, then, will also influence what type of baseline is needed (i.e., the running coach sees the person's problem as a need to lose weight; the participant sees her problem as not fitting into her favorite jeans). She evaluates her success as fitting into her jeans, not losing weight per se. A key point is that to show an accurate picture of what has happened, the same method to assess the baseline is used to assess the results.

What should I do if the intervention has already started and the intervention staff say that no baseline data exist?

In the real world, it is not uncommon to find interventions that do not have baselines—or at least think that they do not have baselines. You have several viable options, depending on the circumstances. One is to help identify baseline data that may exist. After all, someone, at some point, identified the need for an intervention based on something (see Chapter 3 on problem statements). Here are some places to start searching for baseline data:

- Find the people who suggested the need for an intervention or perhaps the initial donors or funders. Asking them how the decision was made to have an intervention may lead to identifying secondary data. For example, someone may remember that a study was done that showed X and Y, and therefore an intervention was developed to address that. Bingo! You have found baseline data!

- Search for external sources of information (also secondary data): census data, school testing results, clinic data, police statistics, or relevant data from other organizations (such as a nonprofit organization, university, or research institute).

These data sources may not provide the whole story; however, they may provide "enough" data to enable you to determine whether the intervention has made progress. A third option is to ask individuals to try to recall what needed to change. Participants or program staff may be able to provide accurate descriptions of what is needed to change, or others who may not be participants or directly related to the program would have likely observed change over time and could also provide useful information. This approach is called establishing a *retrospective baseline*.

Here is my advice on engaging in a conversation with someone who says that no baseline survey or data exist: Ask them, "How did you, or someone else, know an intervention was needed?"

Can you talk more about a retrospective baseline?

A retrospective (literally, looking backward) baseline is obtained when evaluators ask people to describe what it was like before the intervention started. There are three key considerations for using retrospective baseline data. First, it is essential to ensure that whoever is going to use these data, or accept findings based on them, views these kinds of data as credible. If they do not, then do not collect them. Second, it is critical to triangulate the data. Third, consider influential factors, such as time; asking for recall of a situation 10 years ago versus 3 months ago may make a difference, although it depends on the person, the effect of the intervention, and other factors. For example, there may have been a critical event that, when people are reminded of it, improves their before-and-after recall.

Is having baseline data always a better option than having retrospective data?

There are some situations when a baseline is not the best way to assess progress. This is often true when people need to rate themselves. People do not know what they do not know. For example, having people rate themselves on a pre- and postintervention test has the threat of creating *response-shift bias* (Drennan & Hyde, 2008). Let's say that a person thinks he is an expert in evaluation. Before he starts a course on evaluation, the instructor asks him to rate himself on a scale of 1–5, with 1 being "novice" and 5 being "expert." In most aspects of evaluation, he rates himself a 5. He then takes the course on evaluation and realizes that he really did not know about evaluation (and that what he thought he knew was just not quite right). He then rates himself at the end of the training, giving himself mostly a score of 3. If the instructor or the evaluator compared these self-reported data, it would seem as though the evaluation course caused this man's knowledge to decrease. In this case, the instructor or evaluator would have obtained more accurate data by asking him at the end of the course to reflect and rate himself on where he was prior to the course and then to rate himself at the end. This is one example of a situation where retrospective data are useful.

BASELINE DATA

- *Have a few minutes?* Read a succinct post by E. Jane Davidson on the Genuine Evaluation blog (*http://genuineevaluation.com/no-baseline-a-few-tips*), which provides advice similar to that offered in this chapter.

- *Have an hour?* Read pages 388–389 of *RealWorld Evaluation* (Bamberger, Rugh, & Mabry, 2006).

- *Have a few hours?* Check out Michael Bamberger's (2010) paper for the World Bank, which explores why baseline studies are not always conducted, and then outlines strategies that can be used to reconstruct baseline data later in the program cycle (*http://siteresources.worldbank.org/INTPOVERTY/Resources/335642-1276521901256/premnoteME4.pdf*).

WRAPPING UP

Ensuring credible data, credible evidence, and a credible evaluation is an evaluator's responsibility. As part of this process to ensure credibility, the evaluator needs to be grounded in at least one method of inquiry and aware of the other two. This chapter has provided a *glimpse* of what you need to know with regard to qualitative, quantitative, and mixed methods approaches to gathering data to inform evaluative questions. Evaluators need to be able to engage in a technical discussion ranging from how to choose an appropriate form of inquiry, to how to collect, analyze, and interpret data, in an evaluative process. First a researcher is created, and then an evaluator is born.

INTERLUDE

As I was growing up outside New York City, my parents often brought me to see Broadway musicals. I remember the thrill of driving into the city, and then gleefully sitting in a dark theatre watching the show. I delighted in the music, the dancing, the singing, and even the orchestra's interlude—which takes place between the two acts, reminding me of what had already happened while garnering excitement for what was yet to come. I provide my evaluation interlude for the same reason: drawing on what has already been done, while providing hints at what is yet to come. The interlude keeps you fully immersed in what we have covered thus far, while generating enthusiasm for the next steps in the process.

In place of music, my interlude portrays a small story (a vignette), which sets the scene for discussions of linking problem statements, interventions, and results (Chapter 6); results (Chapter 7); theory of change and program logic (Chapter 8); and assessing progress toward and achieving results (Chapter 9).

What We Know Thus Far

We already have a nutshell description of the girls' education intervention we are using as an example (see Chapter 3). Using credible data and credible evidence, we have established that the intervention aims to address a fact-based problem (where we also identify baseline data), have defined the persons for whom the intervention is intended (beneficiaries), and raised the issue of the un-beneficiaries. We have also identified some of the values that inform the intervention and related decisions through understanding key decisions (e.g., what to fund, where to have the intervention, who benefits, and who does not). Everything we have identified thus far will be revisited from a different perspective, and everything we have learned thus far will be used to complete the evaluative journey.

The iterative nature of the journey is core to any evaluative process. It may appear inefficient at first (it is not) and exhausting (it can be). Yet the process is foundational for collecting systematic, incremental data, obtaining verifiable evidence, engaging with multiple perspectives, and valuing the findings.

Figure 5.1 summarizes what we have covered thus far in the evaluative process for the girls' education intervention. Note that the information in Figure 5.1 is provided in a different logical order from the order in which it has been provided in the chapters thus far. This is because what is uncovered is often messy, and out of order, to an outsider looking in. To an insider looking out, it often all makes sense. When the evaluator puts all the information together, it needs to be clear to everyone on the inside *and* the outside.

Now that we are on the same page, literally and figuratively, let's continue.

Problem Statement	Intervention	Beneficiaries
The grand problem in the community is that women are poorly educated and have high rates of unwanted pregnancy, high rates of spousal abuse, and low economic opportunity. The pocket problems are that the community's school-age girl population is double the school-age boy population for the same age brackets; however, few girls attend school (symptom), while all school-age boys attend. Girls do not attend due to issues about their safety (root cause) and the belief held by their fathers or father figures that girls do not need to attend school (root cause). Teachers, community leaders, and school-age girls think that few girls' attending school is a problem. It is a societal problem: Girls' not accessing formal education often leads to these girls' having fewer choices in life, as well as higher rates of abusive relationships, unwanted pregnancies, and poverty than girls who receive education until the age of 18.	The intervention started 3 years ago and will be funded for 2 more years. It focuses on helping school-age girls access education that is freely given in their community. The intervention mostly focuses on convincing fathers or father figures who currently prevent their daughters from attending to support their daughters in getting an education. The intervention also addresses some contextual issues, such as the girls' safety while going to and from school.	The direct beneficiaries are the school-age girls who currently do not attend school. The secondary beneficiaries are the fathers/father figures, and, in a broader sense, the community and society as a whole. The un-beneficiaries need to be explored more, such as by looking at how the boys in the community experience the intervention.

FIGURE 5.1. What we know thus far about the girls' education intervention.

CHAPTER 6
Linking Problem Statements, Interventions, and Results

Start where you are. Use what you have. Do what you can.
— ARTHUR ASHE, professional tennis player

   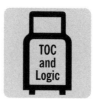

W e have made tremendous progress thus far in our evaluative journey. We have a basic description of the intervention (nutshell description); in general, we know the problems the intervention is aiming to address (problem statement); we know that the problem statement is based on facts; and we know whether the intervention is addressing root causes, symptoms, or both. We know who or what the intervention is trying to benefit (beneficiaries), who may get hurt or who was left out (un-beneficiaries), and who else needs to be involved in the process. We also know that choices exist with regard to how to collect, analyze, and interpret data, and we know that we need to make decisions about our method(s) of inquiry so that evaluation users will find both the data and the evidence credible. This chapter describes how these are all linked together and begins that conversation with a discussion on plausible and evaluable interventions.

THE IMPORTANCE OF A PLAUSIBLE AND EVALUABLE INTERVENTION

An intervention that aims to solve a social problem needs to be plausible. A *plausible* intervention is one that:

- Makes reasonable assumptions about how to address the problem.
- Is designed on the basis of experience and knowledge.
- Is culturally, politically, and socially acceptable.
- Gives thoughtful details about how each tiny part is intended to work and bring about results.

If an intervention meets each of these four characteristics, it is a plausible intervention. A plausible intervention that aims to solve a social problem also needs to be evaluable because an evaluator needs to ask *and* answer questions about what has worked, how, why, when, to what extent, where, and for whom. Part of being evaluable is being able to incrementally assess the intervention.

Incremental assessment is assessment in very small steps, from the problem to the results. Such assessment, when done properly, aims to identify even the smallest changes (or lack thereof). Being able to assess incremental changes is intricately related to understanding how an intervention aims to produce (or does produce) results. At this point in the journey (a journey that started in Chapter 3), a problem statement, an intervention, and intended or desired results are somewhat clear—but the descriptions are probably too broad to enable anyone to effectively assess incremental achievement, or lack thereof, and the links among the three are not yet strongly defined. In this chapter we learn how to break apart the problem statement, intervention, and intended results, and then how to link these smaller parts back together. An evaluator can play a forward-looking role (planning what will happen), a backward-looking role (figuring out what was done and identifying achieved results), or a bit of both in the same process. Note that Chapter 7 focuses exclusively on intended results, and making an intervention plausible and evaluable begins in Chapter 3 and continues into Chapter 8.

Making interventions plausible and incrementally evaluable starts with linking problem statements, interventions, and intended results, and concludes (at least in the first iterative round) with each divided into tiny parts that are linked to each other. Identifying these tiny connected parts helps us do the following:

- Clarify the specific connections among a problem, an intervention, and intended results.
- Identify what can be assessed and when.
- Provide places to collect data to identify why something worked, or why something did not.

BOX 6.1. Plausible and Evaluable Intervention

A **plausible, evaluable intervention** is one in which the evaluator, program manager, or anyone either internal or external to the evaluative process can clearly see (i.e., identify) an explicit, step-by-step link among the problem being addressed, the reasonably believable intervention that aims to fix it, and its realistically anticipated results.

What are some of the practical reasons why assessing incremental change is so important?

Assessing incremental change is important for several practical reasons. First, it can provide real-time data, which means that as something goes right (or wrong), the implementer will know and can address it as needed. Second, imagine that a program implementer (or funder or evaluator) waits until an intervention is coming to an end, and then finds out through an evaluation that the key problem or problems are not solved. That feedback is too late to be helpful to the intervention's beneficiaries, who are still left with the key problems. Third, it is not clear why there is no change, just that there was not (and the opposite is true; if it worked, it is not clear why it worked). At the heart of any intervention (or policy, activity, program, or innovation) is the intention to help someone, or something, in some way; evaluators can serve an important role in supporting implementers *if* incremental data points are identified and assessed. We delve more into this in Chapter 7 with a specific focus on sorting out and understanding results, and continue the conversation in Chapter 8 when we dive into intervention theory and logic.

BOX 6.2. The Cousins: Problem Statement–Intervention–Results Discussion

When imagining a mental image to connect a problem statement, an intervention, and results (which I sometimes call the "three cousins" from now on), it is helpful to picture the intervention in the middle (see Figure 6.1). Then look left to see the problem it is addressing, and look right to see what it aims to achieve. It often takes a bit of time (and patience) to identify all the desired results (or even achieved results), and understand how they connect (if they do) to each other, and then how the results connect to the intervention, and then how these all connect to the problem statement.

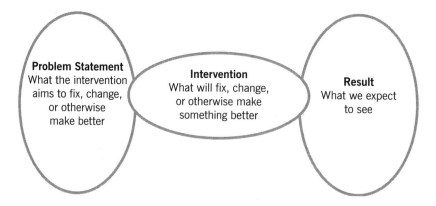

FIGURE 6.1. Linking the three cousins: Problem statement, intervention, and result.

WHAT NEEDS TO BE LINKED

Before we talk about how to link the problem statement, intervention, and results, let's explore the advantages of doing so by looking at an example that demonstrates what happens when we do not (see Table 6.1).

Looking at the example in Table 6.1, can you tell what intervention will address the problem statement and bring about the stated result? I am stumped; are you? The issue is that there is too much buried in the problem and the result statement, which makes it nearly impossible to identify what part of the intervention will fix the problem and lead to that result. If we cannot see how what part of the intervention has influenced or brought about the change, then we do not know if the intervention is contributing to, or bringing about, the result. If the result is achieved (school-age girls' access to education is improved), then we (you and I, the evaluators) cannot tie or link that result back to the intervention, though we could tie it to the problem statement. We need to break down all three (problem, intervention, result), and find the links among them all, to make the intervention evaluable (and in doing so, make the intervention plausible). The next sections will take you through the process to explain how to do this. (If you want to peek at the final product, skip ahead to Table 6.4.). But first, two noteworthy points need to be raised about the example provided in Table 6.1.

Two Noteworthy Points

The first point relates to conducting an evaluation. Sometimes the choice of where to start to unravel the connection is not the evaluator's. For example, an evaluation question may be posed by the funder or government agency, such as "To what extent did the intervention enhance girls' access to education?" The question is well written and appears to be reasonable at first glance. However, at this point it is not clear what the implementer did to achieve, or contribute to achieving, that result. (See Table 6.1 again.) To answer that evaluation question, an evaluator would need to start by asking, and answering, the questions in Chapters 3 and 4, spend a lot of time in this chapter and Chapter 7, and continue until reaching Chapter 10. Keep in mind that while these chapters provide the fundamentals, how those fundamentals are implemented is likely to vary by the evaluation method, framework, or approach chosen; however, I am leaping ahead. (If you want to leap ahead, see Chapter 15 for an introduction to evaluation methods, frameworks, and approaches.)

TABLE 6.1. Problem, Intervention, and Anticipated Result: When They Are Not Linked

Problem (Where we start from)	Intervention (How are we going to get there?)	Anticipated result (Where we want to get to)
Few school-age girls go to school.	?	School-age girls' access to education is improved.

The second point foreshadows Chapter 7's discussion of breaking down all the intended (or achieved) results into small incremental ones, and brings a critical insight to this chapter. There are interventions that have direct results. For example, let's say that a fifth-grade class has been taught to knit (intervention). Now most of the fifth graders know how to knit (direct result). Now that the children know how to knit, they decide to knit blankets for babies in the local orphanage. That result is that all the orphan babies have, new, warm, colorful knitted blankets. The initial knitting intervention has taught the children to knit; however, everything that has happened after that has been a result of the previous result, as well as other contextual factors (e.g., what made the children want to knit blankets for orphan babies and not another benefactor?), and not a direct result of the intervention. (For a longer, more detailed explanation of results logic, read Chapter 7.) This explanation provides another likely reason why it is, at a glance, difficult to understand how to immediately address (and answer) the evaluation question presented above.

The evaluator needs to know what the intervention has been, what its direct result has been, and then how each follow-on result or action has led to another result (and the context in which it happened) to address the evaluation question. Stated another way, the result provided in Table 6.1 is likely not the direct result of an intervention; rather, a combination of results and other actions (and factors) is probably what has brought about that result. The point is critical to remember when you are reading the rest of this chapter—which *only* focuses on direct links, although it lays the foundation to discuss indirect links (which are explored in Chapter 7) and eventually to explore how context, politics, language, culture, and other factors have probably influenced that result (Chapter 13). The remainder of this chapter continues slowly (and incrementally) laying the foundation for more intensive and complicated evaluation questions. As I have noted in "A Conversation with My Readers" at the start of the book, we are the Tortoise in Aesop's fable, not the Hare.

With these two important points noted, let's talk about how to engage in linking the three cousins.

HOW TO IDENTIFY STRONG LINKS AND BROKEN ONES, AND WHY THAT MATTERS

Before starting this conversation, and exploring a two-step process for how to link the three, let's review each cousin. An *intervention* has been implemented (or is being designed) to fix, change, or otherwise make something different or better (this something is summarized in the *problem statement*). By implementing the intervention, an organization (or group of people) wants to achieve at least one, if not multiple, *results*.

Now let's start to break each of these apart and then link the parts together. The problem, intervention, and results need to be linked, or "speak" to each other, at each level. We have talked about problem statements in Chapter 3, and have sorted problems into grand (large) or pocket (small) problems. That same thinking is carried through to results. Grand problems "speak" (are linked) to grand results, and pocket problems "speak" to pocket results. There is a second reason why the terms *grand* and *pocket* are used. The terms are used to remove the ever-present and distracting discussion of labels for results (e.g., *outcome, impact*), which then allows an unfettered discussion on the logic of the intervention. These more common terms for results will be applied when the time is right (which is in Chapter 7); the terms *grand result* and *pocket result* are placeholders that enable an organization to add their own labels later.

We'll start the process by (1) linking a problem statement to its likely intended result, and then (2) seeing how the intervention connects the two. The process encourages a general conversation that will be refined as the process is repeated. It's an iterative process.

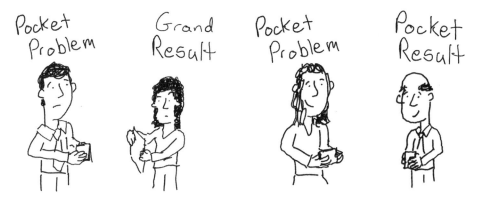

Step 1: Link the Problem Statement and Result

Start by trying to grasp a broad understanding of how the result and the problem statement link (details will emerge as the process continues into Chapter 7). Ironically, four of the easiest ways to identify the link between the problem statement and what the organization intends to achieve do not include directly asking, "So, tell me, what does the intervention aim to accomplish, and how is that linked to the problem statement [though asking that question is perfectly reasonable in some circumstances]?" The four options are as follows:

1. Take any (pocket or grand) problem statement and "flip it." Let's go back to our girls' education example. Here we take "School-age girls *do not* go to school" and flip it; now the statement becomes "School-age girls *do* go to school." In broad strokes, we now know where the intervention started from ("School-age girls do not go to school) and where the intervention aims to reach ("School-age girls go to school"). This method also provides a way to check the program logic; if you "flip" the problem statement, and what is stated does not match what the organization says is its intended result(s), it is the first indication that something is not quite right. (Jump to Chapter 8 for a discussion on program logic.) The process will need to be repeated for all the pocket problems and the grand problem. The process flipping works.

2. Ask this question: What will the situation (or problem) look like when it is fixed (or changed or improved)? Ask each person who is part of the process to describe this in detail.

3. Ask this question: If someone were to visit the site before the start of the intervention, and then to visit the same place at a later point (choose a time frame), what would he observe or notice that is different or changed? Ask each person to describe that verbally, or sign the response. Rephrasing the question, such as by providing different time frames, may yield different answers that can be used later in the process. For example, changes in 5 years are likely to be different from changes expected in 20 years. These kinds of answers provide insight into the expected incremental changes.

4. If the evaluator or her clients are not sight-impaired, providing a visual aid often benefits people's thinking. For some, using a graphic or picture when discussing where the intervention started from (you draw the picture first), and then asking where they want it to get to (they draw the picture), will result in a more fruitful conversation than just a verbal one. Or, the evaluator can ask the client to draw the entire picture (i.e., where the intervention started from and where it intends to go).

Choose a question, approach, and language with which people can engage and that they are comfortable using. Do not try to make your discussion fancy or complicated; it is not a test, for them or you. Keep the questions simple. The key idea is that the problem statement and the result need to meet at the same levels (pocket to pocket, and grand to grand); in this way, they can be logically linked.

BOX 6.3. The Result Is Clear, but the Problem Statement Is Not

There may be a situation in which the intended result is clear, but a problem statement does not explicitly exist. When a person or group has a clear understanding of what they want to accomplish, but not a clear problem statement, just reverse the process. Write what they want to accomplish, and then flip it, thus creating the problem statement. Then identify if the problem statement indeed sets forth a fact (or set of facts), and then move forward and clarify where the intervention addresses the problem (i.e., root causes, symptoms) and how the intervention is linked to the intended or desired results. See Chapters 3–4 to implement that process.

Applying the first option on page 117 (flipping the problem statement) to our girls' education example provides what we see in Table 6.2: Here, flipping the pocket problems has identified anticipated results. The reverse process would also work here—taking the results statement and flipping it to create a problem statement.

TABLE 6.2. Problems Linked to Results by Flipping

Pocket problems	Anticipated results (What the intervention wants to achieve)
Fathers do not permit their daughters to go to school. They think girls do not need a formal education. (Fact.)	Fathers report embracing the importance of educating girls. (Anticipated and yet-to-be-proven result—assumption.)
The road to the school is not safe for girls, for many reasons identified in the research. (Fact.)	Girls can travel safely to and from school. (Anticipated and yet-to-be-proven result—assumption.)

Step 2: Link the Problem–Result Pairing with a Specific Intervention

Now that we have the pocket problem and anticipated result, what is intended to address that problem and bring about those results? Table 6.3 shows the proposed interventions for the girls' education program.

During these discussions, keep in mind what is a fact and what is an assumption. The problem statement is a fact (or set of facts). The intervention is an assumption (or set of assumptions), with perhaps some facts mixed in, of what will work to fix the problem or otherwise change a situation. The intended result is also an assumption (or set of assumptions). The assumptions are the reason we monitor the intervention and its results *because they are not facts*. If it were a fact that the intervention worked to produce the desired results, then there would be no need to monitor the intervention.

When an evaluator is working with an organization in a planning or reflection process, there are three variations of what may be identified in the two-step process. Figure 6.2 is a map of these variations.

TABLE 6.3. Example of the Links among Pocket Problems, Interventions, and Anticipated Results

Pocket problems	What will address these pocket problems? (Interventions)	Anticipated results (What the intervention wants to achieve)
Fathers/father figures do not permit their daughters to go to school. They think that girls do not need a formal education.	Engage with fathers/father figures through peer engagement with fathers/father figures who are supportive of educated women. (Intervention based on assumptions that this will lead to the desired result.)	Fathers/father figures report embracing the importance of educating girls. (Anticipated and yet-to-be-proven result.)
The road to the school is not safe for girls, for many reasons identified in the research. (There are no lights. It is not safe for women and girls to walk on this road, based on previous violence and harassment, especially during early morning and early evening.)	Lights are added to the road, and buses with female drivers take girls to and from school. (Notice that we now have two interventions to address the problem. The problem has been further broken down into more pocket problems.)	Girls have access to safe transport to and from school. (Anticipated and yet-to-be-proven result.)

If the map sends you to Chapter 7, then the links will be completed in that chapter. In Chapter 7, three possibilities are explored for why the problem statement, intervention, and results cannot be linked.

- The results from multiple pocket results need to be combined to reach the grand result.

- To achieve the grand result, more than direct results from an intervention are needed; it is a result of results producing results. One intervention often has multiple, successive results that lead to the grand result.

- It may be a combination of both: Multiple pocket problems and multiple successive results are needed to achieve the grand result.

Table 6.4 shows what has been done thus far (Chapters 3–6). Note that potentially (and likely) even grander problems and grander results can be added to Table 6.4.

Now compare Tables 6.1 and 6.4, and note what has changed between the two. In Table 6.4, there are new, smaller problem statements. Each problem statement has its own facts, its

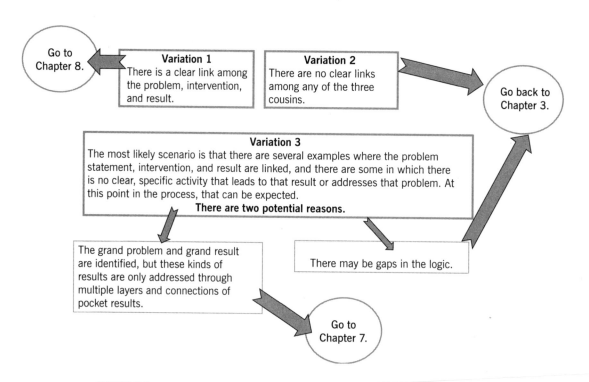

FIGURE 6.2. Three variations in the problem–intervention–result linkage process.

TABLE 6.4. Summary: Key Concepts and Examples from Chapters 3–6

Grand problem	Pocket problems (Where we start from)	Interventions	Anticipated results (What the intervention wants to achieve)	Direct beneficiaries	Anticipated grand result
Few school-age girls go to school. (Fact.)	Fathers/father figures do not permit their daughters to go to school. They think that girls do not need a formal education. (Fact.)	Work with fathers/father figures through peer engagement with fathers/father figures supportive of educated women. (Intervention built on assumptions that this will lead to the desired result.)	Fathers report embracing the importance of educating girls. (Anticipated and yet-to-be-proven result.)	Fathers. (Person or group that benefits directly from the intervention.)	All school-age girls have access to, and attend, school. (Anticipated and yet-to-be-proven result.)
	The road to the school is not safe for girls, for many reasons identified in the research. (Fact.)	Lights are added to the road, and buses with female drivers take girls to and from school. (Intervention built on assumptions that this will lead to the desired result.)	Girls have access to safe transport to and from school. (Anticipated and yet-to-be-proven result.)	Girls. (Person or group that benefits directly from the intervention.)	

own intervention, and its own anticipated result. Each problem statement sets forth a fact (or set of facts), not an assumption. Look also at how the beneficiaries change. By unpacking the problem statements into pocket ones, we can now see what parts of the intervention address which pocket problem, and for whom. Table 6.4 demonstrates how achieving results from each column combines to reach the grand result (i.e., the grand result is not linked to one specific intervention or result, but rather to a combination of them). In doing so, it *begins* to unravel what to assess. In Chapter 7 the results are broken down even further, providing even more details about what to assess, which then support clearer identification of results and expose more of the program logic and theory. (For example, before fathers embrace the importance of girls' attending school, another pocket result occurs, which you will find out in Chapter 7.) Patience. We will get there; look how far we have come.

What are some of the practical problems encountered in the field when the intervention is not clear, and when it is not linked to a fact-based problem statement or clearly defined results?

While eventually an evaluator will face many kinds of challenges when an intervention is not clearly defined or linked to a fact-based problem statement or clear results, having *only* a broad understanding of the intervention is not an immediate challenge; in fact, it is often the starting place of an evaluation (think back to our nutshell description). The evaluator and the implementers may all be clear that the intervention is to educate girls, and that the intervention aims to remove barriers to girls' access to education. The challenge will emerge when the evaluator and implementers are trying to assess and understand how, and to what extent, what part of the intervention directly addresses what problem and brings about what result. Interventions need to be described so that it is clear what they do, whom they aim to reach, and what they intend to address, fix, or improve.

Here is another practical, related example. Asking the person who is designated the "M&E person," or "evaluation officer," or even "external evaluator" to evaluate the effectiveness of a capacity-building program to address homeless youth is akin to asking them to assess a chimera. I have heard discussions where program managers, with poorly described interventions, voice frustration because the evaluator responsible for assessing that program does not know what to assess that will link the intervention to the results. Always keep this in mind: If the intervention is not clearly described, then what to assess becomes anyone's guess. When there is a poorly described intervention, the evaluator can play a pivotal role in clarifying the intervention, problem statement, and results, and linking them together. In this way, the evaluator supports the implementers to clarify how the intervention results are linked to the intervention (or not), and in this way helps the implementers to manage the intervention to achieve their intended results.

Can I assess an intervention without looking at incremental change?

Sure, an evaluator can look at the grand problem and the grand result, and develop a way to assess whether the grand result is achieved, and how and to what extent the grand result has addressed the grand problem. It would probably be impossible, however, to link the result to the intervention without clearly understanding how the intervention has brought about pocket results to address pocket problems, and how all this has led to that grand result. Thus, when an evaluation only assesses the grand result, it is called a *black-box evaluation*. The term suggests that we have no idea what happens between the problem and result, how the result has been achieved, or if it is even connected to what the intervention has done. The whole process is completed inside a black box; we cannot see inside.

Some years ago, when I was working with a program that aimed to prevent youth-at-risk from entering the formal penal system, the intervention was not clear beyond that it was wilderness camping. I kept asking, "But what happens, exactly, to bring about the result? How do children suddenly go from being on the path to the penal system, then attending a camp, to becoming model citizens [their intended result]?" The program manager looked at me and said, quite seriously, "It's our magic." So, in lay terms, we can also call the black box the *magic box*. (I should note that the program was indeed amazing, and that using the process described in Chapters 3–10 made it clear that their results came from thoughtful processes based in social science theory, cultural knowledge, and dedicated staff.) However, magic-box or black-box evaluation is most often trouble by another name. First, the question of how, or if, or to what extent the intervention has brought about those changes (if any) cannot be answered. In other words, how do you link what the intervention has done to the results? Second, if a result is not achieved, how do you figure out what went wrong in the intervention (if anything)? We will continue to talk more about the importance of understanding incremental steps and having clear, explicit logic and theory throughout the book. (Specifically, theory and logic are covered in Chapter 8, though the lessons learned in Chapters 3–10 all support the need for explicit theory and logic.) That said, let's continue in Chapter 7 with unpacking the results.

WRAPPING UP

This chapter has continued the evaluative journey with a heavy emphasis on the importance of having a plausible and evaluable intervention. To untangle a potentially challenging discussion, the chapter has used the terms *grand results* and *pocket results*, which has practically allowed for a logical discussion that connects problem statements, interventions, and results. Again, using the girls' education intervention as the main example, I have demonstrated how linking pocket problems to pocket results, and then linking these to the intervention, also connects the grand problem and the grand result. The process provides foundational information needed to have a plausible intervention that is incrementally evaluable. The next chapter delves more deeply into dissecting the logic of results, which continues to build a plausible and evaluable intervention. Before you leave this chapter, come join me in a conversation.

Our Conversation: Between You and Me

An evaluator can fill many roles. One role that I often fill is when clients engage me specifically to ensure that they have plausible and evaluable interventions. I enjoy being asked to fill that role. At other times, I am hired to evaluate an intervention that is neither plausible or evaluable (and not asked to make it plausible or evaluable). I find that role more difficult, as it is not really a good idea to make a blatant statement to a client, such as, "Hi, thanks for working with me. Your intervention is neither plausible or evaluable." Nope, not a great way to start. If I could, I would start the conversation back in Chapter 3, and use the questions around the problem statement to get the conversation started and then work my way through to Chapter 10. If you were hired to evaluate an intervention that was neither plausible nor evaluable, how would you start that conversation? What would your process of engagement look like for your clients in your context?

CHAPTER 7
All about Results

If you give an evaluator a fact, she will ask you how you know that.
If she asks how you know that, then she will want to talk about assumptions.
If you tell her some assumptions, she will want to look for facts.

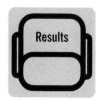

Often people want to start engaging with results before an evaluator even knows what problem an intervention aims to address, or anything else about the intervention. In many ways, this makes sense; after all, most people are often interested in answering the question, "What has happened?" or "Did it work?" So let's talk about results. In Chapter 6, we have laid the foundation for a detailed results discussion by explicating the strong links among the problem statement, the intervention, and its results; we have experienced how useful it is to talk about one of the "three cousins" and actively involve the others. Now we are going to wade deeper into the discussion of results and focus exclusively on those, while not forgetting how results are linked to the other two.

> ### BOX 7.1. Defining the Term *Result*
>
> The term **result** refers to *any level and any kind of accomplishment* that an intervention is trying to reach or achieve. The term is used for two reasons: first, to avoid discussions that often take place too early in the evaluative process about the level of the result; and, second, to avoid arguments about how to label results. To organize the discussion, the general terms *pocket results* and *grand results* are used.

FOUR CRITICAL REASONS TO UNDERSTAND THE LOGIC OF RESULTS

There are four critical reasons to understand, and clearly lay out, the logic of the intended results.

1. *To make results assessable in incremental stages.* It is important to be able to evaluate incremental change (the reasoning of which is first detailed in Chapter 6). If we know what part of an intervention is thought to lead to what pocket results, and what pocket results are thought to lead to what other pocket results, and how that eventually is thought to lead to what grand result, then we know *when to assess what.* By assessing results in tiny steps, we can use our data to show if and when something goes right or partially right (or wrong), so that it is clear what to address, what to continue doing, or what to expand. If assessment or evaluation is only done in large chunks (e.g., school-age girls did not attend school, and now they do attend school), it is impossible to untangle what in the intervention worked, what "sort of" worked, and at what point it went remarkably right or terribly wrong.

Relatedly, when the incremental connections are clear among the results, an evaluator can collect *real-time data* and provide *real-time feedback.* This literally means collecting data, analyzing it, and providing useful information to the implementer as the intervention happens, so that changes can be made immediately as needed. Making informed changes to the intervention (sometimes called *evidence-based* changes, as evidence is used to make those decisions) then positively influences the likelihood of the intervention's achieving its grand result. Or perhaps, based on the evidence, the implementer decides to modify the grand result, take another look at the problem statement, change the intervention, or all three. There is another advantage to clarifying the intended incremental change. See the next point.

2. *To provide the scaffolding for a discussion of theory of change.* As described in the first critical reason, the unpacked results describe the incremental logic, also known as *incremental change.* And here's the cool part: If we understand the logic of the results and the ways the results are intended to work together to bring about change (e.g., improved evaluation knowledge leads to better evaluations, which lead to more-used evaluations, which lead to better-informed programs, which then achieve their results), and all this is tied to the problem statement (e.g., an internal evaluator lacks knowledge about evaluation, evaluations are not used, the program implementers do not have the data they need to make evidence-based decisions), then a discussion that clarifies the program theory, without ever using the word *theory,* can easily begin. All we need to do is ask one starter question: "What makes you think that?" A discussion of program theory, and the reasons why it is important in the evaluative process, can be found in Chapter 8.

3. *To avoid an argument about results labels.* Sorting out and clarifying incremental, logical results allows the evaluator, and everyone she is working with, to discuss the logic of the results and to avoid the age-old argument about results labels. The "It is an output. No, it is an outcome. No, I think it is an impact" discussion often unnecessarily sidetracks and confuses the discussion on the logic of the results. The results discussion should not center around what to call a result; rather, it should focus on whether one result logically leads to another, which informs decisions on when, where, and what to evaluate.

4. *To demonstrate that results bring about results.* While an intervention may bring about a direct result, results also bring about results. So far in the process, we have looked at how the problem statement, intervention, and results are linked. Exploring the results logic shows how one desired result, which is directly related to the intervention, then contributes or leads to the next desired result, and so on. Eventually, the conversation will circle back to how each result (combined with others or by itself) contributes to solving, or entirely solves, what problem, for whom, and how that is related to what part of an intervention.

Whoa. Hold on a second. Did you say that an intervention brings about a result, and that results can also bring about results?

Yes. It is important to know how the intervention is designed to reach its results. For example, there is one activity (e.g., training, mentoring, providing materials) that directly influences one or more direct results. From those few direct results (results directly connected to the activity), many more results are expected to happen. Not all interventions are designed in this way; some have an activity for each result. This is just one realization we can achieve about results when we work through the results logic (as we do in this chapter). It can be illuminating (if not downright surprising) when it becomes apparent that one activity is expected to have one direct result, and that this result is supposed to have a plethora of others. It's a bit like falling dominoes: We only touch the first domino, and if all goes well, the rest of the dominoes will fall.

STARTING THE RESULTS DISCUSSION

A good place to start a results discussion is to return to the discussion on facts and assumptions (see Chapter 4) and situate it in the girls' education example.

School-age girls do not go to school (this is a problem and a fact). Research shows that when girls are uneducated, there is a higher likelihood that they will remain in abusive relationships and have unwanted pregnancies (these are general facts). Thus one problem (not attending school) *probably* (it is an assumption, as it has not yet happened to these specific girls) contributes to future problems for these girls, which are already evident in the girls' community.

Thus, while the literature demonstrates that girls who do not go to school are more likely to remain in abusive relationships and have unwanted pregnancies, it does not mean that these things *will* happen to them. And that is a fundamental difference between problem statements (backward-looking established facts) and intended results (forward-looking assumptions).

The problem statement contains situations that have already happened or are happening, and are confirmed facts. The intended, desired, anticipated, potential, or expected (choose your adjective) results happen in the future. When talking about results, the evaluator has three potential roles: to (1) clarify what is intended to happen (the planning or reflective phase—she is working with assumptions); (2) identify whether the intended results did happen (backward-looking—she is working with facts); and (3) find or recognize unintended results (again, she is working with facts). In each of those situations, the evaluator needs to logically understand how the results relate to each other, and then how they relate to the intervention and to the problem statement; her role in working with the logic of results will depend on where in the process she enters. Regardless of where she enters the process, she needs to understand how to engage with the logic of results. Thus the logic of results is emphasized in this chapter. So let's first explore what it means to think logically.

LOGICAL THINKING IN THE RESULTS DISCUSSION

My dad used to describe people who made seemingly logical decisions as having "horse sense." I am not sure why; maybe it was because we lived in a farming area and horses seemed to have more sense than other farm animals. (Pigs are actually the smartest farm animals.) However, being smart and being logical are not necessarily the same. When I went to university, I often heard the expression "common sense." Now I am not sure why that phrase was used either, because as Voltaire is famous for noting, common sense does not seem to be all that common. Common sense and logic are closely aligned. My more than 20 years of doing evaluation, facilitating, or just plain asking people to explain their intervention's logic have shown me that discussing logic is not often an easy thing to do. Explicit, agreed-upon program logic is not all that common, and either extricating it or building it is often an exhausting (and yet strangely exhilarating) process that is crucial to any evaluative process.

Take the example of a 3-day workshop that I implement, which aims to help organizations clarify their logic (and subsequently determine what to assess, the problem statements, the beneficiaries, and the theory that underpins it all). On the first day, the participants are excited when evaluation terms are clarified, and they start to describe their intervention. On the second day, when I question them—and they question each other—about the logic of their program, they often begin to loathe me (e.g., "How can you question me?" "Of course it is true that it will happen," "What do you mean, it does not make sense?") and sometimes scoff at their colleagues (e.g., "You really think that is how it works?"). When it all comes together on the third day (some groups need more time, but in general this takes 3 days), we are all usually back in each other's good graces. The process that explores the logic of how an intervention is intended to work and what it intends to achieve can be messy and demanding; however, when it all comes together with a clear and shared understanding, it can be immensely satisfying.

AN EVALUATOR'S ROLE IN THE RESULTS DISCUSSION

When an evaluator makes the implicit logic of the results explicit, he will initially work in one of two ways. He will do one of the following:

- *Not work directly with individuals who know the program.* Here the evaluator will work alone or with his evaluation team. The evaluator and his team may need to sort out the results logic through document reviews (program documents), literature reviews, past knowledge, and experience. Sometimes the process can be supplemented with a few key informant interviews (or not).
- *Work directly with individuals or a group of people who know the program.* The evaluator can conduct a workshop or group discussions to make the implicit logic of the results explicit. These discussions often require strong facilitation and negotiation skills to build communication and trust between the evaluator and his clients or colleagues.

Whichever approach is used (and the approaches can also be combined), the evaluator needs to be aware that connecting the dots (which may not be a linear procedure) among the intended results, and linking them back to the intervention(s), problem statement(s), and beneficiaries, is a process tied up in all sorts of unspoken and hidden assumptions grounded in personal knowledge, beliefs, and experiences. As evaluators, we need to make the implicit explicit, often from several perspectives, and likely aim to give equal "air time" or "voice" to each perspective. Often the process of negotiating which results logic will dominate influences the monitoring and evaluation decisions—such as what and how something is assessed and/or valued.

WHY DISCUSSING THE LOGIC OF RESULTS IS (OFTEN) DEMANDING AND MESSY

A discussion on the logic of intended results can be challenging for three reasons. One reason is that it has left the world of facts behind, and entered the world of assumptions about what will happen in the future. That leads to the second reason, which is that assumptions are based on people's life experiences, worldviews, religious beliefs, cultural values, and other potentially sensitive personal ideologies. Thus, when we (you and I, the evaluators) question why people think their intervention will solve the problem, or why they think that a certain activity leads to a particular result, or why this result will bring about that one, we may *think* we are *only* asking them to explain a logical sequence (which can be challenging enough). Yet, in doing so, we are questioning (and some may perceive it as attacking) personal viewpoints.

The third reason is that people use different logics, or ways of thinking, to explore and explain a situation. A person often thinks, and therefore explains logic, more comfortably from either the top down or the bottom up.

- *Deductive thinking* is starting at the top, with a big statement, and working down. An example of deductive thinking would be starting with an anticipated grand result, such as having an environmentally friendly community; when this grand result is unpacked, it shows that one of many necessary pocket results needed to reach that result is to have people recycle their household garbage.

- *Inductive thinking* is starting with a small statement and building it up toward a conclusion. The same discussion of the environmentally friendly community could start at the bottom, stating that people need to recycle their household garbage; this, when combined with other pocket results, would then lead to a higher-level or grand result that leads (or contributes) to an environmentally friendly community.

Some people naturally think inductively, and others naturally think deductively; evaluators need to be able to do both.

Thus the process described next can be used to build the logic (inductive) or take it apart (deductive), or can combine deductive and inductive thinking as necessary. As noted above, in evaluation both types of thinking are often needed. Whichever logic is used, when the logic of the results is completed, take the *other* logic that was not used, and apply it to check the thinking. For example, $2 + 2 = 4$, and therefore $4 - 2 = 2$ (the very logic that we learned in the first grade!).

Our organization has very clear results logic; it is not a mess at all. Evaluators have just arrived to do an evaluation. They do not need to revisit it. Or do they?

When organizations or groups have clearly written and/or pictorial logic for their intervention and its results, it is undoubtedly a good idea to revisit the logic; this logic is core to nearly all evaluative processes. Furthermore, a "well-done logic model" (see Chapter 8 for a description of logic models) does not necessarily mean that everyone (e.g., implementers, beneficiaries, donors, managers) agrees with it, that everyone who needs to know knows it, or even that it is up to date (e.g., things change). It is important that everyone (including whoever needs to implement, assess, and benefit from the intervention) agrees with the logic of the intervention and its results, for several reasons.

Most importantly, different understanding of the logic can bring very different expectations and ways of assessing and valuing results. Even thinking that has slightly nuanced differences can make a difference in what and when to evaluate. (See Chapter 8, Activity 8.1, for a game that emphasizes this point.) When you are working with an organization to ensure that an intervention is evaluable (or working as part of a process to assess results), it can be illuminating to identify whether key stakeholders bring the same results logic (or the same understanding of the logic) to the intervention. If there is not much time to engage in a discussion, perhaps you can try to have a rapidly facilitated process, which is suggested next.

If the group with which you are working has four or more people, divide that larger group into smaller groups of twos and threes. Smaller groups encourage more in-depth dialogue. Provide each group with one or more pieces of flip chart paper, a marker or two, and 10 minutes to discuss and write down answers to the following: What problem is the intervention (or organization) addressing, how, and with what expected results? If all groups bring the same logic to this discussion, and the logic is still relevant, congratulations; you and they have done well! If all or some groups have the same logic but they do not think it is still relevant, or if there are varying degrees of agreement among the groups, or if flat-out disagreement arises, create time to facilitate a process that brings clarity. (See Chapters 1–6, skipping Chapter 5, of this book.)

With that in mind, let's move forward and learn some strategies for how to unpack the anticipated results (anticipated, because they have not happened yet).

STRATEGIES FOR UNPACKING THE LOGIC OF RESULTS: MASTERING THE RESULTS CONVERSATION

The not-so-well-kept trade secret that I will now share with you (drum roll!) is that *output, outcome,* and *impact* (and variations of those words, such as *intermediate result* or *long-term impact*) offer different meanings to different people. There is no common, agreed-upon, concrete, always correct definition. There is a fundamental logic, however, and this is what we are focusing on in this chapter. Once the logic is clear, you can adapt to working with any organization's way of labeling results. (*A side note:* The terms *input* and *activity* are often mixed up in the same conversation. Just to clarify, an *activity* is what is done to bring about a result; it is not a result. An *input* consists of the resources needed to bring about a result.)

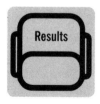

In evaluation processes, some of the most frustrating conversations occur during a discussion about results; a chat about the differences between facts and assumptions is relatively benign, compared to one about, say, outcomes and impacts. I have silently listened to arguments in evaluation courses, circular discussions between colleagues, and ensuing battles between donors and recipients about which is what. The conversation usually starts with what appears to be a very noncombative sentiment (e.g., "I think our program has had some amazing outcomes") or a request ("You need to measure the impact"). Be careful. These seemingly innocent statements about results are fraught with danger. What does impact even mean? How does an outcome differ from an impact?

Avoid Debates about Labels

Do not ever engage in a debate over what is an outcome and what is an impact, or any similar debate about labels. Engage in a discussion that aims to find common ground concerning what is supposed to happen, when, for whom, and how it all connects (which can also be a backward-looking discussion). We can (and will) apply labels later.

As critical as it is to know that different definitions and interpretations of the terms for results exist, the critical conversation involves (and the point on which agreement must be obtained is) the logical flow of the results, not the label. Therefore, when you are working with clients or colleagues, strip off the labels (do not be shy) and engage in a process that describes how the intervention logic moves from here to there. If it helps, and if you first need to see how results labels are sometimes used, there is an example on page 10. Take a quick peek, and them come back here. Below, I give an example of how to talk about results so that you can comfortably engage in, and master, this conversation.

Labels are important. Labels can be useful. But they can also wreak havoc in an evaluative process. Use labels strategically and carefully. Use them only when everyone brings the same understanding of each label's definition. The challenge with results labels is that people often assume they know what the labels mean, that everyone else thinks the same, and that their definitions are right. Move the conversation away from the labels, and toward the important part of the conversation: the logic of the results.

Shh, I have a real secret to share here, not a trade one. Nothing is more frustrating to me than a game of "I call it an impact" versus "Well, I call it an outcome." When this happens, I imagine myself being a cartoon character from *South Park* (Cartman, to be exact) and shouting, "Agh! Please just tell me, what do you expect the intervention to achieve?" The *South Park* visual keeps me calm. Please do not tell my clients.

A results conversation can start with a very straightforward (and common) image. Imagine some stairs. The stairs go up at a slight angle, and all have the same width and height. In this example, everyone agrees that a person starts at the bottom stair and needs to finish on the top stair (the grand result). Using inductive thinking, the conversation starts on the bottom step, or using deductive thinking, the conversation starts on the top step. Let's start at the bottom.

Despite the stairs' not having a label (e.g., *output, outcome*), it is very clear that as the person climbs each new step, he is moving closer to where he wants to be. In fact, everyone watching (monitoring) will agree that he trips on the 4th stair, stops for a bit at the 10th stair, nearly falls off the 17th stair, and finally makes it to the 20th stair (which is the top stair), albeit a bit later than planned. The description given depicts the movement and connection of results. Imagine that an entire group of people can agree on this person's progress without once needing a label. The description of the staircase illustrates the basic premise of a results discussion and shows how removing the labels can facilitate a conversation that then allows a focus on the logic of the results, not the definition of the labels. If you are concerned about the lack of labels, no worries; I will show you how to add the labels back later in this chapter.

Wait. Why would I bring labels back into the discussion?

There are three reasons to use labels. First, my book will not change the real world, and in most evaluation contexts in the real world, people expect to see the results labels. Second, as a final step, once everything is explicit, labels can be useful for succinctly describing the intervention design and what it aims to achieve. And third, let's face it: People like labels.

I work as an M&E officer for a foundation, and my friend is applying for a job at the same place. She needs to know how we use the results labels for the job interview, and if she gets the job, she needs to use them like we do. Should she learn the foundation's definitions?

One of the many reasons why monitoring and evaluation can be challenging is the lack of consistency in how results are labeled. However, it is important for your friend to know how the organization she *wants* to work for (and, let's hope, eventually works for) defines and uses monitoring and evaluation terms. What I would suggest is that you lay out a basic intervention, as we are going to do together in this chapter; then, once it is laid out, apply the foundation's labels on top of each result. Do not only provide her with definitions of the result labels, as these definitions are not often useful in a practical sense (although rote learning may be good for the interview). Also, share with your friend that if she understands the logic of results, she can apply the results labels as needed for any organization in which she works.

THE FRAMEWORK: UNPACKING RESULTS

Guided by the five-question framework on the next page, evaluators can unpack the results. The unpacking can be done by a lone evaluator (reading documents), as a team discussion (e.g., a program team or an evaluation team), or through a larger, facilitated process (e.g., a workshop with an organization).

The five guiding questions are as follows:

1. **What is the very first thing that happens because of the intervention's action?** (*What happens first? This is the tiniest pocket result.*)

2. **What happens next?** (*What happens along the way? We often ask this multiple times, getting more and more responses. These are still pocket results, but slightly larger in terms of achievement.*)

3. **So what?** (*What will it look like when we get there? This is often the grand result.*)

4. **Who cares?** (*This is to be used for answers to each of the first three questions. If results are achieved, who values them? These can be any stakeholders such as beneficiaries, program implementers, or donors, and can also dive into the un-beneficiary discussion. See Chapter 3 for a discussion on these groups.*)

5. **What resources are available to achieve these results?** (*This is to be used for the first three questions, as a reality check to the results identified.*)

Although I walk you through these questions as planning questions, they can also be used once the intervention is well underway, or completed. Just change the verb tense in the sentences (e.g., *is* to *was*, or *will* to *did*). Before we go through the process to unpack the results, be cautioned about two common mistakes:

- Allowing a discussion of *how* to assess a result to creep into the conversation.
- Centering a discussion around if the result can be *asssessed.*

Do not let these topics seep in. *These are separate conversations.* In any part of the evaluative process, always keep the focus on one topic at a time, get clarity, and then move to the next topic. Here we go.

Question 1. *What is the very first thing that happens because of the intervention's action?*

The first question can also be asked in one or the other of the following versions:

- What is the first thing that happens as a result of the intervention, action, or activity?
- Describe the very first thing that can be observed that is directly linked to the action/intervention.

The answer determines what to look for, or what to assess first. For a training intervention, answers may include "People attend the training." For an agricultural program that engages farmers in a community effort to save water, it may be "Farmers came to the community meeting." To return to the peer-to-peer example for fathers/father figures in the girls' education intervention, the answer could be "Fathers attend the peer-to-peer sessions." The very first result is often the easiest result to identify and assess, as it is often tangible, obvious, and directly related to the intervention. Its assessment is often (though not always) considered part of the monitoring, and its data are (almost always) used in the evaluation process. In an evaluative process, these first identifiable results are always *attributable* to the intervention; that is, there is a clear, discernible link between what was done and what happened. *Attribution* means being able to say definitively that this result stemmed from that specific action, in what is commonly called a cause-and-effect relationship. Let's stop and have a brief discussion of the word *attribution* and its partner, *contribution* (further elaborated on in Chapter 8).

Attribution and Contribution

There are all kinds of research techniques to identify attribution (i.e., the intervention causes the result, or the result is definitely because of, and only because of, the intervention). Here, I prefer a more practical discussion.

The level of result that happens directly after the intervention is directly *attributable* to the intervention. Now, when you are engaging in a conversation with program implementers (or their funders/bosses or whomever they report to) about *direct accountability for results* (who is directly held accountable?), look at the very first result. For example, the organization implementing the peer-to-peer groups for fathers has direct responsibility to get fathers to the peer sessions, and to address any reasons why fathers do not attend. Do not misunderstand me; the program staff cannot force fathers to participate. What the program staff can do, however, if fathers do not attend, is to find out why fathers do not participate, and address the issue or issues. There could be contextual issues that prevent fathers from coming, such as lack of transportation, or even cultural reasons. However, the implementers have control over modifying the intervention (based on the reasons that fathers do not attend), or changing what the intervention does, to engage fathers.

When evaluators talk about *contribution*, they are referring to a situation where the intervention also definitely had something to do with the result, but the organization/intervention is not solely responsible for the achievement of the identified result. In the very first result(s), the implementers can almost always show direct attribution, and it is a result they are directly accountable for achieving. I say "almost always," because there is almost always an exception. For example, if two organizations conducted a training session together, the two organizations contributed to the fact that people came to be trained. Although this might seem like splitting hairs, that is sometimes what evaluators need to do. For now, let's look at some common mistakes related to identifying the initial or first result.

Question 1. *Common Challenge A: Skipping or missing the first step in the logical flow*

I find that when people are asked, "What is the first thing that happened after the intervention?", they tend to skip a step ahead in their logical thinking. In terms of the example starting on page 131, they miss a few stairs. Their response is often the second, third, or fourth thing (forgive the use of the word *thing* here; the thing is, it just works so well in the explanation!). For example, if an intervention is held for midwives on the new practices associated with pain relief, people may respond that the first thing that happens because midwives attend is that midwives show *improved knowledge* about various options for natural pain relief during childbirth. The response of improved knowledge is a leap of faith, however; it skips a step or two. Something the intervention has done leads to improved knowledge. What is it? Think about the step-by-step logic: For people to improve their knowledge, something must happen first that creates the change in knowledge. For example, a beneficiary reads a book. To read the book, the person needs to have access to the book. Or, if the intervention is a training, the participant needs to attend the training. Skipping these logical steps (e.g., accessing the book, reading the book, or attending the training) is a problem for any evaluation process for two reasons.

- First, hidden actions and results may actually offer one reason why the higher-level result, such as improved knowledge, is or is not attained. For instance, perhaps knowledge is not improved because no one has purchased the book, let alone read it. Or the book is too technical. Or if the intervention is a training, maybe the training is poorly done or no one attends.

- Second, if we evaluators do not know what is supposed to lead to what, then we will not know where to look to collect data, and it will be more challenging to identify or explain why a higher-level result happens, partially happens, or does not happen at all (or what causes or contributes to this). Hidden steps in the logic obscure what needs to be assessed, and thus obscure answers to evaluation questions. Having the first result directly linked to the intervention provides a very easy place to identify what to monitor and assess, for accountability, attribution, and, in some circumstances, contribution.

A few years back, I was hired to lead a team of evaluators to provide an understanding of why a government's new program, aimed at teenagers to improve their life skills, showed few positive results. The program aimed to teach 10 life skills to youth in specific grades, at specific schools, using new learning material. Assessments of the teenagers showed that they gained very little knowledge. The government asked us to answer the following question: What was the reason for so few changes in the targeted youth's life skills knowledge?

My team developed an evaluation methodology, set up interviews and site visits, and then selected and visited urban and rural sites. What we consistently found in the rural sites was that the training material never arrived; in the urban sites, although the material arrived, it was deemed "too nice" to provide to the students and was literally kept under lock and key. Large amounts of evaluation funds did not need to be spent to solve this mystery. Being explicit and assessing each critical step (e.g., did materials arrive, and were they accessible?) would have identified these issues long before the students' tests showed dismal results. Yet the *most* frustrating part about the life skills program story is not that money was wasted on an evaluation; rather, it is that children did not benefit from something that could have changed their lives.

Question 1. *Common Challenge B: Confusing the very first result with indicators*

Results that are direct results of the intervention are often written as *indicators*. Indicators have not yet been discussed. If you are unfamiliar with indicators, skip ahead to Chapter 9, pages 181–196, and then come back to this section. A brief description is that an *indicator* is a sign, signal, or clue that something is happening or not, and is used to *make the result evaluable*. It is not the result itself (it is just an indication of it). At this stage in the results descriptions, results are often mistakenly written like indicators. For the girls' education example, the error would probably be "number of fathers who participate in the peer-to-peer program." The correct way to write the very first result that happened because of the intervention would be "Fathers participate in the peer-to-peer program." Writing a result as an indicator presents two problems:

- First, the actual result is never clarified (it is hidden); it is only clear what is being measured. Because an indicator is an indication of what is happening or not, this creates a problem. Read more on pages 181–196 for an in-depth explanation.
- Second, writing the result in "number of" (or percentage, etc.) terms shifts the conversation from what you want to happen, into how to assess if something happened; thus the conversation shifts away from what the intervention aims to accomplish, to what to assess. The two discussions are aligned, but different.

These kinds of small changes (e.g., writing a result as an indicator) contribute to confounding monitoring and evaluation discussions. If you see an indicator in the space reserved for a result, simply ask, "What is the result?" While the result may look similar to the indicator, it may also look very different.

In the girls' education example, let's focus on the peer-to-peer intervention. In Table 7.1, we can identify the very first result that happens because of the intervention. Now that we know this result, for one part of the intervention, let's move to the next question.

TABLE 7.1. Answering Question 1:
What Is the Very First Thing That Happens Because of an Intervention's Action?

Problem	Intervention	The very first thing that happens
Fathers do not want their daughters to attend school because they do not think it is necessary for girls to be educated.	Fathers with the same cultural background, who do think it is important for girls to be educated, engage with fathers who do not.	Fathers who do not want their daughters to attend school come to the peer-to-peer session to meet with fathers who support girls' education.

Question 2. *What happens next?*

In the example in Table 7.1, the first result is that fathers/father figures attend the peer-to-peer sessions (a result directly linked to the intervention). Now we need to ask: Because fathers attend, what is expected to happen? And then we need to follow that with three similar questions, as often as necessary:

- What happens next?
- What happens after that?
- And then?

Now we are moving from a result with a direct link to the intervention, to results that are several steps away. In response to these questions, more than one answer is often generated. When working with a partner or group, or even by yourself, write each of those generated results (results that you think should happen) on its own piece of paper. There will probably be a large pile of such results. Then sort these results into logical order, guided by some, or all, of the following five questions. (Some questions are repetitive, and are intended to help you think through an iterative sorting process.)

- Which result happens first? (There may be more than one; see the next question.)
- Which results need to happen at the same time?
- Which results happen at around the same time, but do not need to happen at exactly the same time?
- Which result needs to happen before another result happens?
- Which result happens that is also influenced by more than one previous (or lower-level) result? (For example, do two results need to happen to produce one additional result?)

The results may be ordered in such a way that they show a linear logic (a straight line), or the flow may have various "arms," or it may look more like a spider's web. It is likely that the results will need to be sorted multiple times (e.g., that different logics will need to be tried) before the logic that the implementers, or you as the evaluator, want to use is apparent. Often more results will need to be written (e.g., missing links or missing steps in the logic must be identified) than initially generated, to make the logic "flow" (i.e., not miss any steps).

In answering the "What happens next?" question, you are likely to generate a few results that are potentially better suited for answering the next question (i.e., "So what?"). Therefore, when addressing the next question, you may choose a result already listed in this section (probably the highest-level result from the intervention), or you may decide not to do this. Continuing with the process will make the decision clear.

Using the girls' education example, Table 7.2 has the answers to the "What happens next?" questions.

Question 2. *Common Challenge A: Thinking it can all take place on the computer*

I mention a process challenge first, as it can create a barrier to one's thinking. Do not list all the potential results directly on the computer (in Word or Excel) and then stare at the computer screen hoping that the results will jump into some logical order. Likewise, when results are all written on one piece of paper, or one whiteboard, they cannot be moved around to help you "think through" the logic. Often several attempts are needed before the logic of the results (e.g., results chain, results hierarchy) begins to flow. The process is more like creating a piece of art than building a bridge.

Question 2. *Common Challenge B: Suitcase words*

The most common mistake for Question 2 (though it is often found in answer to every other question) is to use *suitcase words* to describe the result. What are suitcase words? They are

TABLE 7.2. Answering Question 2: What Happens Next (and What Happens after That)?

Problem	Intervention	The very first thing that happens	What happens next?[a]	What happens after that?[b]
Fathers do not want their daughters to attend school because they do not think it is necessary for girls to be educated.	Fathers with the same cultural background, who do think it is important for girls to be educated, engage with fathers who do not.	Fathers who do not want their daughters to attend school come to the peer-to-peer session to meet with fathers who support girls' education.	Fathers learn reasons for educating girls. Fathers learn about the possible negatives for girls who are not educated.	Fathers agree to consider sending their girls to school. Fathers register their girls for school.

[a]We expect these two things to happen at the same time.
[b]Here we expect the first thing to happen first, and then the second thing will happen. These are sequential results.

words that must be unpacked to be understood (much like we are unpacking the suitcases used for our evaluation journey) (Minsky, 2006). Because suitcase words constitute a problem encountered in nearly all evaluation processes, I am going to discuss them in a bit more depth.

Suitcase words can be found in any part of the evaluative process, from defining the problem statement (context) to the intervention (capacity building) to the intended results (empowered). Do not let your clients, colleagues, or even yourself get away with using them when they are not clearly defined. A suitcase word needs to be unpacked so that it is clear exactly what the word means. Suitcase words create angst in evaluation because they do not provide enough information for anyone to know what to assess (think back to our conversation in Chapter 6 with regard to the need to have an evaluable intervention). However, once they are unpacked, these words provide a wealth of information. Examples of suitcase words commonly used for describing interventions and their results include *culture, behavior change, empowerment, capacity building,* and *improved knowledge.* How does one understand culture without defining it? Empowerment of whom to do what? How does one assess capacity building? It is impossible—yet evaluators encounter people who want evaluations implemented with these words haphazardly strewn about, and there seems to be the assumption that the evaluators will magically know what these words mean, and how to assess for their achievement. Evaluators themselves do not escape blame. Evaluators bring their own suitcase words to evaluation, such as *sustainability* and *beneficiaries* (and, dare I say it, *impact*). If suitcase words are encountered (words that do not immediately express their exact meaning to everyone reading them), stop the process, and use one or both of the following prompts, as appropriate:

- You mentioned [insert suitcase word]. Please tell me: What is being done, and exactly what do you expect to see happen? To whom?
- Can you describe what [insert suitcase word] means, without using the word in the description?

An evaluator cannot assess results that lack a clear definition. Once the suitcase word is clarified (unpacked), it should be very clear what is expected to happen, and therefore what to assess. In most cases, unpacking a suitcase word results in multiple items to assess. After all, the suitcase is not being assessed; all the items packed inside are.

Unpacking suitcase words has a multitude of other benefits—for evaluators, program implementers, funders, other key stakeholders, and anyone else interested in or somehow touched by an intervention. Defining and describing *exactly* what is done, and what is expected because that is done, in clear, explicit language, should remove any space for diverse interpretations. If it is left solely to an evaluator to demystify a suitcase word, she may interpret that word differently than, say, a program implementer or a beneficiary does. A different interpretation of the suitcase word by the evaluator has a high likelihood of producing an evaluation that does not assess the actual intervention or its intended results (because she is assessing something else), and that may produce unfavorable, unfair, or just plain irrelevant evaluation findings.

Suitcase Words

Suitcase words create huge headaches for program managers, donors, key stakeholders, beneficiaries, and evaluators alike. An explicit description of exactly what one is trying to make better, what one is doing, what one hopes to achieve, and for whom is critical for ensuring a useful and fair evaluative process—fair because everyone involved has the same understanding of all this.

Now that we have answered the first two questions—"What happens first?" and "What happens next?"—and placed those results in logical order, let's answer the third question.

Question 3. *So what?*

The next question to ask in this sequence of questions is simply this: "So what?" I was raised to think that "So what?" is a very rude question. Forgive me—but try as I may to come up with another phrase, the "So what?" question fits the best, as long as it is asked in a pleasant, inquisitive, and conversational tone.

Let's look again at the peer-to-peer example for intervention with fathers from the girls' education intervention. Imagine that the program implementers provide solid data to support the following statement:

> "The fathers participate in the peer engagements. They have changed their attitudes and perceptions. They now recognize the importance of girls' attending school, and enroll their daughters in the local school."

If all this has happened, what does it matter? Now more girls attend school. "So what?" The response could be that girls graduate with high school diplomas. To which we can ask again, "So what?" And the answer could be "These girls are less likely to be in abusive relationships or have unwanted pregnancies." Remember, this answer brings us back to the flip side of the grand result—what the literature review has identified as the broader societal problems, and what university research has confirmed as community problems. The conversations in previous chapters interlink with what is discussed now.

When looking at the answer(s) to the "So what?" question, an evaluator or evaluative thinker needs to determine whether the progression laid out thus far is plausibly likely to lead to the "So what?" answer(s). Is it realistic, likely, possible (see Chapters 6 and 9 for more on plausible interventions)? And the evaluator needs to determine when to stop asking the "So what?" question—either when agreed upon with the evaluation users; through a discussion among all key stakeholders; on the basis of previous agreements or commitments; or simply through common sense. In other words, to steal a word from systems thinking, the evaluator needs to set realistic *boundaries* for the intervention and its intended accomplishments.

Let's turn once again to our girls' education example, and show how the answer to the "So what?" question is used (see Table 7.3).

Question 3. *Common Challenge: Discerning what level is being assessed and what level is guiding the process*

The one common mistake in answering Question 3 is not distinguishing between an evaluable high-level result and a guiding vision (e.g., a better world). Both are needed. The highest-level result guides the development of all other results; it is something the intervention will always be reaching to achieve. We need this vision to know whether the intervention is moving toward it—but we do not assess it. This is very different from a high-level result that is expected to be achieved, and therefore evaluated (be it in 10 years or 20).

Question 4. *Who cares?*

The fourth question in this sequence of questions is, now that the results are identified, "Who cares?"

Answers to this question provide one of many fundamental places to begin to grasp who values what, and therefore how to develop criteria on which to value the intervention. It identifies (1) whom to ask about the intervention's results, which leads to understanding (2) how different people value what result. Identified stakeholders may have the same

TABLE 7.3. Answering Question 3: So What?

Problem	Intervention	The very first thing that happens	What happens next?[a]	What happens after that?[b]	So what?[c]
Fathers do not want their daughters to attend school because they do not think it is necessary for girls to be educated.	Fathers with the same cultural background, who do think it is important for girls to be educated, engage with fathers who do not.	Fathers who do not want their daughters to attend school come to the peer-to-peer session to meet with fathers who support girls' education.	Fathers learn reasons for educating girls. Fathers learn about the possible negatives for girls who are not educated.	Fathers agree to consider sending their girls to school. Fathers register their girls for school.	Girls attend school. More girls graduate with high school diplomas. The girls in the program who attain diplomas are less likely to be in abusive relationships and less likely to have unwanted pregnancies.

[a]We expect these two things to happen at the same time.
[b]Here we expect the first thing to happen first, and then the second thing will happen. These are sequential results.
[c]The first result in this column could also be listed in the "What happens after that?" column, either separately or in the same sentence as "Fathers register their girls for school," depending on how you decide to assess it. It does not matter, as it does not change the order of the results. The three items in this column are sequential results; the third item lists two separate results that happen in the same time frame.

response for all results, or different responses for each one. Table 7.4 adds the "Who cares?" question to the girls' education example.

Question 4. *Common Challenge A: Forgetting to ask who cares about what*

The most common mistake made in regard to the "Who cares?" question is that people forget to ask it! Yet this is likely to be one of the most critical questions in the process. Furthermore, some stakeholders may value different parts of the intervention differently. Knowing who values what will provide critical information for how to develop criteria to value the results.

Question 4. *Common Challenge B: Suitcase words*

Sometimes suitcase words pop up. For instance, one answer to "Who cares?" may be "Beneficiaries care." To make that response helpful, the evaluator needs to know *which* beneficiaries care—about what. (See Chapter 3.)

TABLE 7.4. Answering Question 4: Who Cares?

Problem	Intervention	The very first thing that happens	What happens next?[a]	What happens after that?[b]	So what?[c]
Fathers do not want their daughters to attend school because they do not think it is necessary for girls to be educated.	Fathers with the same cultural background, who do think it is important for girls to be educated, engage with fathers who do not.	Fathers who do not want their daughters to attend school come to the peer-to-peer session to meet with fathers who support girls' education. Who cares?: Mothers, girls, funder.	Fathers learn reasons for educating girls. Fathers learn about the possible negatives for girls who are not educated. Who cares?: Mothers, girls.	Fathers agree to consider sending their girls to school. Fathers register their girls for school. Who cares?: Mothers, girls, community leaders, funder.	Girls attend school. More girls graduate with high school diplomas. The girls in the program who attain diplomas are less likely to be in abusive relationships and less likely to have unwanted pregnancies. Who cares?: Fathers, mothers, girls, community leaders, funder.

Who cares?

The mothers of the girls, and the girls, value the fathers' supporting girls' being educated and receiving high school diplomas. The funder values the girls' obtaining an education. The girls, fathers, and mothers value the safe transport to and from school.

[a]We expect these two things to happen at the same time.

[b]Here we expect the first thing to happen first, and then the second thing will happen. These are sequential results.

[c]The first result in this column could also be listed in the "What happens after that?" column, either separately or in the same sentence as "Fathers register their girls for school," depending on how you decide to assess it. It does not matter, as it does not change the order of the results. The three items in this column are sequential results; the third item lists two separate results that happen in the same time frame.

Question 5. *What resources are needed to achieve these results?*

Now that we know everything that needs to be achieved, we can ask, "What resources are needed to achieve these results?" In the evaluation context, *resources* include time, money, staff, infrastructure, and other items needed to support an intervention.

An evaluator needs information about how what resources will help the intervention to achieve its intended results. Let me sneak in a label here, *input,* since it is very rare that disagreements appear with regard to this label. Most people agree on what an input is. It is a resource (e.g., time, money, people) that is put into (hence, input) a project, program, policy, or intervention so that it can be implemented and achieve its results. Clarifying inputs provide one critical *data point* (a place or point from which we gather data) that provides part of the evidence needed to answer evaluation questions on *efficiency* (simply stated, comparing what was put in to what happened).

Inputs can provide complications in evaluation for three reasons:

- First, when the intervention's funding derived from different sources, it can be challenging to sort through whose money paid for what part of the intervention, and therefore who can take "credit" for the results.
- Second, sometimes when funding sources change, different funders bring different ideas about results, what and how to assess, and how to value results.
- Third, for international projects, working in different currencies can be a challenge—such as when exchange rates drastically change during an intervention, influencing what can be done.

A few common mistakes are made in discussing inputs. Let's explore these.

Question 5. *Common Challenge A: Beneficiaries seen as input*

Sometimes beneficiaries are labeled as resources; the reasoning behind this is that they are needed for the intervention. However, beneficiaries are not inputs. Beneficiaries are the ones who benefit from the resources that are put into an intervention.

Question 5. *Common Challenge B: Management flow in the intervention flow*

Sometimes the discussion on what people must do to manage the program is placed into the logic of the results discussion. What managers or implementers do to bring about the intervention does not belong in the logic of results. Separating the management tasks and results from the intervention results can be tricky, but it is important. Remember, in the results logic, we are trying to determine how what is being done leads (or contributes) to achieving results for specific beneficiaries. The focus is on clarifying the intervention's logic and the intervention's results.

For example, an organization aims to train young men in computer skills so that they are employable. The computers, training manuals, and classrooms are inputs. *Here, in this process, we are not interested in who built the computers, or how they were purchased, or what the organization needed to do to develop the training manual.* Here is the tricky part, so be careful: If the intended result for the intervention *is* a training manual, that is different. For example, the program aims to develop a training manual that is effective and cost-efficient for a diverse population of young adults who need computer skills. In this case, we *are* interested in that result: the training manual. Furthermore, certain evaluation approaches that look at efficiency and cost will be interested in purchasing prices, for example. However, these kinds of information are not part of sorting out the logic of results.

Question 5. *Common Challenge C: Evaluators trying to be auditors or accountants*

It is not an evaluator's job to examine expenditures like an accountant or an auditor. Evaluators do not, for example, review receipts for items purchased. Evaluators often need to be generally aware of how funds are spent and for what purposes; also, for certain kinds of evaluations (such as cost–benefit or economic evaluations), specific financial information is needed. However, let me repeat that we are evaluators, not auditors or accountants; nor should we be hired or expected to take on this role. See Chapters 11 and 15 for more discussion of how economics, cost–benefit analyses, and cost efficiency float into the evaluation pond.

Bringing Back the Labels

Now let's bring back those labels. After the logic has been discussed and laid out, and everyone agrees that there is a logical, step-by-step flow, results labels can be easily added. In fact, let's play around with those labels, shall we? See Table 7.5.

The question to ask is this: When the labels changed in the boldface column heads, did this change the logic beneath these heads, or the wording of the results? The answer is no. Some donors, organizations, institutes, foundations, and governments may have specific definitions for each label. If so, apply their definitions as needed. Just ensure that first, everyone agrees that one logical step leads to the next.

Although we have laid out the logical steps of our results, the results discussion is not yet complete. The concept of **unintended results,** and the way these results fit into the process, are now briefly discussed. After an intervention is implemented, there is the likelihood of unplanned results. When unplanned or unintended results are identified, they then need to be then plausibly linked back to the intervention. Why would evaluators do that? There are two reasons.

TABLE 7.5. Bringing Back the Labels

	Intervention	The very first thing that happens	What happens next?[a]	What happens after that?[b]	So what?[c]
Problem	Intervention	No labels—"results staircase" is used			
Problem	Activity	Output	Outcome	Intermediate outcome	Impact
Problem	Project	Output	Second-level output	Outcome	Second-level outcome
Problem	Program	Eenie	Meenie	Miney	Mo
Fathers do not want their daughters to attend school because they do not think it is necessary for girls to be educated.	Fathers with the same cultural background, who do think it is important for girls to be educated, engage with fathers who do not.	Fathers who do not want their daughters to attend school come to the peer-to-peer session to meet with fathers who support girls' education.	Fathers learn reasons for educating girls. Fathers learn about the possible negatives for girls who are not educated.	Fathers agree to consider sending their girls to school. Fathers register their girls for school.	Girls attend school. More girls graduate with high school diplomas. The girls in the program who attain diplomas are less likely to be in abusive relationships and less likely to have unwanted pregnancies.

[a]We expect these two things to happen at the same time.

[b]Here we expect the first thing to happen first, and then the second thing will happen. These are sequential results.

[c]The first result in this column could also be listed in the "What happens after that?" column, either separately or in the same sentence as "Fathers register their girls for school," depending on how you decide to assess it. It does not matter, as it does not change the order of the results. The three items in this column are sequential results; the third item lists two separate results that happen in the same time frame.

Sometimes unintended results can be negative ones, causing damage to people, animals, or the environment. Identifying these results and understanding what contributed to them may help program planners or implementers to avoid these negative results in the future or with other similar interventions. At other times, unintended results bring unexpected and welcomed changes; here as well, understanding how and what contributed to these will inform future program designs and increase the chances that the positive results can be replicated.

CONTEXTUAL FACTORS: MESSING WITH THE RESULTS LOGIC

Once the results discussion is clear, a broader discussion explores factors that influence results and are (most often) outside the control of the program implementers—contextual factors. Explore contextual factors by asking:

- What is outside the intervention's control that would *prevent* the results from happening?

- What is outside the intervention's control that would *facilitate* the results happening?

Responses to either question can include tangible and nontangible responses. *Tangible* factors include anything that can be identified by the five senses. Examples include policy changes in education, droughts that affected income or food accessibility, a change in government that brought new priorities, or a reduction in funding for the intervention. *Nontangible* items may include power dynamics, cultural beliefs, or personal factors (e.g., a powerful person just did not like the intervention, or perhaps she did). The questions provide places to (1) look for explanations as to why, why not, or to what extent results were achieved and (2) provide insights into unintended results.

LOGIC AND OUTCOMES

- **Have a few minutes—3, to be exact?** Look at a video in Paul Duignan's Three Minute Outcomes series (*www.linkedin.com/pulse/difference-between-outcome-output-three-minute-4-paul-duignan-phd*).

- **Have a few hours?** Read the Epilogue to Thomas Schwandt's book *Evaluation Foundations Revisited: Cultivating a Life of the Mind for Practice* (2015).

- **Have more time?** Do not read anything else. Take a concrete example and work through the five-question framework presented on page 133, preferably with a colleague. Check the logic: Did you skip steps? Can you see direct links or associations? Then happily apply labels to what is produced (or not).

The activity described next, Activity 7.1, is an organizational intervention. It is intended to be used (1) when a smidgen, or even a mountain, of information suggests that *something* is not quite right with the intervention's logic; (2) when key stakeholders are not in agreement about the intervention and its intended results; or (3) as a capacity- and team-building exercise.

ACTIVITY 7.1. Sorting Out the Results—and Naming Them

Purpose: The activity engages people in a step-by-step process that untangles intervention logic, with an added focus on clarifying the use of results labels such as *output, outcome,* and *impact.*

Materials: You will need a lot of scrap paper cut into small pieces. Different paper colors are useful to keep the steps clear; for instance, all problem statements can be put on red paper, all interventions on yellow, and all results in blue. You will also need flip chart paper and multiple cards for labels (e.g., *output, outcome*). For example, write 10 cards with the label *output,* 15 cards with the label *outcome,* and 5 cards with the label *impact.* The number of each needed will vary by group, and more can be made as needed during the exercise.

Time: Allow from 4 hours to 2 days, depending on the group and on the complexity of the intervention and its results.

Special considerations: The activity brings together lessons covered in Chapters 1–4 and 6–7 (and, to a certain extent, 5). It is a heavily facilitated activity that requires high levels of evaluative knowledge and strong facilitation skills.

The exercise: Ensure that there are no more than three to five people per group. Everyone in the group must be familiar with the same intervention, though different levels of familiarity are acceptable.

The first question I ask is this:

"What is the problem you are trying to solve?"

Write this question on the flip chart. Provide each group with one piece of red paper. When the smaller group agrees on an answer, ask them to write that response on the given piece of paper. (Again, color-coding each step is useful, though the actual color does not matter.)

I then ask:

"How do you know it is a problem?"

Add that question to the flip chart. Allow time for group discussion, if needed. Here, I often bring in the fact-versus-assumption discussion introduced in Chapter 4. Groups must either describe how they know it is a problem (e.g., data exist) or outline the next steps that they will take to clarify that it is a problem (or not). With the problem statement clearly written down, and with clear facts or a plan to get them, I then ask:

"What does the intervention intend to achieve?"

I then provide a pile of small yellow pieces of paper. I ask the participants first to brainstorm with their group and to write down all responses, with each response on its own piece of paper. I ask each person in the group to be responsible for writing their own answer(s), so that quieter members' contributions will not be missed or overlooked. The question should generate a very broad list of potential results at many levels, some of which may end up in the results discussion, and some may not. There are two key rules. If the two rules are skipped or not adhered to, you will be sailing up the proverbial creek without a proverbial paddle.

• *Rule 1: Ensure that no one uses labels.* The mistake often made in this step is that people have a strong desire to label what they write. For example, a person will write "Girls' access to education is improved," and then sneak in "impact" on the same card. It is critical that no labels are used at this point. If you hear people using labels in the group discussion, remind them not to use labels, but to describe results instead.

 What if labels are brought in too early in the activity?

Confusion and arguments will ensue that are difficult, if not impossible, to circumvent. For instance, someone starts an argument by saying, "It is an outcome," to which someone responds, "No, it is an impact." Rather than focus on the result itself (e.g., girls' access to education is improved), the focus shifts to insignificant and useless label squabbles. The process described is designed to solve the labeling argument before it even gets started. Follow the process. (See the earlier lengthy discussion in this chapter.)

• *Rule 2: Each result is written on its <u>own</u> piece of paper.* Writing each result on its own piece of paper is critical for sorting them, having focused discussions, keeping the process untangled, and eventually talking about the logic and theory of the intervention. Even if you are the "lone evaluator" and sitting by yourself going through documents, or have just returned to your desk after conducting multiple interviews from which you now need to sort out all the intended results, do not take a shortcut and write all the results on one piece of paper, type them into one Word document, or use an Excel spreadsheet. You will need to be able to move the results around to create different links and different logic, as needed. This is borne out through the thinking process.

 What happens if someone writes a few connected results on the same sheet of paper?

The challenge is that these results may not be connected, or may have a layer in between them, or one of them is not exactly right. Rewrite the card with one idea per card.

Once the brainstorming is complete, ask the group to place the red card (the card with the problem statement) to the left (either on the table or on a wall space), and then to place their yellow results cards into logical order, moving from left to right. Most likely new cards (the forgotten or hidden results) will need to be written and added to the logical flow. The flow may be linear, or it may resemble a spider web. Some results may happen at the same time, while others need to be sequential. Once the logic is laid out, ask one participant to read the logical flow, using minimal language (not much more than what is on the cards; it should be *that* clear). When the task is complete—and it is complete when the flow is step-by-step and makes logical sense to everyone (e.g., no suitcase words)—provide each group with several cards labeled *output, outcome,* and *impact,* and ask them to label their results. Ask them to place them and then remove them, and ask what difference the cards made (e.g., easier conversation, no difference at all).

Then ask:

"What intervention brings about that result, or that flow of results?"

Provide the group with blue pieces of paper. The responses are written on those blue cards, and each one is placed by the results flow (or specific result card) it intends to bring about. When you are facilitat-

ing this step, remember that different interventions probably have their own results flows, which then likely funnel into one larger, grand result, and there may be other connections along the way. And remember, an intervention brings about intended results, and results also bring about results (see page 126 for an explanation). I then ask:

"Who benefits from what result?"

Provide a green card in a different shape (e.g., a circle) to highlight the beneficiaries. These can be placed next to a specific result, or laid above or below the entire flow to show how the group/person benefits from the entire process. A discussion on unbeneficiaries can also be introduced at this point (see Chapter 3). Eventually, but not too soon, the information can be organized into a format. If a box-like format is introduced too soon, people often try to fill in the boxes and not think through the logic.

When the process is completed (i.e., the logic is laid out, whether it is linear or looks more like a spider's web; it is presented to and interrogated by the other participants; and changes are made as needed), I surprise my group and say:

"You know what to evaluate and when, and can explain your program logic. You can identify gaps or faults in the logic; you know when and where data are needed to test what assumption; you can engage in a results label discussion with confidence; and therefore you can engage in any evaluative process."

When the process is well facilitated, with respect and thoughtfulness, people are often surprised when they can explain their program logic, identify faults or gaps in the logic, engage in the labels discussion as needed, and talk with evaluators regarding what to evaluate when. It is a wonderful feeling for them (and the evaluation facilitator). Furthermore, the process provides the foundation of what is needed to begin to complete the boxes on any type of mandated M&E format (e.g., donor's forms, government forms).

Critical learning points: The problem statement, intervention, and results are connected, and the movement from one to the next needs to be logical to the people implementing, funding, and ultimately receiving the intervention. Most evaluation discussions, from what to assess to what do you expect the intervention to achieve, can be clearly discussed once the logic is explicit. For example, the logic of the results provides insight into what to assess when (e.g., you should not assess for something that is dependent on another result happening first, when that first result has not yet happened). Senseless arguments about results labels are not needed, though results labels can be placed on the logical flow once, and only once, the logic is clear. Understanding how everything connects enables a clear, accessible evaluative discussion for everyone involved.

Learning about the three cousins (problem statement, intervention, and results), how to break them down, and how to link them together is a critical part of being an evaluator. A critical part of that discussion is understanding the logic of the results. The logic of results needs to be explored separately, as it brings its own separate challenges, strategies, and conversations.

WRAPPING UP

This chapter has delved deeply into, and explicated, a nuanced results discussion that reveals the logic of results (also called a *results flow* or *results chain,* among other names). Although at first suggesting a linear orientation, that flow or chain can be represented as a circle, a spider's web, or a host of other logically connected configurations. Although a results discussion is often a messy and demanding conversation, it is at the same time a clarifying and an elating one. Knowing how all the intended results are thought to connect to each other provides pieces of the puzzle needed to link the problem, intervention, and results for a plausible and evaluable intervention. Furthermore, understanding how everything is supposed to connect provides places to find answers for when anticipated results do not occur, and when unanticipated ones do.

The clarity provided in this chapter about results, which has built on Chapters 3, 4, and 6, will support a constructive dialogue that avoids endless arguments over labels (e.g., *output* vs. *outcome*), clarifies the logic of the results, and provides a scaffolding on which to "hang" a theory-of-change discussion. Although Part II of this book focuses on working as an evaluator and doing evaluation, the evaluative logic learned in Part I is critical to the Part II discussion for nearly any evaluation approach, method, or framework.

Now that we have come to the end of this chapter, I want to add a special note. I have written this book to untangle the messy processes in evaluation. To do that requires a fluidly intertwined conversation that ebbs and flows, moves up and down, is turned inside out and outside in, and sometimes produces more questions than answers. Often the conversation needs to veer way off track to stay on track, all without complicating the core discussion. As an evaluator, you need to hold these types of conversations, so that as the evaluative journey progresses with inevitable twists and turns, at the end of the day (or week or month or year), each step described brings clear descriptions, answers, or well-articulated questions. Maintaining the cognitive space for such conversations and skillfully guiding each discussion (even when it all takes place between you, yourself, and the program documents) are critical roles you need to play competently in any evaluative process. Chapters 1–7 provide the guidance to maintain the space for holding such discussions, and Chapters 8–10 and all of Part II make use of it. Before you leave this chapter, come join me in a conversation.

Our Conversation: Between You and Me

Here is a type of situation that you may encounter with regard to the results process. Practicing with these common scenarios will support you when you encounter similar situations in the real world.

A project manager and the funder disagree on what constitutes a program impact, and both insist they are right. You only have about 30 minutes to chat with them and help them reach a mutual understanding. What do you do? For such a thorny conversation, I often find focusing on definitions to be futile; rather, I first try to understand the purpose of the conversation. For instance, I would ask them: Why are they having this discussion? Is it to determine what to evaluate? Is it to agree on the logic of the results the intervention will have? If it is about evaluating something, I would ask them to concretely describe what they want evaluated (e.g., how people act differently or how the community has changed), who is interested in that result, and what they plan on doing with the finding. If it is about the logic of the results, then I would ask them to explain briefly what they expect the intervention to achieve, within what time frame, without using the labels. The key is to shift the conversation from a futile disagreement to a concrete conversation that advances the purpose of the discussion. What would you do? (P.S. I would also consider that maybe there is no relevant purpose to the conversation; perhaps it is just two people arguing about whose impact is bigger than whose. In that case, I would step aside.)

CHAPTER 8

Talking Intervention Theory (and Logic)

> Everything must be taken into account. If the fact will not fit the theory—
> let the theory go.
>
> —AGATHA CHRISTIE, *The Mysterious Affair at Styles*

There are some people who are great at discussing and explaining intervention theory (assumptions about how change is brought about) and theories in general (assumptions about how the world works), and are completely comfortable with beginning a conversation on either. If an evaluative process starts with a client or colleague who says, "We want to work on our theory of change," I suggest responding with "We can do that. Can you tell me about the problem the intervention is meant to address?", and then shifting back to the conversations suggested in Chapter 3 and asking the questions raised in Chapters 4–7. You may end up back at this chapter in a few short minutes, with the client or colleague gleefully chatting about the theory that will inform, or currently does inform, the intervention—or not.

Often, it can be a challenge to have people theorize. Theory can be an intimidating concept, which is why the scaffolding needed to have a useful and thoughtful discussion regarding the intervention theory is laid out in Chapters 3–7. Chapter 8 draws on the preceding chapters to describe how to engage with an important element in any evaluative process: the discussion on the theory of change, its relation to the intervention and its intended (or actual) results, and ultimately its links to assessment and how the results are valued. Carol Weiss, a notable evaluation theorist, titled her seminal 1995 article on program theory "Nothing as Practical as Good Theory," and I could not agree more.

Before you continue, I have a question. What is the difference between a theory of change and a logic model?

Sometimes the terms *theory of change*, *logic model*, and *program logic* (or *intervention logic*) are used interchangeably—yet they should not be. At other times, program logic is labeled a *theory of action* (Donaldson, 2007; Funnell & Rogers, 2011). Program logic, often represented through a logic model, explains the logic of an intervention and its results, and theory of change explains *why* things are done (i.e., why the decisions are made to do what is done). Both aim to explain, in different ways, how activities are thought to contribute to a series of results (see Chapter 7 on results).

What would a standard or traditional logic model look like?

That is a tough question, as there are many different logic models and logic models have changed over time. For example, the United Way of America (1996) provided a handbook on how to do a logic model. This model had four categories: *input, activity, output,* and *outcome*. In 2008, the logic model was expanded and changed substantially, to include *input; strategy,* which now includes *activities, services,* and *outputs*; and *short-term, midterm,* and *long-term outcomes* (United Way Valley of the Sun, 2008). These are just two examples from two divisions of one organization. What has not changed over time is the linear nature of the logic model. Furthermore, this is a structured process, and some people find it too rigid. A third United Way provides an example of one of the more common logic models (*www. calgaryunitedway.org/images/uwca/our-work/supporting-non-profits/Logic-Model-Template-Final. pdf*). These are just a few examples; many more exist that look different.

Any other words of advice?

I have noted above that a logic model is sometimes found to be too rigid and that a theory of change is often not tangible enough to enable people to manage a program, so a hybrid of the two may be created. Chapters 1–7 describe the thinking needed for either a logic model, a theory of change, or a hybrid. This chapter provides a hybrid example, which draws on the girls' education intervention described in earlier chapters. I tend to use hybrids when I have a choice because I find them the most useful.

THREE REASONS TO HAVE AN EXPLICIT THEORY OF CHANGE

When program theory and its related logic are explicit, an evaluator can use that theory and logic to (1) identify gaps in the intervention's design (reflection), (2) inform how to monitor the intervention, and/or (3) guide data collection for an evaluation.

Four Examples of How an Evaluator Engages with a Theory of Change

Here are four ways an evaluator often engages with a theory of change:

1. *Identify the theory of change.* Sometimes, when there is no *explicit* theory of change (i.e., nothing is written down or otherwise verbalized), an evaluator is brought in to clarify what theory or theories have informed the intervention. The word *explicit* is emphasized because there is always a theory, a reason why something is done, though it is often veiled.

2. *Inform the intervention.* Sometimes an evaluator is asked to be a part of the program design process and helps to articulate the theory of change. Here, the evaluator would (1) facilitate the group members in articulating their own theory of change (i.e., only facilitate); (2) participate in the process, bringing in her knowledge of social science theories and her own personal experience (i.e., facilitate and inform); and/or (3) facilitate a group of sectoral, cultural, and other experts in discussing ways to support developing the theory of change and informing the intervention.

3. *Review the theory of change.* By reviewing a clearly articulated theory of change, an evaluator and her team can assess it for any obvious gaps. And/or the evaluator can facilitate a process with internal or external experts on the thematic area (e.g., education, environment), cultural experts, and those familiar with the broader context (e.g., politics, economics) and use these various perspectives to review the theory's likelihood of bringing about change.

4. *Evaluate the intervention.* An evaluator can use the program or its articulated theory of change, can use a general well-established theory of change, or may develop her own theory of change, to evaluate an intervention. To read more about theory of change in evaluation, jump to Chapter 15 to read about theory-driven evaluation.

BOX 8.1. An Evaluator's Engagement with Theory of Change and Logic

Theory and logic often consist of a mix of some or all of the following: personal experience, social science theory, facts, and assumptions. The mix can be magical, benign, or lethal. An evaluator's role can be to identify it, inform it, review it, or use it to evaluate the intervention.

SORTING OUT AN INTERVENTION'S THEORY OF CHANGE: A FRAMEWORK

Engaging (most) people in a discussion about theory, without preparing a scaffolding (clarified links among the problem, intervention, and results, and among all the results—also known as the program logic) on which to base the conversation, is often hard to do. Try to start a conversation out of the blue with the question "So what is your theory of how the intervention works?", and be prepared for blank stares, stunned silence, babbling, and sometimes thoughtful pondering, but rarely a cut-to-the-chase, concrete, explicit description of a refined theory (though it can happen).

The logic of an intervention and its results, sometimes shown graphically through a logic model, is what explains the steps for how to move from the problem that needs to be addressed, to the intended results. That logic draws on, or is guided by, the theory of change. In other words, "Why I think this [theory] informs what makes me do that [logic]." Let's continue from Chapter 7, where the logic of the girls' education intervention has been laid out, and examine how this logic exemplifies a hybrid logic model (as explained on page 152). It is a hybrid because it asks for more than the traditional logic model. Table 8.1 is provided here as a memory refresher on this intervention's logic.

When we look at Table 8.1 and ask, "What makes you think this leads to that?", the implicit theory of change becomes explicit. Some might label this implicit thinking the "underpinning" theory (it is pinned beneath the logic). Remember, asking the question

TABLE 8.1. Hybrid Logic Model: Girls' Education Example

Problem	Intervention	The very first thing that happens	What happens next?[a]	What happens then?	What happens after that?[b]	So what?[c]
Fathers do not want their daughters to attend school because they do not think it is necessary for girls to be educated.	Fathers with the same cultural background, who do think it is important for girls to be educated, engage with fathers who do not.	Fathers who do not want their daughters to attend school come to the peer-to-peer session to meet with fathers who support girls' education.	Fathers learn reasons for educating girls. Fathers learn about the possible negatives for girls who are not educated.	Fathers change their perceptions about the importance of girls attending school.	Fathers agree to consider sending their girls to school. Fathers register their girls for school.	Girls attend school. More girls graduate with high school diplomas. The girls in the program who attain diplomas are less likely to be in abusive relationships and less likely to have unwanted pregnancies.

[a]We expect these two things to happen at the same time.

[b]Here we expect the first thing to happen first, and then the second thing will happen. These are sequential results.

[c]The first result in this column could also be listed in the "What happens after that?" column, either separately or in the same sentence as "Fathers register their girls for school," depending on how you decide to assess it. It does not matter, as it does not change the order of the results. The three items in this column are sequential results; the third item lists two separate results that happen in the same time frame.

"What makes you think this leads to that?" works in the process *now* because of all the thinking and conversations that have taken place in Chapters 3–7, particularly 3–4 and 6–7. The question will likely not work as well (though it could) if these previous discussions and processes had not taken place. Because this thorough process has been conducted, the thinking behind (or underneath) how the problem, intervention, results, and beneficiaries (program logic) all fit together has been germinating, and will be easier to unearth than if the question "What makes you think this leads to that?" had been asked cold.

Having a Nonthreatening Theory Discussion

People can be intimidated by the term *theory,* as in "Hey, can you tell me what theory you used?" Or they may feel threatened when asked to explain an intervention's theory of change, such as when an evaluator asks, "I just want to know the theory of the change . . . hey, wait, where are you going?"

Key to the conversation about a theory of change is *first* breaking down the problem statement and desired results into small pieces (i.e., pocket problems and pocket results), and connecting these to the intervention. These small, tangible, interlinking pieces then provide the concrete words (and often visual aids) needed to discuss and unlock the program theory (i.e., the scaffold needed to have the theory conversation). Once the logic is clear, an evaluator can merely ask, "What makes you think that?", and the theory discussion is launched from stable ground.

Can you explain the difference between a theory of change and a logic model by using a nutshell description, and describe how that relates to implementation?

I like to think about it in this way: A theory of change answers **why,** as in "Why do I think X will lead to Y?" or "Why am I doing what I do?" A good theory tells the story of the intervention. The logic model addresses **what,** as in "What are the steps I need to take (in my intervention) to implement the theory?" The implementation of the intervention has its own theory and logic, and thus needs its own discussion, addressing **how, where,** and **when** something is done. Using a framework that separates these into 10 simple categories, let's apply the barking dog example we discussed on page 63 in Chapter 3. See Table 8.2; start with the complete left column (including entries under both headings), and read toward the complete right column.

Organizing the theory and logic in the manner described above is a way to catalogue or organize the discussion. Sorting through all 10 columns provides an understanding of what to assess, which will eventually inform how to assess. (See Chapters 5, 9, and 15 for how to assess.) The process of understanding (or developing) the theory of change and related logic will vary widely, as will the evaluator's role and those of the stakeholders. When the evaluator is applying the framework depicted in Table 8.2, or engaging in any theory-of-change discussion, her role can be to facilitate a dialogue that will make the theory explicit and

TABLE 8.2. Theory and Logic Framework: The Barking Dog Example

Problem statement (The challenge I need to solve)	Theory of change (Why I think change will be brought about)	Intervention (What is designed)	Implementation theory (How I think change will be brought about)	Implementation logic (Where and when I implement)
The dog is barking (the problem and a fact). The dog is barking because it is bored (it is the cause of the barking, and it is a fact).	If we provide the bored dog (problem) with a toy (intervention), it will play (assumption) and not be bored (assumption), and the dog will stop barking (anticipated result, an assumption).	Provide the dog a toy (it is the step I take because of the theory I am using), or increase the dog's access to toys.	I think that dogs like balls (assumption). When dogs are outside and want something with which to play, it is a good idea to give them a ball (assumption).	I provide a ball for the owner to give the dog when he is let into the yard to play.
Source of knowledge	**Source of knowledge**	**Practical steps I take because of the theory I am using**	**Source of knowledge**	**Practical steps I take because of the theory I am using and my source of knowledge**
Facts are confirmed through observation and hearing.	I have worked with dogs for the past 10 years, have observed this dog, and am familiar with animal behavior theory.	Provide a toy to the dog.	I have a dog, and he likes to play with balls more than other toys when he is outside. Animal behavior books suggest balls as a good toy for dogs.	I have funds to provide a ball, and the dog's owner is available to give the dog the ball when he is let out to play.

logic clear. At times the evaluator may also be left on her own (or with her team) to apply the framework, drawing on documents, literature, and personal knowledge and experience. This is the least desirable option, since in this situation the evaluator (and her team), when attempting to decipher an intervention's logic, must rely on interpretations and assumptions. This reliance then opens doors to allow in misinterpretations and misunderstandings.

COMMON CHALLENGES TO DISCUSSING THEORY OF CHANGE

Even if the evaluative process has produced a clear scaffolding (i.e., the problem statement, the intervention, expected results, and beneficiaries) for a discussion of the theory underlying the expected changes, six common challenges may still be encountered. When there is a challenge to engaging with a theory of change, it is essential to identify that challenge, so that it can be explored and engaged with. Let's count down the six common challenges in reverse:

- *Challenge 6.* Language challenges infiltrate the theory conversation. People use different labels for the same meaning and terms are used interchangeably (e.g., *theory of change* and *logic model*). Or perhaps people are not familiar with some of the terms that are needed to engage (and were not aware of that until the conversation started). As always, ensure that people have the necessary language to comfortably engage in the conversation. (See Chapter 1 on language.)

- *Challenge 5.* Theory is a logical interpretation of facts, propositions, and assumptions, yet not a fact itself, which means that there is no absolutely right or wrong theory (until it is implemented and tested in that context, and proved right or wrong—hence the need for M&E). See Chapter 4, which discusses facts and assumptions.

- *Challenge 4.* The theories people choose to inform an intervention are based on their education, culture, life experience, and other factors. Thus questioning a person on his intervention's theory (e.g., "What makes you think that X will lead to Y?"), if not carefully done, can be viewed as confrontational; it challenges the person's way of thinking, as well as his identity and beliefs. And when people feel that they are being confronted (challenged or cornered), useful dialogue or other fruitful engagement is unlikely.

- *Challenge 3.* The person or group implementing the intervention did not design the intervention, and the theory used to design the intervention was never made explicit. In this instance, the person or the group the evaluator is working with may simply not have clear answers to the "why" questions (e.g., "Why will X bring about Y?" or "What made the program designer think that X will bring about Y?").

- *Challenge 2.* Often people do not want to engage in a theory-of-change discussion, for one or more of many possible reasons; the conversation is therefore blocked, stonewalled, or otherwise ignored. For example, perhaps the intervention is meeting a political agenda or is part of spending down funds, and a theory of change is not relevant (and a discussion of it may be detrimental) to those with decision-making power. Or perhaps the people in decision-making power know that there is only a sketchy theory, and these are not conversations they want to have. Or maybe the person or group implementing the intervention knows that the implicit theory is very unlikely to produce results; however, the intervention is already funded, and nothing can be changed at this point. Or maybe they just find theory intimidating. Or maybe . . . the list goes on.

- *Challenge 1.* Multiple theories, and/or competing theories, are informing the intervention in different ways. All of these theories need to be brought to the surface.

An evaluator's knowledge of theory of change, and his skills in facilitation and often negotiation, are instrumental to engaging with each of these challenges.

*What do we mean by **theory** of change? Is it like a social science theory?*

All interventions draw from someone's knowledge; an intervention is not (we hope) based on a random musing. The knowledge may come from reading social science books or journals, from work or other personal experiences, and/or from cultural beliefs, among many other possible sources. Although social science and natural science have long-established literatures of theories on how change happens, I do not often find that in the real world, people are citing exact social change theories from books or journals (though it does happen) when speaking about an intervention's theory. Often there is an agreement that such a theory exists and that it is acceptable. Most people are comfortable with that type of theorizing, since, as human beings, we draw on theory daily.

When I teach, I draw on adult learning theory, and in writing this book, I have drawn on the same theory. Adult learning theory suggests that adults are more apt to learn when they draw from their own experience and knowledge to apply a new concept, as opposed to learning that new concept through lectures or memorizing definitions. I know that this is an accepted adult education theory, and I know it most often works. I could scour books and journals and find that exact theory, but I do not. Yet when people ask me why I teach the way I do, or what theory informs how I have written this book, they seem to accept my approach readily and do not expect me to cite where the theory is written; perhaps someone might, one day.

What about when someone challenges you, and asks, for example, "Who wrote that theory?" or "Where is that theory documented?"

I would start by trying to understand why that person is asking the question. In my 20-plus years of conducting evaluative processes, and in discussing that exact question with many evaluation colleagues around the world, it has not been our collective experience to have people question an intervention's theory in terms of where the theory is written down, with four exceptions. Here they are:

- When someone suggests a theory that most people are *not* familiar with, it is often questioned.
- When someone suggests a theory that goes against other commonly accepted theories, the theory is often questioned.
- When someone suggests a theory that goes against a popular belief, it is often questioned (consider what happened the first time someone suggested that the world was not flat!).

In these cases, having a documented theory or example of where, when, and by whom the theory was tested proves useful. This leads to the final example:

- When someone suggests a theory that has been tested and not worked, the theory is often questioned.

A theory of change should be grounded in, or based on, explicit knowledge. This means that when an evaluator asks about what theory was used to inform the intervention, the evaluator is seeking to find out what knowledge, facts, assumptions, and propositions explain why the intervention has been chosen and why people believe that it provides a promising pathway to the desired outcomes. Closely related to the discussion of an intervention's theory is theory-driven evaluation. Again, please skip ahead to Chapter 15 if you want to learn more about that approach.

*Does an intervention need a theory of change **and** a logic model?*

A logic model is lost without a theory of change, its best friend forever (BFF), whereas the theory can exist perfectly well on its own. However, a theory living alone, untested in the ivory tower, never gets to live in the real world and prove itself without its BFF, the logic model. Thus they do need each other. The theory of change tells a story: the beginning (the problem being addressed), the middle (why the intervention is doing certain things), and the end (the results). Once the story is clear, we need to think about how to make that story a reality. Thus steps are created, informed by our story, which show what the intervention does at each point to move from the problem statement to the intended results. We name this product the *logic model* or the *intervention logic*, yet it also has other names.

PROGRAM LOGIC AND THEORY OF CHANGE: HOW THEY ARE CONNECTED, AND WHY BOTH ARE USEFUL

Let's expand the girls' education example to two different towns, in order to take a practical look at the connection between theory of change and program logic, and what makes having the explicit theory *and* logic useful (see Figure 8.1).

The Twist: A Difference in a Pocket Problem

The towns have the same grand problem, and similar pocket problems; however, when we break down those pocket problems (i.e., we look at reasons why these pocket problems exist,

Shared problems, theory of change, and results for Town A and Town B (fact)	School-age girls do not attend the local school and do not receive an education.
Pocket problems (facts)	Authority figures in the homes do not support girls to attend school (cultural reasons) and the area between the girls' homes and the school is not safe.
The theory of change (a story drawing on multiple facts, propositions, and assumptions that, when combined, explain what change will be brought about and how)	School-age girls' not accessing education can lead to multiple challenges later in life (education and social theory). Having authority figures who reside in the girls' homes support girls to attend school (gender and education theory); removing cultural barriers (cultural theory); and providing safety measures to address the vulnerability of girls to attend school (cultural and gender theory) will lead to more girls attending school and receiving a high school education. Girls who have a high school education are less likely to stay in abusive relationships or have unwanted pregnancies (education and social theory) and more likely to have greater economic opportunities.
Pocket result (not yet a fact)	Authority figures in the home support girls to attend school, and the area between home and the school is made safer.
Grand result (not yet a fact)	School-age girls do attend the local school.

FIGURE 8.1. Why having an explicit theory of change and logic matters: The girls' education example.

and use facts), it is evident that the reasons for one pocket problem differ: In Town A, there have been violent criminal incidents that make the road to the school unsafe; in Town B, it is not a violent (though still criminal, one would hope) incident or series of incidents, but random verbal harassment of young girls. In Town A, there is a perception based on cultural beliefs that it is unsafe for male teachers to instruct girls in the classroom; that perception does not exist in Town B. Because there are differences in what the term *unsafe* means in practice (see suitcase words, Chapter 7), the program logic and implementation are somewhat different—different enough to influence what to do to bring about pocket (lower-level) results and therefore what to assess—yet the grand result and other anticipated results remain the same. Let's take a look at Town A's and Town B's program logic.

Town A's Program Logic

The intervention in Town A will encourage fathers (authority figures) to support their daughters' school attendance as a result of a peer-to-peer mechanism; provide buses and female bus drivers to drive girls to school; and provide female teachers to teach girls (addressing vulnerability and cultural appropriateness), which will contribute to more girls' attending school. Notice the buried theory in the peer-to-peer activity: It is theorized that fathers are influenced by their peers (peer-to-peer intervention, which draws largely on a theory that people are heavily influenced by their peers).

Town B's Program Logic

Program implementers for Town B decide to apply the same theory, yet they apply a different logic because the pocket problems are similar, but not quite the same. In Town B, while walking to and from school is not considered safe when girls are alone due to random verbal harassment (and furthermore, it is perceived as culturally inappropriate for girls to walk alone), walking with a parent or adult relative creates a safe space and is deemed culturally appropriate. Instead of purchasing buses like Town A, the focus is on organizing parents to escort the girls on different days. The challenge with fathers not permitting their daughters to attend school is found to be the same challenge as in Town A (though for slightly different reasons), and the peer-to-peer intervention logic remains the same.

What to Monitor and Evaluate in Town A and Town B

In Town A and Town B, an evaluator would likely assess (at a minimum) to find out if authority figures in the homes now support girls' school attendance, if the girls and their parental figures now find it safe to attend school, and if school-age girls attend the local school. Yet in each town, the specific monitoring would be slightly different. For example, in Town A, some questions would focus on the bus intervention; in Town B, there would be no questions on buses, just questions on the effectiveness of having parents walk girls to and from school, which would also probe to find out if it addresses cultural challenges. In Town A, questions would look at the safety of the classroom, where in Town B, the monitoring would not. Breaking the problem statement down into smaller pieces enables the logic to be made explicit and appropriate to the problems in each location. This in turn enables the logic and implementation of the intervention to test the same theory in different circumstances, and ensures relevant data collection. In a nutshell, this example illustrates how making the theory and logic explicit has two advantages. First, it makes intervention evaluable. Second, the intervention can be managed to achieve its intended results because relevant data are collected (see Chapter 9 for more on what to assess).

Remembering That We Are the Tortoise

An intervention that has well-thought-out theoretical foundations and clear step-by-step logic does not happen overnight, or often even after a few weeks. A theory of change and its associated logic need personal and organizational commitments in terms of both time and resources. If it is important for multiple parties to have widespread understanding and agreement on the intervention and its results (e.g., more people than the program director or program implementers), then broad participation in the process to develop the theory and logic is needed. (See Chapter 12 on values and Chapter 15 on participatory processes.)

THREE THINGS WE KNOW WHEN THEORY OF CHANGE AND LOGIC ARE CLEAR

Here are three basic scenarios that are useful to think about when conducting an evaluation, or when explaining to a colleague or client reasons for having an explicit theory of change and clear program logic (Donaldson, 2007; Funnell & Rogers, 2011; Patton, 2008).

- *The intervention is implemented poorly, with few or no results.* In this scenario, the evaluator cannot tell if the logic or the theory is not correct. Take our barking dog example: Let's assume that the ball is purchased, but the owner forgets to give the dog his ball. In this example, nothing is tested. The intervention is implemented poorly. *Implementation failure.*

- *The intervention is implemented well, with no results.* In this scenario, the logic is tested because the components are all implemented well, but there are no positive results. The dog plays with the ball, but also continues to bark. A logical conclusion could be that the theory of change is not appropriate to this context. *Theory failure.*

- *The intervention is implemented well, with good results.* In this scenario, the data show that the implementation (intervention logic) of the idea (theory) produces the expected results. The dog plays with the ball and stops barking. An evaluator will test this carefully, as she will need to show contribution or attribution of the intervention to the result (i.e., the action contributes to or causes the result). For more on contribution and attribution, read Chapter 7. *Success.*

BOX 8.2. Implementation Tests the Logic and the Theory

Implementing an intervention tests both the logic (what is done) and the theory (why it should work). Only if the intervention is implemented well can the logic, and therefore the theory, truly be tested. For example, if an intervention is not implemented, then the theory and logic are never tested. If the intervention is implemented well, with fidelity to the logic (meaning it does what is says it would do), and relevant contextual factors are taken into consideration, and yet few or no positive expected results are identified, then probably the wrong theory of change has been used to address that specific problem, in that specific context, in that time frame, for those beneficiaries (Pawson & Tilley, 1997; Westhorp, 2014).

THEORY AND LOGIC: INFORMING WHEN TO MONITOR AND EVALUATE WHAT AND WHERE

Having a clear theory of change and program logic provides excellent ways to understand what to monitor and/or what to evaluate because an explicit theory of change and clear program logic transparently demonstrate when and which results are likely to happen (Funnell & Rogers, 2011). Thus they are invaluable in that they show us *where* to look for *what* results, and give an indication of *when* (e.g., one result happens before another); they heavily inform all aspects of monitoring and evaluation. Here is one example of when a theory of change and logic are useful in an evaluation.

A funder mandates that an evaluation takes place, and no results are found. A clear theory and logic can identify whether the results have been searched for much too soon, and/or perhaps in the wrong place. I see this a great deal with what are commonly called *impact evaluations* (see Chapter 15), when higher-level results (such as grand results) are expected to be achieved far too early in the intervention's implementation process. However, if there is no explicit theory of change and clear program logic, a program implementer is in a very precarious position from which to argue (likely after the evaluation is done) that the reason no results are found is that the evaluation has occurred too early in the process.

Thus choosing the wrong time to evaluate may have incorrect, and possibly dismal, consequences for an intervention. I am blissfully ignoring the fact that when a boss, manager, donor, or other person to whom you are accountable tells you, "Evaluate now," you must obviously evaluate now. How theory influences when to assess something is demonstrated in Activity 8.1, a game that compels participants to think through how theory of change influences what to assess and when. An expanded version of the Evaluation Logic Game, with graphics for the game cards, is available on this book's companion website (*www.guilford. com/podems-materials*).

ACTIVITY 8.1. The Evaluation Logic Game: Thinking Through When to Evaluate What

Purpose: To learn how different ways of thinking about an intervention's logic influence what to assess and when.

Materials: Graphics for three sets of cards are provided on the companion website. Each card has one result written on it, and when all the cards in the same set are combined, they provide a chain of results. However, *at least two groups need the same set of cards* because you will compare the orders in which the groups place the cards. Laminate the cards if you plan to use them more than once, and print each set of cards on its own color of paper (e.g., one set green, one set pink, and one set white). This will enable you to organize them quickly when the exercise is complete.

I have provided one set of cards in Figure 8.2 as an example of what a pile would look like before the game. I then use a different set of cards later (see Figure 8.3) to demonstrate how the game is played. So, for example, if there are three groups, have three sets of the *same* set of cards, and provide each group with the same set. If there are four groups, then ensure that two groups have the condom use example provided in Figure 8.2, and the other two groups can use the girls' education example provided in Figure 8.3. Note that each set has one input card.

Time: Allow approximately 10 minutes for groups to sort the cards and choose a presenter, and at least 20–25 minutes to play the games and discuss learning from the games. Total approximate time: 30–35 minutes.

The exercise: A sorting game is a practical way for groups to understand how logic works and how it influences monitoring and evaluation. I have mentioned earlier in this book the importance of not choosing an example that is familiar to the group, as you want the focus to be on learning the idea or concept, not the specific details of the actual example. Ensure that each group has three to five members (although two in each group would work), and that each group has one set of cards. Do not let the groups see any other group's cards (which, for at least two groups, are the same). Provide these instructions:

"In the stack of cards I will give you, there is one input card, and the rest of the cards each have one result."

"Put the cards in what you believe to be the correct order."

"The input card goes first, and after that there is no wrong or right order, as long as group members can clearly and defensibly explain their logic to the other groups."

The exercise is designed with minimal instructions and requires no further instructions from you as the facilitator. Do not answer any questions about the order or about how cards need to be laid down. Do not provide an example. Often when you provide an example, groups are likely to copy what you do. For example, if you say, "One suggestion is to lay them in a straight line," everyone will have them in a straight line. This takes away the thinking that maybe, just maybe, the cards should not go in a straight line but should be in a circle or other formation. If people ask for further instructions, just keep repeating, "Put the cards in an order or position that is logical to you."

Once the groups have finished sorting, have the different groups present their cards, and have each group's presenter read *only* what is on each card (no long stories, no ad-libbing), in the order the group members have laid the cards out. Groups with the

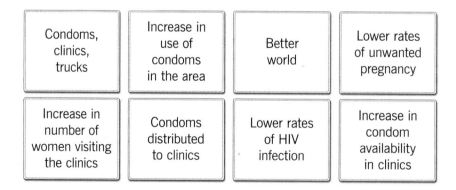

FIGURE 8.2. A set of cards for Activity 8.1 before the game begins: An example of an intervention to promote condom use. For an actual game, the cards should be of different colors (see the "Materials" section on page 163).

Group 1

Reading books; tutors	Girls 15–16 years old attend reading class	Increase in girls who are taught reading skills	Reading skills of same girls increase	Decrease in unwanted pregnancies in the same girls	Girls attain high school education	Fewer of the same girls abused by their partners
Year 1	Year 1	Year 1	Year 2	Year 3	Year 4	Year 10

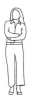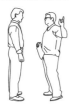

Group 2

Reading books; tutors	Girls 15–16 years old attend reading class	Increase in girls who are taught reading skills	Decrease in unwanted pregnancies in the same girls	Reading skills of same girls increase	Fewer of the same girls abused by their partners	Girls attain high school education
Year 1	Year 1	Year 1	Year 2	Year 3	Year 4	Year 5

Group 3

Reading books; tutors	Girls 15–16 years old attend reading class	Increase in girls who are taught reading skills	Reading skills of same girls increase	Girls attain high school education
			Decrease in unwanted pregnancies in the same girls	Fewer of the same girls abused by their partners
Year 1	Year 1	Year 1	Year 2	Year 5

FIGURE 8.3. A set of cards for Activity 8.1 once the game is completed: The girls' education example.

same sets of cards are likely to place the cards in different orders or in different formations. (*Note:* If all the groups have exactly the same order, change one group's cards after they present their logic, so that a different order can be presented by you.) When groups are done placing their cards in order, ask the following facilitation questions:

"How does the different logic of these cards influence monitoring or evaluation?" (Answer: It determines what is assessed when.)

(Move the order of the cards, or move to a group with a different order, and ask:) "These are two different logics. How does that influence what gets assessed when?"

"What are some of the consequences of not making logic explicit for monitoring? For evaluation?"

Figure 8.3 is an illustration, using the girls' education example, of how this exercise may look once the piles of cards are sorted. I have added the consideration of times when things happen, as some groups may have the same logic but different ideas of how long the results will take to achieve. Having cards labeled "Year 1" and so on is not necessary. Once the order is decided by the group, time can be discussed as part of the game's facilitation.

Critical learning points: There are several key learning points.

- Different people have different ways of seeing the world. And different theories or understandings of human action also involve different understandings of how change happens. This is why people place the cards in a different order or in a different configuration (e.g., a star or a spider's web). Implementing that logic tests the theory. As long as the logic can be explained before it's tested, no one logic is better or "more right" than another.

- The group may agree that the logic starts with the same result (e.g., girls attend school) and ends at the same place (e.g., girls are less likely to be in abusive relationships), and yet what happens to get from the first result to the last may look very different. The difference in that thinking then changes what to evaluate when because the logic, and likely the theory, are different.

- Based on one logic, the timing of when to evaluate for the result is right; however, based on another logic, the evaluation takes place before results are likely to have occurred. The order of the cards (the logic) essentially determines when to look for what change. If the order of the intended results is not clear, this could lead to one of two types of problems:

  o Looking for a result too soon and not finding it may lead to the wrong evaluative conclusion (e.g., the intervention is not successful).

  o Waiting for one result to happen before assessing for the next linked result, but getting the order wrong, may result in collecting data that are not timely.

- Having different potential logical orders may provide clues to when to look for different potential results, as these orders provide different ideas that are all possible.

- The conversation about why the cards are placed in a certain order provides a good place to start asking "What made you think that?" questions, which lead to discussion of the theory—the theory that underlies the logic of the results. Thus the game can illustrate the difference between theory and logic and provide an informal space for learners to engage with both.

The activity emphasizes how clear and explicit theory and logic support evaluative thinking and an evaluation process.

I thought a theory of change was much broader than what has been described here.

There is no official description or definition of a theory of change. At this point in the book, this lack of agreement in the evaluation field should no longer surprise you (see Chapter 1). In this book, I describe a theory of change as a story of how an intervention moves from the problem it is addressing to the results it wants to achieve. Always ask someone what she expects to see in a theory of change, and who will use the theory of change for what purpose. In other words, invest time and effort in a good, open, clarifying discussion. Ask for examples of theories of change that the group finds useful; these examples will provide a good indication of what is expected. A person may indeed expect a theory of change that is broader than what I have described thus far, and if so, please read the next section.

The Broader, Messier Theory of Change

In practice, people may expect a theory of change to be broader and messier than what is described above, and to show a larger picture of various ways in which change can be brought about (and in which it may be prevented). Let's look at another understanding of a theory of change. Theories of change can be drawn to represent, or written to explain, the complexities of economic, cultural, social, and political influences that are often hidden when we are exploring social change. A theory of change may also depict different pathways (called *causal pathways*) that may lead to the same change, even ones that are not related to the intervention on which we are focused. The theory of change may also describe the contextual issues that may prevent or influence those pathways. Such a theory can help us situate an intervention within the bigger picture or the larger context.

In doing all this, a broader theory of change will be more explicit about what will prevent or facilitate change that is beyond the reach of the intervention. These can be cultural, political, social, or other factors that may have significant or even small influences on the intervention's ability to achieve success. For instance, an intervention may rely on a certain policy's not being changed, or the economy's remaining stable, or the government's supporting certain aspects of the intervention. Having a larger theory of change can be useful, as it provides more information on how to shape the intervention, and enables us to understand why an intervention achieved (or did not achieve) its intended results.

How much information needs to go into a broader theory of change?

How much information should go into a broader theory of change is a tough question, much akin to how long a piece of string should be (answer: as long as you need it to be). For this response, I turned to a renowned theorist, Patricia Rogers. Rogers shared her understanding and experience with using theory of change. She writes (and I have edited this with her permission):

. . . I've also seen some [theories of change] where the assumptions are about the context in which the causal connections are understood to work. For example, watering plants will help them grow, assuming they also get adequate sunshine. This form of using assumptions looks quite like a realist approach to understanding causality—identifying the contexts in which causal mechanisms do and do not operate—and has important implications for monitoring and evaluation. Obviously, we should be collecting data about the extent to which these assumptions were met, and whether there was the expected variation in results where they were not (e.g., those plants that were in the shade did not grow as well as the ones in full sun). But I also wonder how these are identified and how wide we should go . . . (personal communication, November 9, 2017)

In this reflection, Rogers is focusing on the important characteristics of the *contexts* in which an intervention is implemented as a key part of the theory of change. The practical use of a theory of change is not likely to permit the listing or explanation of all assumptions, and even the top theorists in the field, such as Rogers, struggle with the question of what to include. Here is where the concept of *destroyer assumptions* (see Chapter 9) provides guidance (though by no means perfect answers) in making decisions about what to evaluate, and what to keep an eye on more casually.

What are **causal pathways,** and how is following such pathways different from taking a sequential look at a program?

A causal pathway is simply a way of demonstrating how one cause will lead to a change in something else (i.e., what the cause is that nudges A to move to B). A series of such changes is seen as a pathway (like a road) to change. The causal pathway often describes the broader picture (though not always) and explains or shows the way that various factors (are thought to) interconnect and relate to each other. It is a way to look sequentially at a program or intervention. Thus the terms *causal pathway* and *sequential examination* are referring to the same process or kind of understanding. Sometimes the term *outcomes hierarchy* is used as well; such a hierarchy also shows how one outcome (is thought to) lead to the next.

Can you summarize the benefits of having a good theory of change?

Several benefits have been noted by Huey Chen (1994), Stuart Donaldson (2007), Sue Funnell and Patricia Rogers (2011), Michael Patton (2012), Carol Weiss (1998), and others. A detailed theory of change does the following:

- Explains clearly why and how an intervention logic should work, and allows for an explicit critique of why it may not.

- Clearly identifies causes and expected effects.

- Provides explicit places to question when something does not work, or when something does.

- Ensures that program managers, implementers, and their donors (or others to whom they are accountable) are all on the same page with regard to what is expected to happen and when (though perhaps not necessarily in agreement), thus removing any ambiguity about the intervention and its potential pitfalls and results.

- Related to that, allows for a practical discussion on what can be evaluated and when.

- Provides an unambiguous explanation to someone who needs to evaluate the intervention, and thus informs the evaluation design: what to ask, who to ask, when to ask, and where to look for answers and explanations for why and how something happened or did not.

How is a theory of change written or presented?

Theories of change usually include two types of explanations, often used together. A narrative offers a written explanation. A diagram (or picture) illustrates the relationships among different components of the theory. What is challenging with a diagram is that the arrows or links from one item to the next are often not understandable without the narrative, so that the diagram is often not answering the question of why we think X leads to Y; it is just showing us that X does (is thought to) lead to Y. Sometimes when there is just a picture or diagram with no written assumptions, it is labeled a "pathway of change" or even a "causal pathway" because it shows the path, but it still does not explain why someone thinks that path will lead to change. With labels being what they are, as we have discussed throughout the book, it is always good to ask what the diagram or picture is meant to represent, and then to identify what other information is needed for a full understanding (and effective monitoring and evaluation) of the intervention.

If there is a graphic picture of the theory of change, but no narrative that describes it, consider having the program manager, designer, or other person you are working with draw a picture of his thinking—stick figures or circles with words in them (no one needs to be an artist!). As he draws this picture, have him narrate it. Trying to draw the theory provides something concrete (the visual) with which to explain (verbalize) the theory.

What is presented in this chapter seems so old-fashioned and linear! What about other ways of looking at theory and logic?

Ah, yes, the process I have explained may be considered old-fashioned and linear. However, in my 20-plus years of experience, the basic thinking presented can be used with any approach, even a systems approach. A basic logic (and theory) is inherent in all interventions, even complex ones. Although the final product may end up looking like a spider's web, or even abstract art, it all starts with a simple idea.

Sue Funnell (2000) has introduced a slightly different way to think logically. Funnell's approach focuses on the outcome level; then she has the organization describe what actions will lead to each outcome, and allows for discussion on contextual facilitators and challenges. To organize this thinking, she uses a matrix that includes a description of what success would look like; program factors and other factors that are likely to affect the program in different ways; and different levels. While her approach involves a broader contextual discussion, at its heart it still follows the very basic step-by-step logic presented in this chapter (and this book). Another example is *outcome mapping,* developed by Canada's International Development Research Centre (Earl, Carden, & Smutylo, 2001). Outcome mapping provides another way of explaining intervention logic and introduces new language and labels. Again, however, at its core can be found the same step-by-step logical reasoning. (See Chapter 15 for more on outcome mapping.)

The ability to unpack any intervention, policy, program, project, or activity into basic step-by-step logic is critical to understanding what will, can, or should be evaluated, and where to look for explanatory data. Remember, even a spider's web starts with the spider's spinning one silk string.

Are there any other challenges in using a theory of change to inform an evaluation or to better understand a program, or just other points to be aware of?

No approach to determining what to evaluate or understand in an intervention is infallible, even one that just seems perfect. Evaluation constantly engages with very real human beings; as such, with humans just being human. As humans, we tend to look for and interpret information that confirms how we view the world—a tendency commonly called *confirmation bias* (Heshmat, 2015; Nickerson, 1998). Plain folk call this "jumping to conclusions." People tend to interpret what they see according to their own theories of how the world works. For example, a person arrives in a new country with a very different culture, sees something confusing, and then searches for an explanation (in other words, takes the data and interprets information) that confirms their own worldview, when a different worldview would offer a more appropriate explanation. That is another potential challenge in using a theory of change.

The second potential challenge is that having one theory of change encourages a focus on *that* theory of change only, which may be like wearing blinders and may promote tunnel vision. In this instance, the evaluator may neglect other potential theories (sets of facts and assumptions) that could equally contribute to, diminish, or just better explain the result (or lack thereof). Considering alternative explanations (e.g., worldviews, theories) is critical (Scriven, 2008). Finally, a caution relevant to any data collection and interpretation process is that having a good theory of change, and valid and credible data, does not mean that your audience or key stakeholders will accept the findings. When a theory is presented with valid and reliable evidence, the findings may still be ignored because the theory of change (regardless of the stellar data) does not resonate with the very people to whom you are providing the evidence.

THE THINKING FOR THEORIES OF CHANGE AND LOGIC MODELS

- **Have 3 minutes?** Check out this TED Talk from ecologist Eric Berlow on simplifying complexity (*www.ted.com/talks/eric_berlow_how_complexity_leads_to_simplicity*).

- **Have 30 minutes or more?** Follow Patricia Rogers's theory-of-change blog on the Better Evaluation website (*www.betterevaluation.org*). She provides tips, explanations, and various resources on theory of change. Feeling a bit more scholarly? Read this timeless article by Carol Weiss (1995): "Nothing as Practical as Good Theory: Exploring Theory-Based Evaluation for Comprehensive Community Initiatives for Children and Families."

- **Have a few hours a night for the next few months?** In 2011, Sue Funnell and Patricia Rogers published a book called *Purposeful Program Theory: Effective Use of Theories of Change and Logic Models*. Read at least part of one chapter per night.

- **Have some more time?** An enduring book by Carol Weiss is *Evaluation Research: Methods for Assessing Program Effectiveness* (1972).

WRAPPING UP

Chapters 3–7 (and to some extent Chapters 1–2) laid the necessary groundwork for informed conversation on theory and logic. The preceding chapters aimed to clarify why the intervention is being implemented; which cultural, political, and contextual reasons may play roles in its success (though these are covered in more depth in Chapter 13); what the intervention aims to achieve and how it aims to do it; who or what the intervention intends to benefit; and who or what the intervention can potentially hurt. This chapter has built on these elements to then explore what makes people think something will work and why people do what they do; in other words, what their theory and logic are. A good theory offers guidance in the design of the intervention, clarifies what to expect from the intervention, guides data collection, and offers explanations for why something might work (forward-looking). At the same time, a good theory can be used to explore why something has or has not worked (backward-looking). Thus separating the logic (what is done) from the implementation (how it is done) from the theory of change (why that should bring about results) provides a framework for exploring the potential of an intervention, and for evaluating it once it's implemented. Before you leave this chapter, come have a conversation with me.

Our Conversation: Between You and Me

Here I describe some situations you may encounter with regard to discussions of logic and theory. Practicing with these common scenarios will enable you to deal with similar kinds of situations in the real world.

1. A client comes to you and says, "We spent weeks developing our logic and theory, with beneficiaries, implementers, partners, and some local experts. Now we are being criticized by other key stakeholders." There are three common scenarios when such criticisms are raised:

- **Data suggest that the logic or theory is wrong.** Someone brings data showing that some of the assumptions are not true. Engage with these data. Perhaps your group does not find the data credible, or the data are dodgy. For instance, in a country where I worked on a national evaluation, we were relying on census data. We later found out that the census data had been miscalculated. This was a case of dodgy data. On the other hand, the data may be strong, and provide useful insights that result in redesigning an intervention. The intervention will now have a higher likelihood of achieving its intended results. Thus keep an open mind, and engage with the data provided from various places.

- **Someone says that the theory and logic do not make sense.** A person who is asking for clarity may be pointing out that there are some jumps in the logic or the theory, or perhaps there are a few suitcase words remaining. Check for these, and if you find them, sort them out. Sometimes an outsider brings useful insights, as your group may have done what is often called *groupthink* (i.e., everyone in the group starts to think alike). While this may be good in some ways (e.g., it encourages teamwork), it also brings in the danger of not seeing what is obvious to an outsider. On the other hand, the person asking for clarity may make different assumptions and think differently from your group. This does not make him right or your group wrong; the new insights may provide an alternative approach to understanding the intervention. Considering this person's vantage point may help to strengthen the intervention.

- **A new funder does not like the logic.** Think about this very, very carefully. The scenario is tricky (e.g., politics and power; see Chapter 13 for more on the topic). First, ask him for concrete examples of what he expects to see in a logic model or theory of change. He may bring a different understanding of what is a theory of change or logic model. If you are in agreement as to what they are, probe and find out what, exactly, the person does not like, ask what makes him think that, and encourage a dialogue. Finally, ask him to present his own logic, or invite him to a facilitated session to discuss the logic.

For each response, it is key not to be defensive. Ask questions. Listen to answers. Hear different perspectives. Think about how the different perspectives may improve the intervention or its evaluation. Finally, consider how to move forward so that whoever, or whatever, is intended to benefit from the intervention is best served.

2. A colleague shares this story: "I confirmed that the problem statement was a fact, and the program logic and theory of change were validated by experts, but we are not getting the results we expected. I don't understand it." What do you do to help him? I would point out that while the problem statement was a fact, the intervention is an assumption of what will work to bring about what results, not a guarantee. Furthermore, while the theory may have seemed appropriate, it was, after all, a theory. As long as the results are not causing harm to people, animals, or the environment (such harm might be a reason for a bit of panic), remind him that the intervention is testing a theory and logic of what the organization *thought* would work to bring about certain results. The fact that it has not, and he knows it has not, is a good thing. I would commend his monitoring and reflection. I would then suggest considering an implementation evaluation (for an explanation, see Chapter 15) that explores what has gone right (it is very rare that *something* does not go right) and what has gone wrong or differed from expectations. Perhaps the results were not the ones expected, but maybe they are still helpful to the beneficiaries or another group. *What would you do?*

CHAPTER 9

Assessing and Evaluating Progress

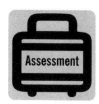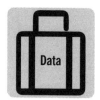

Two questions I am often asked when brought into an evaluative process are "How do we know whether there is progress?" and the often-related query "What should our indicators be?" Chapters 3–8 have smoothed the way for a captivating and informative discussion of what someone needs to know to make decisions on how and when to assess for progress. To understand which method of inquiry to use, read Chapter 5. To understand what to assess and when, keep reading this chapter.

 I have a few trade secrets to share about these conversations. Well, to be perfectly honest, I have sort of a few trade secrets *and* advice combined. No one knows automatically exactly what to assess; a perfect indicator does not exist; and indicators are not always necessary. Phew. So the secrets are out. When someone asks a question regarding how to assess if an intervention is moving toward what it aims to achieve, reframe the conversation. Do not be pressured to give an automatic response, or think that you should be able to do so. To have an informed discussion about how to assess for change, influence, or progress, the program theory (including the problem statement) and the program and its logic (including intended results, how the intervention is being implemented, and the social, political, and cultural contexts) need to be clearly laid out. If this has not been done, reframe the conversations around the discussions and processes in Chapters 3–8. If the conversations raised in those chapters are clearly understood, then it is time to have the "How do we assess for progress?" discussion.

Before we have the conversation, let's clarify the difference between measurement and assessment.

MEASUREMENT AND ASSESSMENT: THE DIFFERENCES

In Chapter 1, I have talked about how some terms have specific meanings (e.g., *causal inference*) and others have varying definitions (e.g., *evaluation*); in these latter instances, we need to negotiate their meaning. **Measurement** and **assessment** are tricky words, as they have specific meanings that are often used rather loosely in the field. Thus if someone asks you to measure something, or to assess it, stop for a moment and clarify what they mean. It is useful to distinguish between these two words, to encourage a clear understanding of what is expected in the evaluation process. Let's examine the two words a little more closely.

We use quantitative data to measure something. We measure how tall we are with a measuring tape, and how heavy we are with a scale. *Measurement* gathers data that simply quantify *what is*. So when a client asks you to measure, he is telling you that he wants information described with numbers. Or maybe not: Because the word *measure* is used commonly in everyday conversations, he could also be asking you to assess something qualitatively—so it may be worth taking the time to ask him what he wants. Measurement can be objective (e.g., determining how well someone performs on a test) or subjective (e.g., determining what people report feeling or experiencing). Measurement refers to something that is quantified (Huitt, Hummel, & Kaeck, 2001; Stake, 1995).

This leads us to the word *assessment*. When an evaluator assesses something, she is gathering evidence, which can be qualitative or quantitative. Thus assessing an intervention means that the evaluator is collecting data that will be used to understand it better. Some people use the term *assessment* to mean that there is a comparison against a norm or standard; however, that is not always the case. For example, a baseline assessment gathers evidence that is used as a reference point *to* assess for any change; the baseline establishes a "base" for comparing the situation before and after an intervention, which is then used to assess the intervention's effectiveness. (For more on baseline assessment, also called a *baseline study* or just *baseline,* see Chapter 5, pages 106–107.)

While we are here, let's toss back in the term *evaluation*. Although different people define evaluation in different ways, its core definition is agreed upon: Evaluation is a systematic, transparent process that values something, and it is political. To evaluate is to determine the worth, merit, and significance of something. (To refresh your memory, return to Chapters 1 and 2.)

So if we say we measure something, it is about numbers. I get that. Then when I do a qualitative evaluation, I am assessing something and valuing it, but I am not measuring anything. Is that right?

In qualitative inquiry, we do not measure because we do not collect numbers. We are reporting what happens in a program, what we observe, or what people say. When an evaluator is asked a question that is suitable for qualitative inquiry, he constructs an approach to answer that question by collecting words from people through interviews, words from documents, and observations (i.e., he gathers evidence). These are not numbers; they are words in the form of descriptions, observations, and stories. To make sense of these words (which are also data), he interprets them by identifying patterns and themes; he aims to understand their meaning. He uses these data, and his understanding of the data, as evidence to assess the intervention against the evaluation question, or even against standards and norms; he just does not assess it against a set number. He could also use a mixed methods approach—gathering data to measure by means of numbers, and then using those quantified data to assess the intervention. So assessment can involve either qualitative or quantitative data.

If we had all the resources in the world, everything could be assessed. However, most likely, limited resources exist. When assessing for progress, a program manager, donor, or evaluator is interested in finding out whether an intervention is moving toward its intended results or away from them. In monitoring, the most popular way to assess if something is moving toward its intended results or not is to use an indicator. More recently on the evaluation scene are *progress markers*. Outcome mapping (which uses progress markers) and most significant change (MSC) do not use numbers to monitor for change; they assess change through gathering words and understanding their meaning. These qualitative approaches are described later in the chapter.

Again, indicators are quantitative measures. They also do not measure every single tiny part of an intervention. Indicators provide *enough* data on certain items to let us know if the intervention is moving toward its intended results, moving away from them, or standing still. An indicator can have many synonyms, such as clue, signal, or sign. That is a very brief explanation, and we talk more about indicators later in the chapter. However, before we talk about indicators in depth, we need to be clear about how to choose *what* is assessed.

WHAT TO ASSESS

Three kinds of factors come into play in evaluating progress: (1) *practical* factors, (2) *use* factors, and (3) *technical* factors. At times, these types of factors can overlap (e.g., what is practical is useful, or what is useful is technical). Although it is critical that an evaluator consider all three sets of factors when deciding what should be assessed, they rarely all have equal weight. In some cases, one practical factor may outweigh all the use and technical factors combined. Sometimes the practical and use factors "team up" together against the technical factors; at other times, technical factors become the most important. In an ideal world, all factors would inform a decision equally, but that is not how it often happens in the real world. Let's look at how practical and use factors can influence decisions on what to assess, and then have a longer discussion of the technical ones.

Practical Factors

There are many different practical factors to consider in deciding what to assess. These factors can include *resources*. For instance, there may not be enough staff to collect all the data that are needed to assess a result. Or certain data may require a statistical software package that is too expensive to purchase, or necessitate a skill set that no current staff member possesses. Practical factors can also include *timing*. For instance, the most useful data may be secondary data captured by another organization; however, these data are collected far less frequently than is ideal for monitoring. Another set of practical factors may involve *accountability*. If a program is committed to assessing something in exchange for funding, then it needs to be assessed, even if the resulting information is not useful to inform program management decisions. Practical factors can include *politics* as well: What needs to be assessed may be what external people or groups expect to see. Finally, practical factors can include *ethics*. For instance, it might be useful for the local health clinic and educators to know how many children in the community school have HIV, so that appropriate care can be given to them; however, it would not be very ethical to test them.

Use Factors

If those are practical factors, what are the use factors? A basic premise for deciding what to assess is to assess what is useful to whoever will use the data. However, the use factor is not as straightforward as it first appears; use can be a funny thing. Managers use data to manage their programs—to identify what is going wrong, what is going right, and what needs immediate attention. However, there are other uses besides informing management decisions. Sometimes, the usefulness in collecting data is to provide information to whoever funds the program; it is for accountability, perhaps, or maybe it is just what evaluators refer to as *check box* or *tick box* use (for more on check box/tick box evaluation, see page 230) that keeps funding flowing.

Technical Factors

Last but not least, there are the technical factors that influence what to assess. The technical factors often overlap with the use factors, and sometimes overlap with the practical ones; when they all overlap, it is like winning the lottery. The technical factors are discussed after I share a melancholy trade secret.

The "sad but true" trade secret is that sometimes in the real world, when a more powerful someone tells you what and how to assess, that is often the end of the discussion—even when what is to be assessed, or how, does not make sense or is not useful to those who implement, need to manage, or benefit from the intervention. Recognizing and engaging with the fact that this happens can help keep evaluators (and those who manage a program) sane. In *monitoring,* one solution is to collect (additional) data that are relevant and useful (if possible) to those who need to manage, or otherwise make decisions about, the intervention. In an evaluation, when not given a choice about what and how to assess, the evaluator needs to explain the decision-making process in the methodology section (more specifically in the limitations section) of the report, at a minimum. It is important to recognize that power and politics influence every part of the evaluative process, including what, how, and when to assess. (Power and politics in evaluation are covered in Part II, especially Chapter 13.)

Technical factors in decisions about what to assess require that an evaluator or program manager have a thorough understanding of the problem–intervention–results links (the program logic) and the theory of change. The "what to assess" decisions focus on the intervention (what is done—the action) and the results (what happens—the result). A useful way to frame the discussion is to use a modification of the concept of so-called "key" and "killer" assumptions, taken from the logical framework approach (United States Agency for International Development [USAID], 1980). I find "killer" to be too abrasive, and the "key" part to be unnecessary, so I have slightly changed the name and the process. Briefly, because of the nature of an assumption (it is not a fact), an evaluator needs to assess whether an assumption has become a fact through the implementation of the intervention. One way to sort out what and how to assess that is to break the discussion into two categories of assumptions: assumptions around action, and assumptions around anticipated results. Deciding what to assess is connected to when to assess. An evaluator must first check the assumptions about action (i.e., make sure that whatever was supposed to be done was done), and then assess for anticipated results in their anticipated order (i.e., make sure that what was supposed to happen happened, when it was expected to do so).

Assumptions about Action

Identifying action (i.e., whether something has physically happened) is logical, although a step can easily be missed (e.g., by assuming, "Of course it happened"). Here are two key questions for addressing assumptions about action:

1. Was the intervention implemented? (Do not assume that actions happen.)

2. Was it implemented as planned? (If so, this is often called **fidelity.**)

In terms of action, knowing what to assess can be drawn from the implementation theory and program logic, which explain what needs to be done, when, and where to achieve the intended results. If the intervention or program was *not* implemented with fidelity, this does not automatically suggest a negative finding. For example, perhaps changes were made to the initial program design that ultimately contributed to the intervention achieving its results. Knowing that the intervention was not faithful to the original design, knowing what changes were made (no matter how small), and discovering that the intervention did achieve its results are useful findings (if we think to assess them). At the same time, knowing if an intervention was implemented with fidelity is a critical part of some evaluation designs, such as randomized controlled trials (RCTs). An RCT is

> a way of doing impact evaluation in which the population receiving the programme . . . is chosen at random from the eligible population, and a control group is also chosen at random from the same eligible population. It tests the extent to which specific, planned impacts are being achieved. . . . The strength of an RCT is that it . . . [helps] evaluators and programme implementers to know that what is being achieved is as a result of the intervention and not anything else. (White et al., 2014, p. 1)

For that reason, RCTs require an intervention to be implemented with fidelity, so that results from different (randomized) groups can be compared. Thus assessing the action of an intervention is critical both to managing a program (e.g., informing changes along the way) and to evaluating one.

Assumptions about Results

The second category of assumptions consists of the results at all levels. (See Chapter 7 for examples of different levels of results, and of how results link to each other.) Now, because an action happened (it is confirmed), the next decision is to choose what anticipated result(s) to assess and when. Common sense tells us that according to our program logic, one result must happen before the next one, and sometimes several results need to happen before the next one (i.e., no result should be assessed or evaluated before its time). For instance, people need to gain knowledge and skills before they can apply these. Technically speaking, all results should be assessed, yet practical factors (e.g., it is too expensive) prevent that from happening.

Action and Results Assumptions

In this section, I lump action and results assumptions together, and explain how to determine what is likely to be more important to assess than something else (from a technical perspective).

These assumptions (action and results) can be divided into two groups. I call these the "do not worry too much about me" assumptions, and the "destroyer" assumptions (i.e., the ones that have a lot of risk associated with them). The "do not too worry too much about me" assumptions are (1) those in which, if something goes wrong, it is not likely to destroy the program and (2) those that are highly unlikely to be wrong. For example, it is safe to assume that people will act in a civilized manner when attending a training on evaluation; the chances that the participants will cause a riot are very slim. Simply stated, "destroyer" assumptions are ones that are critical to the intervention, that may well be wrong, and that are more than likely to result in the intervention's failure if they are wrong. These are the assumptions on which data should be formally collected, at set points in time.

For example, in our girls' education program, we assume that fathers who do not support their daughters' school attendance would be willing to attend a peer intervention activity (action assumption). That is a destroyer assumption. Why? If the fathers do not attend the peer-to-peer session, the intervention will fall apart. Directly addressing fathers is a critical part of the intervention theory and logic. Collecting data on whether fathers participate in the peer-to-peer sessions is thus critical. If the implementer knows that fathers do not attend, then there is the option to address that challenge (e.g., by meeting one-on-one with fathers). Or perhaps fathers *do* attend the peer-to-peer sessions, but the peer-to-peer intervention does not change the fathers' perceptions. In this instance, the intervention is also likely to fail, as changing fathers' perceptions about girls' education forms a large part of the intervention theory. Here the theory will would need to be revisited, along with a closer look at how the peer-to-peer activity was implemented (i.e., was the theory wrong, or was the peer-to-peer activity poorly implemented?). The extent to which the peer-to-peer interaction changes fathers' perceptions is a critical assumption to be assessed. These are some examples of how, if an assumption is not assessed and is a wrong assumption, it can destroy a program. In other words, there are three items to assess: (1) whether the fathers attend, (2) what the quality of the peer-to-peer intervention is, and (3) whether the fathers' attitudes change. All three are based on destroyer assumptions.

Applying Destroyer Assumptions to the Rest of the Evaluative Process

Before we leave the discussion on destroyer assumptions, let's consider how such assumptions apply to *all* aspects of the evaluative process. Can the evaluators safely assume who benefits? What about assuming who values what, and how? What about assumptions made with regard to politics, culture, or the economy? Which political, cultural, social, economic, and other contextual assumptions should be monitored closely, and which ones can we pay attention to through more informal means (e.g., hallway chatter, newspaper articles, Twitter)? For all assumptions in every part of the evaluative process, there are some that will immediately present themselves as destroyer assumptions. It may seem as though *all* the assumptions are destroyers, and though that may be the case, it is more likely that several will "bubble to the top" through a facilitated discussion on them. Once more, the ultimate decision on what to assess is influenced by each intervention's particular mix of practical reasons (which includes ethical, political, and accountability ones), choices about use, and technical decisions.

The Use of Informal Information

Informal data collection takes place almost constantly. Newspapers, radio shows, Twitter, hallway discussions, an email or a phone call, or simply observing something that suggests the intervention is not working (or is working in unexpected ways) should not be ignored. Simply because we choose not to formally assess something does not mean ignoring data that suggest (or even whisper about) a problem or an unexpected achievement. Furthermore, if we do decide to assess something, and our formal data tell us one thing and the informal data tell us another, the informal data should be considered.

The sections starting on page 177 have clarified three ways to make decisions regarding what to assess: considerations of practical factors, use factors, and technical factors, some of which may overlap. Once it is decided what to assess and when, decisions need to be made about how to assess. One of the most popular ways to assess progress is to use indicators.

HOW TO MEASURE PROGRESS

What Is an Indicator?

Now that we have decided what to assess to see if the intervention is making progress, and when to assess it, let's talk about a common concept: the illustrious **indicator.** Indicators are sometimes called *performance indicators* (as they measure performance), are sometimes labeled *key performance indicators,* and are sometimes given other names with slightly nuanced definitions. Whatever label is used, indicators are one of several ways to measure an intervention's progress (or lack thereof). So what is an indicator? Indicators are just what the word suggests: indications, signs, signals, ideas, pointers, or gauges that an intervention is moving toward or away from its intended results, or simply standing still in its quest to achieve these results. An indicator is not a result; it is an indication of a result. Think about some common indicators in your own life. When your stomach growls, it is an indication, sign, or signal that you are hungry. Or maybe not: It might be indicating that you ate bad food, or that you feel sick. However, a growling stomach does not definitively mean that you are hungry, or sick, or ate bad food. It merely suggests what could be happening. However, an indicator at the lower level is often very much like a result, but not quite the result itself (it is a closely related measure of achievement); the indicator makes the result measurable. Table 9.1 shows three illustrations drawn from the girls' education example.

There are several other labels that often have the same meaning as *indicator* (in addition to *sign, signal, gauge,* and *clue*), such as *measure* or *metric.* At this point in the book, multiple labels for the same concept should come as no surprise. However, sometimes a *metric* is only used when it refers to a specific number, which is also called a *target.* (A later section of this chapter provides a further description of targets and benchmarks.) The often-repeated advice in this book applies here as well: Clarify terms, labels, and definitions before embark-

TABLE 9.1. The Indicator: Making Results Measurable

	The very first thing that happens	What happens next?	What happens after that?
Result	Fathers who do not want their daughters to attend school come to the peer-to-peer session to meet with fathers who support girls' education.	Fathers learn reasons for educating girls.	Fathers send their girls to school.
Indicator	Number of fathers who attend X number of peer-to-peer sessions.	Number of fathers who can articulate the importance of educating their girl child.	Number of girls previously kept from school by their fathers who are registered to attend school.

ing on a discussion about how to implement the concept. (See Chapter 1 for a discussion on the importance of language in evaluation.)

Indicators are quantitative? My donor is asking for qualitative indicators; what are those?

Ah, the old qualitative indicator. It's a bit of a contradiction, really. I do engage with qualitative indicators in this chapter because I know that donors and governments, among others, ask for them, and they are used in the real world. An example could be "quality of health care as perceived by teenagers." Essentially, a qualitative indicator is one for which data are collected via qualitative inquiry approaches, and then the data are quantified. If a donor or manager asks for qualitative indicators, ask him for what purpose these data should be collected. If it is to provide deeper insight, introduce the MSC or outcome mapping's *progress markers* (both discussed later in this chapter) as optional choices.

Here is an example of what you might find in the field. A health organization wants to measure the quality of its service at local health clinics. To measure quality, the evaluator develops measurement items, such as collecting data on how long a patient waits to see a doctor, and how patients rate the friendliness of the nurses on a scale of 1–5. These quantifiable data then provide indicators of the service quality at the health clinic. However, the evaluator could also collect stories from the patients and assess those stories to better understand the quality of care at the clinic. Since you asked, let's delve a bit deeper into the distinction between qualitative and qualitative indicators.

A Discussion of Qualitative and Quantitative Indicators

Quantitative indicators are very straightforward: The data are collected with a closed-ended approach and often provide a simple number, percentage, or ratio. One exception would be with policies, where moving from a *green paper* (initial thoughts) to a *white paper* (final paper) would be an indicator that a bill is moving toward being approved. Qualitative indicators—

well, I would say there are no such things, but as I just noted, I have seen them with my own eyes. When these are requested, providing them can be challenging because qualitative data need to be quantified as suggested on the previous page. Look at the following example of indicators that draw from qualitative data:

- Number of people who report feeling good.
- Number of people who report feeling bad.

An open-ended question can be used to gather these data. For example, "How are you feeling today?" would be an open-ended question to gather data for these two indicators. The responses could include "good," "great," "awesome," "very good," "super," "not so well," "terrible," and "awful." These data are then analyzed (see Chapter 5 on qualitative data) into themes of "good" and "bad." The indicator data are as follows: Five people reported feeling good, and three people reported feeling bad. In rare cases, qualitative indicator data stay in words and are not quantified; as such, they do not fit the true definition of an indicator, but they exist. Indicators are intended to measure something and provide a quick glance that shows if an intervention is on track or not.

A final, general note on indicators: Indicators are often used in the politics of making certain groups visible or making them disappear. *Disaggregating* data (meaning separating it) by sex, age, marital status, and other characteristics that make a difference is extremely important. It is important because if data are not separated, their aggregation can mask trends that are different. (See more on these kinds of discussions in the Resources on page 196.)

BOX 9.1. Progress Markers

A **progress marker** is a bit different from an indicator. Used in outcome mapping (discussed in Chapter 15; see also the Resources feature at the end of this chapter), progress markers are qualitative data collected to mark progress and show a result. A progress marker must be descriptive and therefore qualitative in nature. An example for the result "More participation by disabled persons at community meetings" would be collecting data by observing disabled people attending, speaking at, and being listened to at the meetings. In contrast, an indicator could be "Number of disabled people at the community meeting," which would *signal* that there is more participation by disabled people at the community meetings. Progress markers are always qualitative, and show results through describing what happens through progression (Earl et al., 2001). With some programs, it is sometimes useful to combine the two approaches (indicators and progress markers) in a hybrid approach, and perhaps even to add a third, MSC, for a three-way hybrid. Again, MSC is discussed in more detail later in this chapter.

A Good Indicator Is a Useful Indicator

A useful indicator is one that provides credible data (for more on credible data, see Chapter 5) to inform a management decision. Based on the data collected, the decision might be "Everything looks great; let's keep moving," or "Something is not right here; let's check it out." Different organizations use different ways of examining indicators to see if they are "good" indicators, so it is important to find out what those criteria are. However, general criteria for indicators include that they are *reliable, accurate, useful, feasible,* and *timely.* Here are some examples of how these words are used:

- *Reliable:* If different people were to use the data collection tool, would they get the same result? *Reliable* doesn't mean *right* (e.g., a broken scale could consistently tell you that you weigh 200 pounds when you actually weigh 150).

- *Accurate:* Does the indicator give the true value (e.g., you do indeed weigh 150 pounds and the scale shows that you do weigh 150 pounds)?

- *Useful:* Does the information gleaned from the indicator help in managing the program, or is it collected and just put to the side?

- *Feasible:* Can the data be collected with the available human and financial resources, or is the collection process too complicated or too expensive?

- *Timely:* Can the data be collected when they are needed? *Timely* also refers to having the data when decisions need to get made.

You may hear the acronym SMART when people talk about critiquing indicators. The acronym stands for S̲pecific, M̲easurable, A̲ssignable, R̲ealistic, and T̲ime-bound, though sometimes the letters in the acronym are used differently. SMART is often associated with Peter Drucker (1995, 2007), an organizational theorist who popularized it in connection with his "management by objectives" approach. It is a somewhat tired acronym. Here is a more basic and quite sensible way to determine how "good" an indicator is. Test it and, after gathering the data, ask these three questions:

1. Were the data collected with a reasonable amount of resources?

2. Did the indicator measure what it was supposed to measure?

3. Were the data used?

Common Challenges in Using Indicators

Here are nine challenges evaluators often encounter when using indicators to measure progress, and some advice on how to engage with each challenge.

• *Challenge 1.* The program only collects indicator data. The larger picture, and the other program components not measured through indicators, are often forgotten. This reliance on only a few indicators leaves big gaps in understanding what is happening, and creates the potential for things to be missed that may influence the achievement of results.

Engage with all available information. Consider introducing multiple approaches, such as progress markers or MSC. Formative evaluations by external evaluators who can bring a different view to the program might provide some additional insights. If formal changes are not acceptable, consider gathering data informally via a less structured and more holistic approach, such as at meetings or workshops.

• *Challenge 2.* Indicator data and other data sources provide contradictory information. For example, indicator data suggest that the program is moving along in the right direction; however, other data suggest multiple problems. The other data are ignored.

Again, engage with all available information. Imagine that an airplane is spiraling out of control and heading toward the ground, even though all the indicator instruments on the control panel say everything is fine. Indicators are just that—indications of something happening or not happening—and sometimes they are wrong. If other signs or signals tell you a different story from the one told by your indicator data, consider them carefully.

• *Challenge 3.* There is no agreement on what the indicators should be. Arguments ensue about identifying indicators, with little knowledge of the program logic or program theory.

Find common ground. Avoid discussions of indicators until the program logic and underpinning theory are clear and agreed upon. Even after the theory and logic are clear, arguments may still ensue. Consider using a framework (e.g., SMART, the organization's own criteria, or ones the group agrees on) to assess the indicators, so that the discussion is organized and clear. If there is still no agreement, consider bringing in one or more experts in the field.

• *Challenge 4.* The indicator is useful to the donor, government, foundation, or other funding sources, but not to the implementer. Often funding to an organization or government department comes with indicators attached. Sometimes these indicators do not adequately (or sometimes even closely) measure what the organization or department is doing. For example, an organization accepts money based on an agreement on the grand problem (e.g., HIV/AIDS, global climate change, human rights). Later, the implementing organization realizes that the mandatory indicator(s) do not even remotely measure the organization's intervention, which addresses vastly different pocket problems.

Explore the options. In this situation, there are at least four options. The first is to give back the money or stop accepting the funds (painful choices, but options just the same). The second is to negotiate a change in the indicators through a facilitated discussion between the implementer and the funder, which explores the intervention, the pocket problems it addresses, and its intended results. The third option is to change the intervention. The fourth option is for the organization to meet its contractual obligation (providing data on a required indicator) and then collect additional data to manage the program.

• *Challenge 5.* Indicators state, "Change in . . . ," but there is no baseline. Whenever there is an indicator that begins with "Increase in . . . ," or "Decrease in . . . ," or "Change in . . . ," baseline data are needed. To measure any change, an evaluator needs to know this: A change from what?

 Again, explore the options. There are several strategies. First, consider that there might be baseline data existing within, or outside, the intervention. See Chapter 5 for how to identify an existing baseline. If there are no documented baseline data, consider collecting retrospective data, as also described in Chapter 5. A third option is to remove the indicator and replace it with one that is feasible to measure.

• *Challenge 6.* A qualitative indicator is mandatory. It is not clear why qualitative indicators are needed; however, it is mandatory that they be collected.

 Consider who wants qualitative indicators, and for what reason. It is possible to quantify qualitative data (as discussed earlier in this chapter). Find out why these data are being requested. Understanding why they are requested will bring insight into what the donor, government official, or whoever mandated collecting them wants to know. Once it is clear what this person or persons want to know, alternatives might be possible. For example, MSC could provide a viable option.

• *Challenge 7.* The intervention has started and is well underway, and then a new person to whom the program manager is accountable (e.g., the donor, a government department official) changes the indicators. Sometimes, when new people with decision-making authority join an organization or take on a new position, they change the indicators, or refine their definitions.

 Identify the reasons for the change. There could be very good reasons (e.g., the new person realized that different indicators, or refined definitions, would be more useful, or the funding stream has shifted and necessitated the reporting of different data for accountability reasons). On the other hand, perhaps the new person did not like the old indicators for some reason, and just decided to change or refine them. Regardless of the reason, it is important to take stock and understand the impact that changing one or several indicators (or their definitions) will have on data collection and other resources. Furthermore, it is critical to understand the extent to which these new indicators are useful to program management, and to consider different options if they are not useful. For instance, is it possible to continue collecting data on the old indicators (i.e., are there enough resources)? While the new indicators may not be as useful as the old ones (to the program manager), are they useful "enough" to enable the implementers to continue managing the program effectively?

- *Challenge 8.* The intervention changes, and the current indicators are no longer appropriate.

We live in a rapidly changing world. Problems shift, interventions shift, and intended results may shift. Whenever something shifts, it is critical to reexamine indicators to ensure that these signs or signals are still relevant to the intervention. Sometimes indicators cannot be changed, even when they are no longer relevant. For instance, an intervention's funding may be based on certain accountability measures; the indicators are sealed in stone. In such a situation, document that the indicators are no longer relevant, and give clear reasons (e.g., the intervention is doing something different because the problem being addressed has changed). Provide these reasons to the person(s) to whom you are accountable, and encourage them to meet with you to discuss changing the indicators. Recognize, however, that sometimes indicators cannot be changed for any reason during a funding cycle; in that case, roll your eyes upward (make sure no one is watching) and collect those data.

- *Challenge 9.* There are 394 indicators (or some other huge number) for one intervention. Unless it is an extremely large and enormously well-resourced intervention, it is unlikely that collecting data on all of these indicators will be useful to manage an intervention.

It is highly unlikely that one person, or even one group of people, can realistically monitor 394 indicators. Those are a lot of signals or signposts to keep an eye on. Thus consider the extent to which each one is necessary. To do so, consider the following process. Identify which indicators are mandatory. The mandatory ones are likely to be related to funding (which could be related to political reasons) and need to be set aside in the "keep" column. Then review the ones that are left. Group them as, for example, quality indicators, process indicators, and results indicators. You could even break down the results indicators into output, outcome, and impact indicators. Then decide how many in each group are "enough" that are feasible to collect and provide adequate signals that something is going right (or going wrong). How many are enough? It may take a few trial-and-error efforts to identify the "magic" number, but experience is often the best guide. As noted earlier in this chapter, consider what it means not to collect certain data, or not to disaggregate it; if this is not done, what will remain hidden or not known? Find someone who has knowledge, experience, and familiarity with the intervention (or a similar one), and ask for advice.

If that is an indicator, what is a target?

A *target* is something an intervention aims to achieve, or (to keep the target metaphor) something to shoot for and aim to hit. It is almost always a number. The reason to keep discussions about targets and indicators separate is that they are truly different discussions. Imagine the following discussion. One person says, "I think the intervention should measure if 75 girls attend school in the fall semester." Someone else says, "Well, I do not agree with that." My question would be this: "You do not agree with what? The indicator [number of girls attending school] or the timing [in the fall semester] or the target [75]?" Discussing the indicator, the timing, and the target will call for entirely different conversations. Table 9.2 shows four examples of indicators and their targets.

TABLE 9.2. Different Kinds of Indicators and Their Targets

Indicator	Target
Number of fathers who attend peer-to-peer sessions and stay longer than 30 minutes.	By the end of the first year of the intervention, 75 fathers attend peer-to-peer sessions and stay longer than 30 minutes.
Percentage of girls between the ages of 14 and 16 in the community who attend school.	75% of girls between the ages of 14 and 16 in the community attend school.
Percentage of girls who achieve at least 95% attendance in school.	90% of girls maintain at least 95% attendance in school in the first term of the year following the intervention.
Percent change in the number of fathers who regard girls' attending school as important.	25% more of the fathers regard girls' attending school as important.

Keeping conversations streamlined will support a clear discussion, help everyone to reach an understanding, and eventually (as needed) foster agreement. Furthermore, targets can change while the indicator remains the same. An interesting demonstration of how they relate to each other and to the entire evaluative process is provided in Chapter 10 through an interactive game (which is also an activity and a process).

If that is a target, what's a benchmark?

These words are sometimes used interchangeably. The best advice is to ask whomever you are speaking with how they use this term. In general, a **target** is a specific number. We could aim to get 75 women (a target) to attend the university's agriculture course in the fall semester, and then 50 women (another target) in the spring, and so on. **Benchmarks** are normally taken from the literature or from another similar intervention in a different site, or even from the same intervention in a previous year; they provide numbers or statements with which to compare the intervention's progress. Or, in some interventions in health or economic interventions, for example, some benchmarks are calculated according to formulas. Some of you may be reading my example and thinking, "Wait, that is not how my organization defines those terms." Heavy sigh. Be clear on how the terms *target* and *benchmark* are being applied in your situation.

Choosing to use qualitative or quantitative indicators, progress markers, or some other form of assessment that gauges progress depends on what types of data will provide the most useful, feasible, accurate, cost-effective information for learning, improving and/or judging the program, and making management decisions. The needs for these types of data are then balanced against cost, time, and the skill sets and knowledge required to collect and use the data. Mixed into those decisions are considerations of what data are most credible and needed by those to whom the evaluator (or program manager) is held accountable. It is most often the evaluator's role to facilitate a discussion and help the program manager (or the person who needs to engage with the decision) make the best decision possible, with what is known at that point in time.

Critiquing Indicators

No indicator is perfect, and most indicators can be, for lack of a better description, ripped to shreds. An evaluator needs to be comfortable interrogating indicators and, at times, supporting a process that interrogates indicators. Facilitating the Party Game (Activity 9.1) introduces the concept of an indicator and the different kinds of indicators, and it shows how to develop indicators and how to tear them apart; in so doing, it demonstrates that no indicator is perfect. The Party Game, with a graphic for the invitation, is available on this book's companion website (*www.guilford.com/podems-materials*). Let's have a party!

ACTIVITY 9.1. The Party Game: Developing Indicators and Spotting Their Weaknesses

Purpose: To become comfortable with indicator development, use, and refinement through learning how to develop, write, and critique one.

Materials: You will need one or two copies of the invitation in Figure 9.1 for each group, printed on one piece of paper apiece. (See the invitation on the companion website.) Each group needs blank paper (it can be scrap paper) to write their answers, and a pen or marker with which to write. As the facilitator, you will need a flip chart and marker to note critical points.

Time: Groups need approximately 10–15 minutes to construct their answers. The sharing of the indicators, and the learning process, take approximately 20–25 minutes. The total approximate time is 30–40 minutes, depending on the number of groups, the interaction, and the discussion of each question.

The exercise: To play the game, divide the participants into equal groups of no more than four people per group. If the same people have been sitting together in previous activities, mix them up. Provide

each group with one to two copies of the party invitation and blank paper on which to write their responses. Read the introduction on the party invitation, and ask each group to provide one indicator for each question.

There are two rules. First, an indicator cannot be repeated. For example, a group cannot have the same indicator for the third and fourth questions. Second, each answer must be written like an indicator.

Some groups might need an explanation of a proxy indicator. A *proxy indicator* is an indirect indicator; it is used when a result cannot be directly measured. For example, to know how many people come to the party, a person cannot count the number of people (this is a direct indicator). A proxy indicator could be the number of coats hanging in the closet or the number of shoes at the door.

Give the groups about 10–15 minutes to develop one indicator per question. When they are done, they should have developed six indicators. Have the members of one group read out their indicator for the first question only. Ask if anyone has the same or a similar answer. Then allow the other groups to critique that indicator. Use critical facilitation questions such as these:

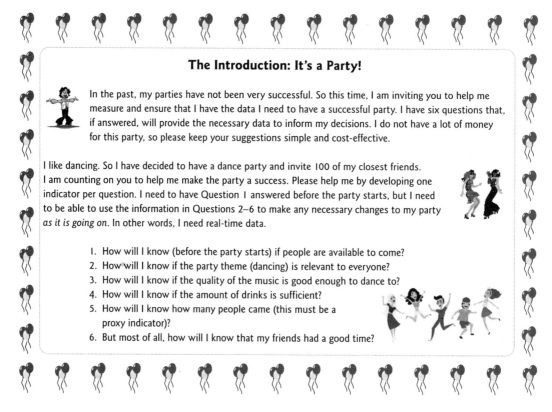

FIGURE 9.1. Party invitation for use in the Party Game (Activity 9.1).

- What else might that indicator be measuring?
- How might that be difficult to measure?
- How realistic/feasible is that?
- What could go wrong with that indicator?

Continue until all six indicators are discussed.

The game requires extremely good facilitation skills, for two reasons. First, although it can be lots of fun, it is your job to listen carefully and draw lessons. While I have listed the main lessons, many more lessons will emerge from playing this game. Second, you need to be able to pick up the mistakes, correct them, and offer solutions, all while keeping it fun; it is a party, after all. Table 9.3 (pp. 192–193) lists each question, some potential responses to each question, and the key lesson and specific facilitation tips for each question.

Critical learning points: An indicator is an indication, sign, or signal of a phenomenon, and most can be torn to shreds. There is no such thing as a "perfect" indicator. The game has four aims. Participants should:

1. Be comfortable discussing indicators.
2. Understand that indicators have advantages and challenges.
3. Understand the role of an indicator.
4. Understand that there are different types of indicators.

The game enables participants to develop a basic knowledge and understanding of indicators, as well as of the role played by indicators in the evaluative journey.

Is there anything else we need when using an indicator, or just the indicator itself?

Sometimes an indicator seems simple—it is one sentence. However, there is often a whole lot more going on behind that indicator and its one sentence, which is needed to ensure that the indicator is useful. For instance, a program manager or evaluator needs to understand what data should be collected, when and how the data should be collected, how the indicator value will be calculated, who will analyze the data, when it needs to be reported, and so on. Also, sometimes indicators include suitcase words, which are often used for brevity (see the discussion of suitcase words in Chapter 7). The attached indicator sheet should define each such word so that it is measurable (e.g., *empowerment, capacity built, pass rate*). The indicator's details need to be clear to ensure clarity, transparency, and credible data.

Finally, government departments, donors, foundations, and nonprofits often have their own format for clarifying indicators (sometimes called an *indicator specification sheet* or an *indicator reference sheet*). This format needs to be used to ensure that the indicator meets the organization's needs. Ask the organization that you work with, or for, to provide you with its template. See the next question to understand further what happens when only the indicator statement (i.e., one short sentence) is written.

Our organization has gone through long discussions to select what are likely to be good indicators. Once the indicators are selected, what else can go wrong in measuring progress?

Quite frankly, lots can go wrong, despite having well-thought-out indicators (and the same holds true for progress markers). Let's talk through some possibilities. Knowing what can go wrong prepares an evaluator to prevent it from happening. Let's pretend that it is your job to provide evaluation support to seven environmental nonprofit organizations, each located in a different country (or county, state, or province). You are hired 3 months before the nonprofit organizations need to provide the first report to their donor (funder); this report focuses on providing data from one mandatory indicator. Let's see what could go wrong.

You decide to bring representatives of all seven organizations together in a nice conference hotel to host a 1-day facilitated dialogue with them. Each organization has the same program logic and the same donor-mandated indicator. You review the one indicator with them, which is "Number of national parks and protected areas with adequate management." The donor has not provided any guidance on the indicator or its data collection. You note that *adequate* is a suitcase word (again, see Chapter 7). So you ask the representative of each organization how that group defines *adequate*. Five of the seven different nonprofits have defined this word so that it has meaning to them and is evaluable. The representatives of the two groups who do not have a definition ask to move to another room and work together to define the suitcase word. As you are pressed for time, you agree.

You now have five nonprofits represented in the room. It is not clear how the data are being collected, or where the data are coming from, so you ask how this is happening. All

TABLE 9.3. Questions, Potential Responses, Key Lessons, and Facilitation Tips for the Party Game (Activity 9.1)

Question[a]	Some potential responses (there are many)	Key lesson and facilitation tips
1. How will I know (before the party starts) if people are available to come?	Number of people who respond, *disaggregated* (i.e., broken down) by yes or no responses. Number of people who respond positively.	People want to state the data, such as "yes or no," or "98 people." These are not indicators; these are *data* for an indicator. It is a good learning point to distinguish data from indicators. People want to put in *methods* here, and will respond with "Twitter/Facebook responses," "email responses," or "phone calls." These are ways to collect data on the indicator, not the indicator itself. People want to add in *targets*. Targets are generally numbers, as discussed in a question and answer in the chapter text (p. 187). We are not setting targets in this discussion, or at least not yet. If someone says, "75 people respond," they have jumped one step ahead. Remove the target (actual number).
2. How will I know if the party theme (dancing) is relevant to everyone?	Number of people dancing. Number of people who say they like dancing.	Here the question concerns "relevance." I want to know if the theme is important to the matter at hand (which is my party). So let's look at two ways to challenge these common answers: • Why might people *not* be dancing? • Why might people say they like dancing, when they really do not? There are always alternative explanations available (often funny ones!).
3. How will I know if the quality of the music is good enough to dance to?	Number of people dancing. (The group may have already provided this answer to Question 2; if so, it is a repeat indicator, and the group needs to choose another.)	Here the question involves "quality." Remember that each group has its own set of answers, and that the group members cannot repeat their *own* indicator. One indicator cannot measure two phenomena. Otherwise, we will not know which question is being answered (or which result being measured is being achieved).
4. How will I know if the amounts of drinks are sufficient?	Number of people holding each type of drink.	Here the question concerns "sufficiency." Do the amounts of drinks meet everyone's needs? The lesson often drawn from this discussion is about time: At what point in time is this measured? It is different

	Number of each type of drink available. Number of drinks per person.	if people complain that there are not enough drinks when the party is almost over, as opposed to an hour after the party has started. This then leads to the question "Hey, wait, how long is this party?", which begins another discussion. When questions arise about indicators, they also begin to arise about the intervention (in this case, the party). Thus lots of conversations start out with "What is the indicator?" or "How will we measure this?" and evolve into discussions of program logic, program theory, or program action. Do not discuss the theory and logic for the party; make the point that indicators often lead into these kinds of discussions.
5. How will I know how many people came (this must be a proxy indicator)?	Here answers are often the most creative, and the easiest to attack. Some responses may be the number of coats (if it is cold), the number of umbrellas at the door (if it is raining), or the number of plates used.	This question requires a *proxy indicator*, which is a way to estimate when you cannot directly measure what you want to measure. So, for example, a response *cannot* be "Number of people who came through the door." That would be a direct measure. How might any of the answers in the middle column not give a good indication of how many people were at the party? For example, some people may not wear a coat, or they may not take it off. Or someone may use one plate more than once, while another person will take five plates. The key lesson here is that we do tend to rely on proxies, yet look how easy they are to pick to apart!
6. But most of all, how will I know that my friends had a good time?	Number of people who stay after the official time of the party is over. Number of people who report having a good time.	Why might some people stay after the party has ended? Some reasons might be that they are too tired to go home; they have missed their bus; or their Uber driver did not arrive. The key lesson in this discussion, however, is that having one indicator to measure a very large and critical result is often not enough to fully understand the result (in this case, whether and to what extent people enjoyed my party). This is probably a question that is better answered with an evaluation (in-depth questions) than with having just one indicator. While the other indicators would help me make changes (buy more drinks, change the music) to improve my party, the final question probably requires more information. For example, I do not want to have an indication that everyone had a good time; the party is important to me. I want to know *why* they had a good time (or if they did not have a good time) and what made them enjoy themselves. A simple "Most respondents reported having a good time" would leave my information needs unsatisfied. Thus indicators are great for monitoring, but not so much for some important aspects of evaluation (e.g., valuing and judgment).

a Remember that Question 1 needs to be answered before the party starts, and that Questions 2–6 are to be answered after the party starts, to provide real-time data.

five representatives respond that The Nature Conservancy, a large organization, collects these data in each country. You breathe a silent sigh of relief and, as the day is over, end the meeting. Several weeks later, you follow up with the representatives of the two nonprofits who did not define the word *adequate*. They report that they never did reach agreement and they will get back to you, but they do not.

It is critical that no suitcase words exist in the indicator *unless* they are unpacked in another document (e.g., indicator specification sheet). If suitcase words do exist, define them. While defining the word can seem like an easy task, at times it can be formidable. Here, an evaluator would draw on her facilitation skills to support groups to define such words so that each word or concept is assessable and meaningful (or bring in a knowledgeable other to support the process; see Chapter 1).

A month later, you contact the representatives of the five nonprofits that defined their indicator to check on their data collection and see if they need any support. Only three of the nonprofits have the information they need. "What happened?" you ask the representatives of the other two. One representative tells you that the Nature Conservancy in her group's country is extremely large and the group did not have the name of the person who captures these data, so she was just passed around and around, and was unable to get the data the group needed. The other representative had the name of the person who was responsible for the data that were needed, but when he called her, she said they only collected the data annually (the data are needed semi-annually). Now there are only three nonprofit organizations that have access to the data they need. But wait: Now the representative of one of these organizations calls you back and says, "I have a slight problem. The data we needed are available, but many other organizations have identified the secondary data as inaccurate and untrustworthy." Oh, dear.

There are three critical lessons here. First, when a program manager of a nonprofit (or any organization) is depending on another organization to collect necessary data, the program manager needs to ensure that there is a clearly identified contact person who will provide the data (or access to the data). Second, although secondary data can be very useful, as such data can save a nonprofit (or any organization) time and money in data collection, these data must be accessible when needed. Third, the secondary data must be credible.

BOX 9.2. Primary and Secondary Data

Primary data are data for which you have control over how to collect the data, where to get the data, and from whom. Secondary data are collected by someone else who has control over how it is collected and from whom. *If you have no control over the data's credibility, then they are secondary data.*

There are now only two nonprofits writing their reports using their indicator data. But now a representative of one of these nonprofits calls you and tells you that a big argument has ensued about whose responsibility it is to analyze the data and turn it into a report. The argument seems to be rooted in two overlapping problems: The organization has no staff who are confident to interpret the data, and no one will take responsibility.

The critical lesson here is to ensure that the person responsible for reporting on the data understands how to analyze the data and turn it into a report—or that the nonprofit has the resources to access a team or an individual who can support the group in doing so.

Now only one nonprofit remains that has no complications. This nonprofit has several staff people who understand and can analyze the data; facilitates the use of the data by presenting it to the management team for reflection; and then provides the findings to a staff member who writes a well-constructed final report.

Sigh. One out of seven nonprofits has submitted a report including the mandatory information. Do not despair; it is through mistakes that we learn. This example demonstrates how little pitfalls can turn into gigantic, gaping holes in the evaluative process. In working with any organization, client, or colleague, thinking through these kinds of details (long after choosing or being given an indicator, progress marker, or other way of assessing) is critical to having a useful evaluative process.

In the chapter you talk about other ways to assess progress or change besides the indicator, such as progress markers and MSC. Can you talk a bit more about MSC?

The indicator is the most popular method of measuring progress. The progress marker has its own small following. The *most significant change* (MSC) approach has a core group of supporters, including me. Sometimes called the *story* approach, it is an approach that does not use indicators; rather, data are collected throughout the intervention's implementation through storytelling, which then provides data on results, usually at the higher level (i.e., not the activity or output level). So, for example, stories are not collected to indicate that an intervention took place, but rather to describe what happened because of that intervention, with a specific focus on providing contextual details and specifics (such as who did what, when, and why). A key part of the inquiry is to learn *why* a person is telling that story because the answer to this question makes it clear how that story is important, and thus what makes it an example of "significant change" (Davies & Dart, 2005).

I am working with a program that needs to develop indicators. We have a clear theory of change, and that is helpful to determine what to assess. However, is guidance available on the typical or necessary indicators in certain fields (e.g., education, health, environment)?

There are global initiatives such as the UN Human Development Index, Education for All, the Convention on International Trade in Endangered Species of Wild Flora and Fauna, to name a few, and even the UN's Sustainable Development Goals can provide guidance. Some of these indicators can be mandatory for your intervention, or they can provide guidance on what kinds of indicator data can be useful. Furthermore, government departments and large organizations often have data indicator sets; be sure to ask whomever you work for or with, if any such guidance exists.

INDICATORS, PROGRESS MARKERS, AND MSC

- **Have a few minutes?** Check out a page on the Centers for Disease Control and Prevention (CDC) website for a quick description of indicators (*www.cdc.gov/std/ Program/pupestd/Developing%20Evaluation%20Indicators.pdf*).

- **Have 30 minutes or more?** Glance through more information about MSC on a document available on the Overseas Development Institute (ODI) website (*www.odi.org/ publications/5211-msc-most-significant-change-monitoring-evaluation*).

- **Have some more time?** For indicators, read the Performance Monitoring and Evaluation Tips provided by USAID (*https://pdf.usaid.gov/pdf_docs/pnadw106.pdf*). For outcome mapping and progress markers, look at *www.outcomemapping.ca* for an explanation, a free book, training materials, and a community of followers. For MSC, Rick Davies manages a website named Monitoring and Evaluation News (*www. mande.co.uk*), which provides a wealth of information on all kinds of M&E topics; the information on MSC includes links to papers, descriptions, blogs, databases, and trainers (*www.mande.co.uk/special-issues/most-significant-change-msc*).

WRAPPING UP

An evaluator needs to prevent people from jumping straight into discussions of indicators, or of how to assess an intervention, without first giving attention to everything else that influences these decisions. Having a discussion of what and when to assess is intricately intertwined with the program logic and theory of change, which are in turn affected by three types of factors: practical factors, use factors, and technical factors. After deciding what and when to assess, an evaluator must then consider how to assess progress; indicators constitute the most common quantitative approach, and progress markers and MSC are slowly gaining ground on the qualitative side. A conversation on how, when, and what to assess should not be mingled with a discussion on targets and benchmarks; as in any evaluative discussion, it is important to keep the conversations focused on one topic at a time. In this chapter, we have also played the Party Game and learned in this activity about developing and critiquing indicators. We have also filled the role of an M&E expert and learned several critical lessons on things that can go wrong in monitoring a program, and ways to mitigate them. Before you leave this chapter, however, I invite you to have a conversation with me.

Our Conversation: Between You and Me

Here I describe one situation that may be encountered with regard to indicators, and I share a trade secret. Practicing with this common scenario will help you as you encounter these kinds of situations in the real world.

At the beginning of an intervention, indicator sets are mandated by the donor or government agency. These indicators are not helpful in managing the program, and they cannot be changed. The program manager does not mind collecting the mandated data, but she still needs data that will inform her management decisions. How should an evaluator advise her client?

I am going to provide a more in-depth response than the one I have provided earlier in the chapter, and in doing so, I share a trade secret. When an indicator is required (e.g., a manager or board of directors mandates it for accountability purposes) that is clearly not useful for managing a program, it is acceptable to create additional ones that do—and thus to have two sets of indicators or other ways to assess progress. I am *not* suggesting that as evaluators, we should act like dishonest accountants who keep two sets of books, one of which is undisclosed. We are not hiding data; rather, data are collected and used for different purposes and for different users. It is acceptable to collect data that are not used by the donor or others to whom a program is accountable. Indeed, I recommend letting the donor or others know that you are collecting additional data. Should anyone want to see these data, then by all means share them.

To be a bit more specific, there are different audiences for different data. More simply put, different people want or need to know different stuff, and sometimes at different times. Sometimes broad accountability measurements are needed by the funder on a yearly basis. However, the program manager needs monthly data that are very specific and frequent. For example, knowing the number of people (disaggregated by gender) who attended a training could be "enough" information for your donor. However, to manage the intervention, the program manager needs data on which geographic areas the attendees came from, and how well the topic was presented.

So that was a monologue, not a dialogue. Here is the conversation: What happens when there are no additional resources to collect more data, and the data being collected are not useful for day-to-day management of the program? Now we (the evaluators) are invited into the discussion. How should we support the program manager? First, we commiserate with the group or person. Second, we identify the reason(s) why the indicator is irrelevant. Third, we identify new indicators, or determine what else can be done to assess change over time. Fourth, we present and negotiate a change in indicators or in how progress is assessed. These four steps may not result in a change, in which case we revert to the first step. *How would you start a conversation where someone approached you about an indicator that did not provide useful data?*

CHAPTER 10

Thinking Through an Evaluable Intervention

Pulling It All Together

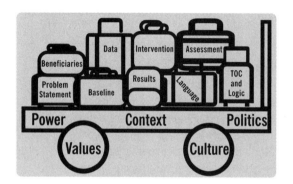

We have covered a lot in our evaluative journey, unpacking and repacking our suitcases along the way. Now it is time to collect our suitcases to see where our journey has led us. This chapter introduces a game that seamlessly brings together everything we have learned. Of all the games (and activities and processes) described thus far, the one described in this chapter thinks that it is the best. Now do not tell the others this. First, they might get jealous; and, second, what the conceited game will never admit is that her success is dependent on two factors: (1) her predecessors' doing their job very well, and (2) the level of facilitation provided during the game. The game (which is also an activity and a process) has been successfully used with a multitude of people, including (but not limited to) university professors, health clinic nurses, women's groups, farmers, managers of trade programs, early childhood development teachers, community strengthening advocates, nonprofit managers, foundation staff, sex worker advocates, and environmental activists, as well as evaluation colleagues.

This game is unfailing in its ability to pull together everything discussed thus far. It provides a basic format for discussing nearly every question, issue, and idea raised in the book, and likely a few more. For such an important game, it has a rather silly name. In writing the book, I felt tremendous pressure to rename the game, which has been called the "Baby

Game" for the past 10 years. The main reason I call it the Baby Game is that the only part of the initial game that still exists, after multiple testings and revisions, is the picture of a baby. There are two more practical reasons. First, is that, well, calling it the "M&E Framework Basic Demonstration Game" (yawn!) does not convey how fun the game is, how illuminating, or how easily it enables an evaluator to engage people in thinking through how to have a plausible and evaluable program. Second, the title is neither scary or intimidating; who's afraid of a baby? Thus it encourages people to engage.

THE BABY GAME

The Baby Game provides a framework that pulls together the basics for how to assess and evaluate an intervention (i.e., it brings together Chapters 1–9). In doing so, it lays out the basics for any evaluative process (monitoring or evaluation), and provides space for in-depth discussion. The game needs to be played, however, only *after* participants have gone through the content covered in each previous chapter, or the game becomes a frustrating challenge for everyone; **this is a wrap-up activity (and game), not a warm-up.** The complete version of the Baby Game, with graphics for the appropriate cards, is available on this book's companion website (*www.guilford.com/podems-materials*).

I also describe an optional step for practitioners: Once the basic game is played, the other game cards are removed (or one row can be left to be a reminder), the framework cards (i.e., the "header" cards) remain, and two more cards are added (i.e., a card each for the activity and beneficiary). The participants then complete the framework, using details from their own program. The game thus provides a practical approach that enables participants to engage in describing a plausible and evaluable intervention through an interactive and nonthreatening activity.

Let's play!

ACTIVITY 10.1. The Baby Game

Purpose: Again, this activity takes all the parts that have been discussed and puts them all together in a holistic picture that forms the basis for any evaluative thinking process—completing M&E formats or frameworks, or thinking through a plausible, evaluable intervention and related evaluation. After playing the game and clarifying terms, the participants can apply the framework to their own intervention.

Materials: A complete set of the Baby Game has a total of 42 cards (seven header cards, and then 35 game cards). So, a room of eight people or less would need one set of cards. A room of 16 people needs to be divided into two groups (with each group having its own Baby Game, each of which consists of 35 game cards plus seven header cards). Make as many sets as needed, and laminate the cards if you will be using them multiple times.

Time: As the facilitator, you will need 5 minutes to lay down the header cards and read each card to the groups. All participant groups will have 10–15 minutes to sort their pile of cards. You will need approximately 15–20 minutes to highlight teaching points once cards are sorted. The total game time is approximately 25–35 minutes, though times can vary based on the learning conversations.

Applying participants' program results to the framework: If, once the game is played, participants then apply one or two of their own results (and all their related information as required) to the framework, it solidifies learning and enables participants to understand how each of these terms applies to their own program(s). To apply one or two results to the framework, allow an additional 30–60 minutes, and provide the two additional cards for the activity and beneficiary.

The exercise: This is a sorting game. It is most useful when there are at least four people in each group and no more than eight (each group with its own header cards and then 35 cards/game pieces). One small group can play the game, or several groups can play at the same time. If there is more than one group, each group needs its own set of cards (i.e., each group has identical cards). When there is more than one group, make it a fun competition to see which group can sort the cards first.

As the facilitator, you will lay the "title" or "header" cards in a straight line on the ground (again, this is a sorting game, so people need space on the ground or on a large table), as shown in Figure 10.1. Each group needs its own header cards, as each group will sort an identical set of Baby Game cards. (If an or-

ganization uses a different label for any header card, change that card's name as needed, or have that relevant discussion.) Furthermore, the header cards can be in any order that makes logical sense to you and the group.

- *Briefly* (this is not a lecture), review each of the header cards, reminding the groups of the meaning of each word: For example, "This is the problem statement; it contains a problem supported by facts. This is the baseline; it's where the intervention starts from," and so on. If people are "fuzzy" on what the terms on the cards mean, or the differences among terms, *do not reteach or clarify anything at this point.* Do not answer any technical questions. Ask them to trust the process and continue with the game. *The game will do the reteaching.* For some groups, it is not necessary to review the header cards. As the facilitator, you will need to make that decision.

- Hand each group a set of identical cards, which are not in any order (i.e., they are shuffled). The set of 35 contains five problem statements. For each problem statement, there is a corresponding baseline, indicator, indicator tool, target, result, and time frame. Ask the group to sort the cards into the correct columns and rows under the header cards (you have laid down the header cards for them). Do not help them. Do not provide hints. *Your advice is a crutch that is not needed.* The group members will sort the cards, and their discussions will help them learn.

- When the groups think they are done, check the cards. If two or more are incorrect, just tell them that some cards are incorrect. If they are completely stuck, tell them which column or columns have incorrect cards. The group then discusses and

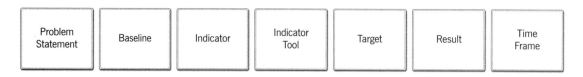

FIGURE 10.1. Title or header cards for the Baby Game.

identifies the incorrect cards. Once the order and layout are correct, if there is more than one group, bring all the groups together to look at one game, and facilitate the following questions.

Figure 10.2 shows what the shortened version of the game looks like once the cards are sorted. Please see *www.guilford.com/podems-materials* for the game in its entirety.

Facilitation questions: You can now use the Baby Game to ask some questions and help the participants understand how the different columns are connected. The more comfortable you become with the game, the more questions you can ask. For now, let's start with these:

- Turn over the card with the picture of the ruler (so it is now blank) in the "Baby" row (the row with the card depicting a baby saying, "I need to grow"). Ask the participants, "If a ruler were no longer available, what else would need to change?" (Answer: The baseline, target, and indicator, since the tool to assess all of these is now gone). Point out as well what would not need to change. Then ask, "How else can we assess if the baby is growing if we do not have a measuring tape or ruler? If we use that option, what else changes in the row?" Ask when or how this can happen in a real-life situation. Give some relevant examples, and/or ask the participants if something similar has happened to them (and, if so, what they did). Now put the ruler card back with the ruler showing.

- Turn over the card that says "Gain 15 pounds" on the American version or "Gain 10 kilos" on the British version (so it is blank), and ask, "If the target were to change to [suggest a number], what else is likely to change?" (Answer: If the number is much higher or lower, then the time frame is likely to change. Does anything else change? No.) Give some relevant examples, and/or ask the participants if something similar has happened to them (and, if so, what they did). Now put the target card back with the target showing.

- Turn over the card with the baseline for any example (so it is now blank), and ask, "What else is likely to change?" (Answer: The target, as we do not know where we have started from.) Then ask, "What are other options if we do not have a baseline?" (Retrospective data would be one answer.) Give some relevant examples, and/or ask the participants if something similar has happened to them (and, if so, what they did). Now put the baseline card back with the baseline showing.

- Turn over the card depicting the baby *or* the person with a fever (so it is now blank). Ask, "What else is likely to change?" (Answer: Everything, or perhaps the result could stay.) But how can there be an intended result with no problem statement? When could this happen? Drawing heavily on Chapters 3–4, discuss how programs sometimes have results with no clear problem statement. Give some relevant examples, and/or ask the participants if something similar has happened to them (and, if so, what they did). When the example is played in the game, participants can see how silly the idea of a result with no problem statement is; however, when they were reading Chapter 3, it probably did not seem as silly, just matter-of-fact. Now put the problem statement card back with the problem statement showing.

- Point to the terms on the header cards, and discuss what other labels could be used for each card. (Changing the label *Result* to *Intended result* would be one answer.) Ask what other columns can be added that could be helpful in their situation. Re-emphasize that the reason we have a column for each category is that the card in one column can change, while the rest could remain the same, or information on one card can change that nearly changes the whole row.

- Ask participants if they have any other questions or additional insights. The game is complete.

Optional step for practitioners (applying real-life examples): Now pick up all the playing cards, leaving the header cards, or you can leave one row of the

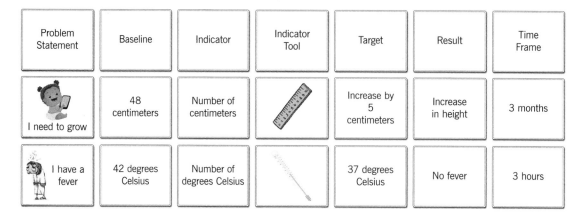

Problem Statement	Baseline	Indicator	Indicator Tool	Target	Result	Time Frame
I need to grow	48 centimeters	Number of centimeters		Increase by 5 centimeters	Increase in height	3 months
I have a fever	42 degrees Celsius	Number of degrees Celsius		37 degrees Celsius	No fever	3 hours

FIGURE 10.2. The 21-card version of the Baby Game, with two rows completed.

game cards as reminders. Add two cards to the header row: *Activity* and *Beneficiary*. It does not matter where these cards are placed in the header row. Now ask the group members to choose one of their results, its corresponding problem statement, and labels for any other cards (e.g., indicators) that they have developed throughout the process that respond to the result card they have chosen (Chapters 1–9), and place them into the Baby Game framework. Where there are empty columns, have them take a blank piece of paper, write the answer, and place it into the Baby Game framework, or note that the information still needs to be determined. Then, when the row is complete, have the participants present it (with no extra wording; they must present the title of the column and then what they placed underneath). They can present from left to right. Alternatively, an approach I find useful is to have them present the activity and beneficiaries; then the problem statement and the result; then the baseline, the target, and the time frame; and then the indicator and the tool. When the cards are presented in this way, it is often easier to see what does and does not make sense. Ask them questions about the logic of what they have done (e.g., "Does it make sense?") and about the potential challenges (e.g., "Where are the challenges?"). Here are some specific facilitation questions:

- Does the problem statement match the result? Look for potential challenges (e.g., pocket problems are matched to grand problems; see Chapter 7).

- Does the activity lead to that result? Does the activity address the problem?

- Evaluating for progress can be discussed: Does the indicator measure progress? Do we need to use something else to assess change (e.g., progress markers, MSC)?

- Who is benefitting from that activity? The answer then opens up a dialogue on whose values matter and whether that is an identified problem for that group, among other discussions.

- Is there a baseline? If not, how was the target set?

- If there is a specific baseline, ask if there are data to support that. If a target is named, ask how that target was set.

- Are any suitcase words used? (These are often found on the cards for the problem statement, result, and beneficiary.)

As the results move to higher levels, there will be fewer cards, and the format will probably (though not always) begin to look like sets of stairs, as one activity often has many intended results. (See Chapter 7's explanation of how results bring about results.) Once the basic information is laid out, further discussions are possible:

- *Logic* can be discussed. Ask, "Do the intended results address the identified problem?" (Refer to Chapters 3–7.)

- *Theory* can be discussed. Ask, "What makes you think that will happen?" (See Chapter 8.)

- *Assessment* can be discussed. Ask, "How useful is that indicator? Do other options exist?" (Refer to Chapter 9.)

Critical learning points: While the game cards help to reinforce the practical use of each concept, the actual placing of an intervention into the framework is an exercise that demonstrates how these concepts work together to support having a plausible and evaluable intervention.

The process that leads up to the Baby Game, and the Baby Game itself, are best implemented before completing any M&E frameworks, performance-monitoring plans, log frames, logical frameworks, or any other form that has little boxes, checklists, or summaries.

COMMON CHALLENGES WITH M&E FRAMEWORKS

"Here Is a Form; Fill It Out"

To summarize or assess a program, many donors, funders, government departments, or others to whom or which an intervention is accountable provide a form or format. And when a format with boxes is provided, people often laboriously attempt to fill it in, empty space by empty space. In a sort of zombie-like trance, people think "There. Is. Empty. Box. Must. Fill. In." Thus a form is filled in, box by box, with information often squished into too small a space. At best, filling in the form results in continued funding or meeting a management accountability need; at worst, it changes the program to reflect perfect answers instead of actual ones that will be appropriately used to assess the intervention and inform further decisions about it. Form completion promulgates an age-old belief that "M&E" is an add-on process that is done for the funder, the boss, the "higher-ups," or the M&E people. Yet, when used to summarize a thoughtful, well-laid-out evaluative process (see Chapters 3–9 and the Baby Game description in this chapter), summary formats can be very useful indeed.

Facilitating the Process, Not Filling Out the Form

So what is our role as evaluators? We (you and I) move the form to the side, find a comfortable place to sit, and ask, "So tell me about the intervention; what problem is it intended to address?" or "What do you expect from the monitoring [or the evaluation or the M&E process]?" (For guidance, refer to Chapters 1–9.) The role of an evaluator is to prevent people from *immediately* filling out a form, providing words in a box, or adding numbers to an Excel spreadsheet that aims to sum up the intervention before the intervention is fully understood. And let me do some "myth busting" here: A myth exists that an evaluator or M&E person knows instinctively how to fill out all M&E forms. Um. No. While evaluators should understand the terms and concepts used on the form, and technically what is needed on the form (though again, maybe not, as terms and concepts can vary by organization; see Chapter 1), they do not automatically know what to fill in—unless they have answers to the questions raised in Chapters 1–9. When these forms or formats are filled out to "look pretty," it often thwarts the very process and thinking that the format is trying to capture and assess.

When an organization, donor, or other person provides a data indicator sheet, a logical framework approach (LFA), a results framework, or anything else that has check (tick) boxes and blank lines, stop. Do not pass Go. Do not immediately attempt to fill out the form. Facilitate a calm evaluative process (as described in the preceding chapters) to guide and support the thinking, discussion, and reflection needed to complete the form *eventually*.

Facilitating Necessary Discussions Before Filling Out an M&E Form

In Figure 10.3, I have provided a checklist (the irony is not lost on me) to summarize the steps in an evaluative process that ensure a well-thought-out, evaluable intervention. (While the last two boxes on the list are raised throughout Part I, I elaborate on them in Chapters 12 and 13.) If these discussions have not taken place, facilitate the conversations described in each cross-referenced chapter, and wrap up the discussions with the Baby Game.

M&E FORMS

- **Have a few minutes?** Take a whirl through a page on the Better Evaluation website (*www.betterevaluation.org/en/evaluation-options/logframe*), which provides definitions, examples, and tips on using an LFA. Do not forget to look at the critique written by Chambers and Pettit (n.d.), to which a link is provided on this webpage. If you have a few more minutes, skim through USAID's Performance Monitoring and Evaluation TIPS: Building a Results Framework (*https://www.ndi.org/sites/default/files/ Performance%20Monitoring%20and%20Evaluation%20Tips%20Building%20a%20 Results%20Framework.pdf*). A results framework is different from an LFA, as it focuses more specifically on results. Look at these two resources and compare the similarities and differences.

- **Have 53 minutes?** Sit back and watch a video with a practical use of an LFA, as explained by Engineers without Borders USA (*www.youtube.com/ watch?v=OHEPVS2TAHk*).

Question	Yes	No
Is the monitoring and evaluation **language** clear? Are all the key evaluation words being used in the same way, such as *monitoring* and *evaluation*? How are evaluation words used differently, and how does that influence the evaluation process, if at all?		See Chapters 1 and 2.
Is the **problem statement (grand and pocket problems)** clearly defined, with defined and clarified suitcase words? How do we know that the problem is a problem? Who thinks it is a problem that needs to be addressed?		See Chapter 3.
Have **baseline** data been collected? Are they needed? If not, why not?		See Chapter 5.
Is the **intervention** clearly explained, with no suitcase words? Is the intervention linked to results? Back to the problem statement? Who thinks the intervention is valuable? Who designs, who implements, who values, and who judges the intervention? What is the context in which the intervention is implemented?		See Chapter 6.
Have the **results** been clearly defined, with no suitcase words? Are the results linked to each other and back again to the problem statement(s)? Is the pathway from one result to the next clear? Are results linked to the intervention?		See Chapter 7.
Are the **beneficiaries** clearly identified? The client? The audience? The actors? The un-beneficiaries? Any other stakeholders?		See Chapter 3.
How will the intervention be assessed? Are the **indicators**, **progress markers**, or other clear ways of assessing progress defined? Can these be changed or modified? Have data been collected on the indicators, progress markers, or other methods of determining change? Were the data useful? Who used the data to make what decisions? What is known about the program because of these data? What is not known?		See Chapters 4 and 9.
Have **targets** and/or **benchmarks** been set or discussed? How were these set? Who set these? Can they be changed, if needed? Are time frames clear?		See Chapter 9.
Have an explicit **theory of change** and **program logic** been articulated? Are there multiple theories or logics at play? Who has what different ways of thinking about the theory or the logic? Have the implementation theory and logic been discussed and made explicit?		See Chapters 7 and 8.
Is it clear who can make decisions **(power and politics)** to change any of the answers above, and what are some likely scenarios if those answers change?		See Chapters 3–9 and Chapter 13.
Is it clear whose **values** influence what decisions, and how these decisions in turn influence M&E decisions?		See Chapters 3–9 and Chapter 12.

FIGURE 10.3. Thinking through an evaluable intervention: A checklist for support.

WRAPPING UP

This chapter pulls together all that we have learned so far in Part I of this book.

- Chapter 1 has laid the initial groundwork for any evaluative discussion by describing how to have a conversation about monitoring and evaluation terminology, and has clarified related discussions.

- Chapter 2 has distinguished between an evaluator and a researcher by contrasting evaluation and research.

- Chapter 3 has started us on the evaluative journey: sorting out the problem statement, recognizing its importance in the whole journey, and introducing a discussion on stakeholders and the many roles that fall under that broad description (such as beneficiary, client, audience, and un-beneficiary).

- Chapter 4 has asked us how we know what we know and how they know what they know and engaged us in a conversation about facts and assumptions. It has also acknowledged that while an evaluator needs an academic understanding of research and evaluation, practitioners do not often need to use academic language.

- Chapter 5 has provided a look at methods of inquiry, and engaged us in thinking about credible data, credible evidence, and credible evaluations.

- Chapter 6 has shown how linking the problem statement, intervention, and results lays the foundation for a plausible and evaluable intervention.

- Chapter 7 has been all about the results; it has shown the logic and usefulness of breaking down results, determining how interventions produce results, and highlighting that results produce results.

- Chapter 8 has brought in the theory of change and has shown how the program logic and theory of change are BFFs.

- Chapter 9 has explained some basic decisions that need to be made about assessing and evaluating process and demonstrated how to make them.

- This chapter, Chapter 10, has brought it all together with the Baby Game.

We now know the importance of, and how to engage in, a multifaceted discussion about the intervention. We have an idea of what different levels of results look like, and we know the importance of knowing who informs all of that. We know that it is essential to identify and link results to the intervention and problem statement, and to discuss the theory behind, and the logic in front of, each of these discussions. We know how to figure out the basics of what to assess, how, and when. Finally, we know how to take all that information and pull it together in a holistic manner—a process that also identifies gaps still needing to be addressed. Along the way, we have learned to listen–speak–listen, ripped off labels, had a party, and filled the role of an M&E advisor.

In short, Chapters 1–10 have ensured that we are speaking a language that we all understand and have illustrated how to help others speak the same language. We know strategies to employ when facing typical challenges in any evaluative process, and we have built a strong, practical evaluative scaffolding to use as we shift to the book's next section. In Part II, we focus on working as an evaluator and exploring evaluation. Before we leave Part I, however, I invite you to join me in a conversation.

Our Conversation: Between You and Me

Here I provide two situations often encountered with regard to using M&E frameworks, or being asked how to assess an intervention. Practicing with these common scenarios will help you engage with these kinds of situations in the real world.

1. You are asked to fill out a few different M&E forms for your organization. However, the implementation team and the manager do not have time to engage with you. They are really busy. Yet what the intervention aims to address and achieve, how, and for whom (beyond a generic group of beneficiaries) are not clear. Often an evaluator is hired for the specific reason of "taking care" of the M&E, which is often seen as fulfilling a role that reduces work for the rest of the program management team. In some cases, that can certainly be true. However, just to begin to figure out what to assess and how to do it, the evaluator often must ask a lot of questions: what the intervention aims to improve, fix, or otherwise change; what the related assumptions and facts are; who aims to benefit and who may get hurt; what the theory and the logic are; who needs to use the data for what purpose and when; and so on.

To answer these questions, the evaluator can encourage discussions and support iterative processes that are not necessarily met with tears of joy from the management team (though tears could be involved if the evaluator is left on her own to fill out a form on a project she does not understand). The evaluator could be viewed as creating work (which, let's face it, we are doing, at least initially) and/or as not understanding the intervention (OK, that is probably true too, which is why the evaluator is asking so many questions).

There are several ways I might approach this situation, which depend on the amount of time, the budget, and the staff's willingness to engage with me. Often people do not understand the nature of monitoring and evaluation and what is covered in Chapters 1–9; I would suggest a short meeting to introduce how assessment is interlinked with the program logic (and theory) and how, when done correctly, it can greatly assist in management decisions related to learning, improvement, judgment, and broader knowledge generation. Sometimes, once people realize how monitoring and evaluation and the intervention are interconnected, they are very willing to engage in evaluative discussions and processes. And at other times? Not so much. When the approach described does not work, the game described in Activity 7.1 (see Chapter 7), which demonstrates how critical it is to know which results to assess when, can be helpful. *What would you do if you had very little time to produce an M&E framework, knew very little about the details of the intervention, and were also meeting with resistance?*

2. The intervention is given money by three different donors: a bilateral organization, a government department, and a foundation. They all require different M&E frameworks, different data collection tools, and different reporting timelines for collecting data. Moreover, they all use evaluation terms in different ways. First, familiarize yourself with each approach and its associated terms, tools, and timelines. Identify any overlaps or similarities. See what can be tweaked so that there is overlap. For example, the foundation wants the outcomes assessed, and the government department wants the impacts assessed. However, reviewing the program logic brings the realization that changing the name of the results label is needed, as both bodies are focusing on the same result (just using a different label). Another option is to speak with the funders and ask if there is any flexibility in what data are collected, their reporting format, or the timing of the report. Sometimes everything is carved in stone; at other times, there is flexibility.

Once it is clear exactly what needs to be done, then work with the organization that has hired you on designing an approach that meets its accountability needs. If the organization you are working with has any time and energy left over (and budget), engage its staff in a discussion to identify whether its internal learning and management needs are being met. If not, identify how those gaps can realistically be filled. *What would you do?*

PART II

WORKING AS AN EVALUATOR AND EXPLORING EVALUATION

In this second part of the book, I shift away from describing an evaluative process; I focus on what it means to be an evaluator and explore the field of evaluation. I know that it can be a personal choice to be an evaluator—or maybe you stumbled into being one, perhaps you were assigned the evaluator role, or maybe you are still contemplating the whole idea of evaluation. Regardless of where you find yourself at this moment in time, the next chapters bring you through a thoughtful, reflective process of what it means to be an evaluator, which can be backward-looking, forward-looking, in the moment, or all three. One cannot talk about being an evaluator without also discussing the multitude of evaluation approaches, theories, and methods that exist in the field; exploring the complexities of designing and implementing an evaluation; and sharing real-life experiences. Thus, Part II moves between being an evaluator and discussing the various ways of thinking about evaluation. I conclude this part of the book by sharing some of evaluation's "dirty laundry."

MY STORY

"Deciding what and how to write about evaluation was guided by my own evaluation story. Let me share a bit about my journey."

My path to being an evaluator started as a lucky accident. After I obtained a master's degree in public administration, I applied to the Peace Corps to volunteer in Mongolia or in any African country, and was accepted as an agricultural volunteer in Guatemala, where, among other things, I learned colloquial Spanish. When I returned to the United States, I was hired because of my colloquial Spanish by a research and evaluation company as a field worker; my job was to collect data from Spanish-speaking agricultural workers. I traveled around the United States, and on one of my trips, I was asked to stay an extra week and collect data for an evaluation. Because of that small experience in evaluation (which was just data collection), I was then trained by the company to do basic evaluation to support AmeriCorps programs. During that time, I applied for a fellowship with the United States Agency for International Development (USAID) in the Dominican Republic. I was accepted to the program and was sent to South Africa for an initial 9 months as a USAID Gender Fellow. Because I had some experience with evaluation, I was also asked to support the program department, where I learned about USAID's approach to evaluation. After the fellowship ended, I was hired to work on a South African–based M&E project funded by USAID, because I understood USAID's evaluation approaches and organizational culture, and likely because I was in the right spot at the right time.

Now, this whole time since my university days, my dream had been to be a foreign service officer; it just seemed so romantic and adventurous. One day my dream came true: I was accepted! So I went to Ethiopia to celebrate (it had been on my bucket list) before my training would begin in the United States. On the second day of the tour, my taxi had a head-on collision that was fatal for some passengers—though by fate or luck, I only sustained broken ribs, a split-open head, and some bumps and bruises. Lying in a clinic in a rural town in Ethiopia, where I waited 2 days to be medically airlifted to Nairobi, I had a lot of time to think. And I had an epiphany (among others): I no longer wanted to be a foreign service officer; I wanted to be an evaluator.

So I wrote to Michael Quinn Patton, whose book I had read, and explained who I was, what I believed, and that I wanted to get a doctorate focusing on evaluation. I also wrote to Jennifer C. Greene, whose work I had also been reading. Well, it turned out that there was no such thing at the time as a doctorate in program evaluation. So I explained the kind of evaluator I wanted to be, and the university to which Dr. Patton was attached allowed me to create my own program that offered what I needed to know to be the evaluator I wanted to be; it included course work in sociology, anthropology, organizational development, research methods, and evaluation theory. Dr. Patton became my dissertation advisor, and since I was required to have one external doctoral committee member, I invited Dr. Greene, who graciously accepted. Several years later, I graduated with a doctorate in interdisciplinary studies. Dr. Patton's and Dr. Greene's influences on how I think about evaluation permeate my work today.

Throughout graduate school, I continued to conduct small evaluations, and upon graduation I started a one-person consultancy for no other reason than to allow me to continue living (legally) in South Africa. Although I have since realized that I am not really a businessperson, I did realize that I loved the business of evaluation. Since then, I have tried out different methodologies and dabbled in many thematic areas; have made tons of mistakes and have had as many successes; have worked with various kinds of clients and evaluation teams in over 25 countries;

and along the way have been mentored by many people, to whom I am very grateful. I have published articles (and have been turned down with the most horrible, personal, and soul-crunching criticism); have presented at evaluation conferences (and have had presentations rejected); and have lectured at four different universities. During it all, I have been praised and ripped to shreds, have laughed (sometimes hysterically), and have cried (sometimes from happiness). I have stood up to figures of authority when I thought they were being bullies (and lost contracts and income as a result; see my earlier statement about not being a businessperson!)—and, yes, have sometimes stayed silent. And, slowly, I have thus become the evaluator I am today, all of which inspired me to write this evaluation book. Throughout it all, self-reflection, peer feedback, reading, writing, teaching, being mentored, and mentoring others have kept me moving forward. Yet, truth be told, I am *still* on the path of being the evaluator that I want to be, and while I see multiple paths that I can take next, I also know that circumstances will play a huge factor in deciding which path I take. That is my story, which I hope is far from being over.

CHAPTER 11
The Personal Choices of Being an Evaluator

How wonderful it is that nobody need wait a single moment
before starting to improve the world.
—ANNE FRANK, German-born diarist

WHAT TYPE OF EVALUATOR DO YOU WANT TO BE?

Let's face it, sometimes we (you and I) just end up in the jobs we end up in. So perhaps you
are thinking how to shift your path slightly into an evaluation role that galvanizes you, or
maybe you are an evaluator who has more flexibility and wants to make more informed
choices about how to move forward in an intentional manner. Perhaps you are still finding
your feet as an evaluator. Or maybe you are still deciding if you want to be one. Regardless,
it is time to discuss the many roles that exist for an evaluator, and what kind of evaluator
you *want* to be.

I know that reading about evaluation can be inspiring, interesting, and—let's face it—
at times a bit boring. At least it can be these things for me. So, in the next few sections,
the text is peppered with key evaluation terminology, while at the same time whisking you
through the various discussions on what it can *mean* to be an evaluator. It is a splendid way
to have inspiring, self-reflective conversations while learning about evaluation and its terminology. To initiate these conversations, let's start with a rather large brainstorming of the
many potential roles an evaluator can fill.

BEING AN EVALUATOR: AN ABUNDANCE OF ROLES

Framing an Evaluator's Role

Evaluators do lots of things and can fill many roles. What we do, and how we do it, can
often be the topics of long, convoluted discussions. Every time (and I mean every single time)
someone casually asks me what I do for a living, it gives me the "deer in the headlights"

syndrome. I often say something vague about social change, and then quickly try to turn the conversation around by saying something such as "Well, enough about me, what about you?" What? People like to talk about themselves. And I do too—which is why my vague answer is sort of an odd response, considering that I love being an evaluator. I *could* talk about what I do for hours (and hours)—and that is at the core of it: The conversation would take quite some time.

Skolits, Morrow, and Burr (2009) describe many possible roles of an evaluator, some of which overlap with lists developed by Mathison (2005) and others (Mark, 2002; Morabito, 2002; Patton, 2008; Volkov, 2011) Table 11.1 shares many of the roles suggested by these authors, and a few more.

When I shared the Table 11.1 list with my evaluation colleagues, they identified other roles that evaluators can fill. Four more commonly mentioned roles included therapist, advisor, philosopher, and scapegoat. One colleague recounted that many times interviews "feel like therapy sessions, and the respondent answers way more than I asked and just seems so relieved to talk to someone." At the same time, colleagues commented that throughout evaluations, others view the evaluator as an advisor; for instance, the evaluator advises on how to address evaluation culture within the organization, or serves as an advisor through the role of providing recommendations. Several colleagues mentioned the philosopher role, and spoke about the many "what if" discussions they have been involved in.

The fourth role is not so nice, and is a role that is always given as opposed to chosen: scapegoat. Try to avoid that role. A *scapegoat* is a person who is blamed for all that goes wrong. The role sometimes seems to emerge out of the blue. For example, an evaluator provides somewhat critical findings, and others respond that those findings were his fault; he was using biased methodology (otherwise the results would be positive), or he was only looking to find problems or he just did not understand the intervention. The potential to be labeled (or at least treated as) a scapegoat can sometimes be seen a mile off, such as when an evaluator's initial and subsequent meetings are met with hostility, or the evaluation seems to be a not-so-nice surprise to the implementer. When someone else designates the evaluator as the scapegoat, it is often a defensive reaction; understanding that person's position can help the evaluator to better engage with being assigned that role. Or not. It is a tough one.

The particular roles that make evaluation exciting and meaningful to me are that of educator, facilitator, and negotiator, which is probably evident from how I have explained the evaluative process in Chapters 1–10. I recognize that not all evaluators fill these three roles, and not all evaluations need them. The importance of these three roles will depend on how you view an evaluator's role in society, on the types of evaluation you conduct, and on the kinds of organizations and people with whom you work.

- *The educator role.* The educator role does not refer to being an evaluation lecturer or university professor, though those are excellent roles. Here the focus is on being an educator *during* an evaluative process. The educator role can be subtle, such as recommending an

TABLE 11.1. Some Possible Roles of an Evaluator

Interpreter. Evaluators can explain evaluation terms in the appropriate language for everyone involved.

Advocate, change agent. Evaluators can encourage use of the evaluation findings to bring about social change.

Anti-bully. An evaluator takes on this role through providing clear processes, clear language, and clear explanations to all involved or touched by an evaluation.

Critical friend, collaborator, coach. An evaluator can provide information, and then support an organization in engaging with it.

Cruciverbalist. A *cruciverbalist* is someone who solves crossword puzzles. An evaluator often uses these skills to sort out M&E frameworks and other evaluation forms that have small boxes to fill in.

Developer. An evaluator can work with intervention staff to design an evaluable program.

Diplomat. An evaluator can act as intermediary between a funder and a program, or an implementer and the community.

Learner. Evaluators can be reflective and thoughtful about their own practice, which strengthens their own knowledge and skills.

Logician. An evaluator can serve as an expert in logic.

Manager. Throughout all of the stages of the evaluation process, an evaluator can be a manager.

Scholar. Evaluators can publish and present their work.

Lecturer/professor. An evaluator can choose to formally teach evaluation and thus support new and emerging evaluators.

Detective, sleuth. The evaluator can explore the context of the program and identify evaluation needs.

Describer. The evaluator can describe the intervention, what problem it aims to solve, and what it aims to achieve (or what it does or did achieve).

Designer. The evaluator can develop a feasible evaluation plan that will simultaneously produce accurate and useful information.

Reporter. Evaluators can communicate and disseminate findings.

Novelist, writer. An evaluator can write reports that are engaging, or edit other people's reports.

Researcher, social scientist, methodologist. Evaluator can develop research designs and can collect, analyze, and interpret data.

Judge, magistrate. Evaluators value an intervention.

evaluation blog, article, book, or webinar to key stakeholders or those from whom data are gathered (i.e., the people interviewed or observed). Or it can be more overt, such as describing methods of inquiry or explaining evaluation approaches to colleagues or clients. One example of when an evaluator can fill the educator role is when clients or colleagues are challenged by evaluation terms in an evaluative process (see Chapter 1), or are not aware of the plethora of evaluation options that can provide appropriate processes and designs for their evaluation question (see Chapter 15).

• *The facilitator role.* The facilitator role can vary greatly, from helping stakeholders (all those who have a stake in an intervention; see Chapter 3 for further discussion) to develop or refine evaluation questions, to aiding them in developing theories of change, to conducting data analysis workshops and interpreting results, to ensuring use of evaluation findings.

• *The negotiator role.* The role of negotiator emerges when an evaluator is faced with diverse viewpoints, such as when key stakeholders have different needs from an evaluation. Examples of topics that often need at least some negotiation include evaluation questions, focus of the evaluation, budget, time frames, persons to interview and not to interview, data collection methods, and ways to disseminate the findings, just to name a few.

These three roles—education, facilitation, and negotiation—are often mentioned with regard to interactions with and among clients, participants, and beneficiaries. However, these three roles are also often critical to leading, or being an active member of, an evaluation team.

The role of evaluation *ambassador* is critical to the evaluation field and one that I enjoy filling, both formally and informally. It is a role that an evaluator can fill all the time, not just when evaluative processes are being conducted. An evaluator fills the ambassador role by promoting evaluation; educating others on its standards and ethics; and raising awareness about evaluation societies, groups, and other organizations that are relevant to the contexts in which evaluators work. Remember, when you label yourself (or others label you) as an evaluator, you represent us all.

Can you give some ideas of how to be an ambassador, both formally and informally? That sounds interesting.

Let me start with formal ways. Join an evaluation association and become an active member. To my knowledge, you can join any evaluation association; it does not need to be in the country in which you reside. For example, I have lived in South Africa for more than 20 years and am a U.S. citizen by birth. I belong to the South African Monitoring and Evaluation Association (SAMEA) and the American Evaluation Association (AEA), and because I am a member of SAMEA, I am automatically a member of the African Evaluation Association (AFREA). I am also a member of the European Evaluation Society (EES). After becoming an active member, consider running for your association's board. Informally, volunteer to give webinars, blog, Tweet, or otherwise promote ethical and culturally sensitive evaluation in public forums. Make people aware of evaluation and its relevant topics.

Although it is useful to know that a multitude of different roles exist, how does one choose? As noted, sometimes it is not a choice, rather it is circumstance. Evaluators develop identities that are shaped by the roles they fill, skills they use, types of evaluations they perform, skills they possess, places they work, aims they pursue, and attributes and dispositions they bring to the work. With that understanding, the next sections explore some evaluation terms, and intertwine discussions of evaluator roles from different perspectives and in relation to varying purposes.

AN EVALUATOR'S ROLE BY EVALUATION PURPOSE: FORMATIVE, SUMMATIVE, AND DEVELOPMENTAL

Evaluation has many typologies and framings. Here I introduce one approach, which categorizes evaluation into **formative, summative,** and **developmental** types. Some evaluators may gravitate toward one type of investigation, and some evaluators may implement all three. While an evaluator often fills a multitude of roles in each, some roles are far more common to one type of investigation than another. *Formative evaluation* has a focus on informing and shaping programs. *Summative evaluation* focuses on informing judgments, and *developmental evaluation* aims to actively inform innovative programs that are still taking shape (i.e., still being developed). Michael Scriven coined the terms *formative evaluation* and *summative evaluation* in 1967 (see Scriven, 1991), while Michael Patton conceived *developmental evaluation* later (Patton, 2010). People sometimes mix up the term *developmental evaluation* with *development evaluation,* which refers to implementing evaluation in the context of the developing world or emerging markets; this broad category (development evaluation) can refer to an evaluator's filling any type of evaluation role imaginable.

> ### BOX 11.1. Formative, Summative, and Developmental Evaluation
>
> Formative evaluations collect data that aim to inform or improve an intervention. A summative evaluation aims to inform a decisive judgment, such as to continue to fund or not to fund the intervention. Whereas formative and summative evaluation can take place at any time during the life of an intervention, developmental evaluation informs an innovative intervention as it takes shape.

The simultaneous conversation on roles and concepts begins with describing formative and summative evaluation, as they suggest a clear-cut division, which may help to describe the many different roles that are often associated with each kind of evaluation. But do they? In reality, the distinctions between the evaluation roles filled in formative evaluation, and those filled in summative evaluation, can be more nuanced than their definitions suggest. Let's look at this closely by exploring some misconceptions about these two umbrella terms.

Some roles commonly associated with formative evaluation include critical friend, coach, collaborator, detective, describer, designer, methodologist, facilitator, educator, and . . . judge. You may be asking about the last one, "Judge?" One common misconception is that an evaluator, when using formative evaluations, does not judge a program—probably because an absence of judgment is implied in the definition. Yet, when I am practicing formative evaluation in the real world, it is not exactly how I would describe it. If you thought that conducting formative evaluation removes the judgment factor, think again. Deciding to conduct only formative evaluations does not get an evaluator out of the judgment role. After all, before a suggestion is made to improve something, some sort of judgment is made that an intervention needs to be improved. It is how the term *judgment* is used in formative evaluation that is different from how it is applied in summative evaluation. In formative evaluation, an evaluator (and perhaps his team) would judge that something was not working, was not working well enough, or was missing in the intervention. He would then make suggestions aimed at improving the intervention so that it would be more likely to produce the intended results. And this type of judgment is not necessarily all negative; evaluators also identify what is working well and what should be expanded on, replicated, or adapted. In this way, judgment still exists, and it is used to inform the intervention or other related decisions.

With summative evaluation, there is no intent to improve the intervention. Rather, the evaluator (or his team, or others) makes a final statement and declares the intervention good, bad, or perhaps a mix of both; this statement both includes and informs judgment. In doing so, the evaluator can identify what works well and what does not, and can specify what should be expanded on, removed, amended, replicated, adapted, or otherwise learned from. Summative evaluation usually includes the roles of judge, detective, designer, describer, methodologist and . . . educator and facilitator. Surprised? Conducting a summative evaluation does not preclude an evaluator from taking a participatory approach, filling a learning or capacity-building role, or engaging in process use. (For more on process use, read further in this chapter; for more on participatory processes, see Chapters 12 and 15.) Thus choosing to focus a career on doing formative evaluation does not get you out of the judgment role, and choosing to do summative evaluation does not always remove you from personal interaction and engagement.

In formative or summative evaluation, the evaluator often has a clear understanding before the evaluation begins of the roles he is likely to play in that evaluative process. There is often an evaluation design in place, or some kind of formal (or even informal) agreement is reached, before the evaluation process begins (for more on evaluation design, see Chapter 15); this design or agreement details what is meant to happen, and therefore indicates the roles the evaluator is likely to fill (I say "likely," because life is full of surprises). Although some unanticipated roles can arise during the evaluation process, it is not that common. In developmental evaluation, the situation is a bit different: Because the intervention has not yet taken shape, the agreement between the evaluator and client is less structured. So much is still unknown that it is not always very clear which roles (and associated knowledge and skills) will be needed throughout the process. Thus the evaluator who practices developmental evaluation needs to be comfortable with having roles shift over time (which could mean weekly), and in some cases will need to have ready access to multiple knowledgeable others to do effective work. (For more on knowledgeable others, see Chapter 1.) In developmental evaluation, a role the evaluator always fills is partner, and other likely roles include educator, facilitator, methodologist, coach, describer, and advisor.

How an Evaluator, or Evaluation, Is Perceived

How an evaluator's role is perceived is another conversation, which is tied up in a discussion about how an evaluator is received by clients, program managers, or beneficiaries. The client, program manager, or beneficiary could perceive that a formative evaluator is a helper, that a summative evaluator is a judge, and that a developmental evaluator is a partner. In the real world, how respondents are likely to engage with an evaluator (i.e., respond to her questions and interact with her) can change, depending on the evaluation's intent *and* on the person's perception of the evaluator's role. This does not imply that people are untruthful. Imagine these three scenarios:

"Hi. I am here to help improve the intervention." (formative)

"Hi. I am here to make a definitive judgment about your program's merit and worth." (summative)

"Hi. I am your partner." (developmental)

It is conceivable that people may respond differently to these three distinct scenarios. And because of that response, an evaluator may need to draw more on her facilitation skills in a summative evaluation because people are running for the hills or are paralyzed with fear, than in a formative or developmental one. I'm just saying.

This brings me back to the importance of an evaluator's filling the ambassador role, combined with the educator role, in all types of evaluation. The more evaluators can take on these roles, the higher the likelihood that clients and other people involved in an evaluation will have a clear understanding of the evaluation and clear expectations of what it can achieve. Furthermore, the three scenarios above highlight the need for an evaluator to be an active (as opposed to passive) educator about whatever type of evaluation she is conducting. She needs to explain to all those touched by the evaluation, at a minimum, what will happen (the process); how the findings will be used, by whom, for what purpose; and who could be hurt (i.e., the un-beneficiaries; see Chapter 3).

How an Evaluation Is Used

Before leaving the discussion of formative and summative evaluation, I want to mention that neither label always accurately portrays an evaluation's *actual* use, either. If a formative evaluation falls into the hands of a decision maker who, based on that evaluation, decides to end the program, the formative evaluation has just been used as a summative one. Contrarily, if an evaluation intended as summative is used to improve a program, it then also becomes a formative one. There's a third area for consideration when one kind of evaluation is intended, and another use occurs. Imagine that during an evaluation process, the evaluator has told the organization (and those she has interviewed or otherwise interacted with) that the evaluation's purpose is to improve the intervention, and then a decision (which is out of the evaluator's control) is made to decrease funding. Consider how that experience will influence future evaluative processes in that organization. Furthermore, consider how that could also influence the evaluator's credibility, and her role as a coach, critical friend, or collaborator. These things do happen.

AN EVALUATOR'S ROLE BY EVALUATION PURPOSE: FOUR MORE OF THEM?

Why the question mark in the heading above? For three reasons. First, different evaluation theorists (and therefore books on evaluation) do not always categorize and describe an evaluation's purpose in the same ways. Melvin Mark, Gary Henry, and George Julnes (2000), Marvin Alkin (2011), and Donna Mertens and Amy Wilson (2012) are a few of the evaluators who have published books that categorize, and recognize, an evaluation's possible purposes differently. Sometimes the differences are nuanced; sometimes categories overlap by name; sometimes, when you look at descriptions and definitions, one theorist's differently labeled categories are very similar to someone else's; and some categories are unique. These different ways of thinking stem from how these evaluators view the roles of evaluation, and of an evaluator, in society. As Carol Weiss (2006) has noted, because people see the world differently, "it is not surprising that we have such disparate perceptions of an evaluation purpose" (p. 34).

I think it is fascinating that there are so many purposes for evaluation. I would like to be involved in that debate.

It is indeed a fascinating and interesting discussion. I do not really think that it is a debate per se; it is more a case of different theorists suggesting different categories and others saying "Oh, hmm, interesting. I think another way." If you are interested in thinking more about how to categorize evaluation, or providing another way to define an evaluation's purpose, I suggest reading the three books mentioned in the previous paragraph (among others), practicing evaluation for several years, and moving on from there. Evaluation needs thoughtful, insightful people to contribute to evaluation theory.

Wait. Before you move on, does the present book touch on different roles as described by Alkin, Mertens and Wilson, and Mark and colleagues? What about those roles?

Alkin (2011) looks at a variation of formative and summative evaluation, so the roles associated with his evaluation purposes have been mostly covered in the section starting on page 217. Mertens and Wilson (2012) has a stronger focus on social justice, which is covered in multiple chapters of the present book (including Chapters 14 and 15, which talk a bit about Mertens's theory and other social justice theories). Mark and colleagues' (2000) main contribution is separating causal inference/judgment from accountability. Causal inference is covered in Chapters 4, 5, and 15 of this book, so the reader can infer the evaluator's role in those situations. The four purposes selected to frame the next discussion provide a broad and widely accepted understanding of evaluation, and an evaluator's role in society, and are based on Patton's (2008) view. Knowing that these constraints on the conversation exist (I am not covering all different possible categories), let's have a go anyway, shall we?

Exploring the next four purposes for evaluation creates another platform for exploring evaluators' potential roles. These purposes are (1) program improvement, (2) knowledge generation, (3) accountability and judgment, and the more recently identified (4) development of an intervention. (Although developmental evaluation has been discussed, it fits into the discussion here as well, and therefore has been included here.) Different evaluation purposes are *likely* to influence the roles fulfilled by an evaluator—but sometimes not. Sometimes an evaluation's purpose may overlap or seamlessly combine with another purpose. This convoluted answer (along with the plethora of roles already mentioned) explains my "deer in the headlights" syndrome mentioned at the start of this chapter.

There are two more reasons why the heading on the previous page has a question mark. What an evaluator does can be fluid, and even when it is clear what she does (the approach I have taken when explaining formative, summative, and developmental evaluation), explaining it does not necessarily get to the core or the heart of what an evaluator is. Therefore, the next discussion takes a different approach from the discussion of formative, summative, and developmental earlier in this chapter. It explores four purposes of evaluation with a focus on what a person enjoys and is good at doing, and on how this could influence (if it can; not everyone has a choice) how an evaluator focuses her career.

A person who relishes engagement with different people; is comfortable being a critical friend, coach, collaborator; and likes the role of facilitator and capacity builder may appreciate being an evaluator for an evaluation that aims for **program improvement.** These roles are also common in participatory theory-of-change processes (see Chapter 8 for further exploration), which may or may not be a part of the program improvement process. If a person has these qualities, *and* is good at logical thinking and understanding how others think, leading a theory-of-change process is probably a nice fit. An evaluator who enjoys a more scholastic role may appreciate conducting **knowledge-generating** evaluations. These evaluations attempt to identify generic principles about program effectiveness that aim to inform practice (Patton, 2008, 2012). It is theory testing with a focus on what makes a program effective, to inform the wider practice. A person who has a particular passion (e.g., about women's rights or the environment) may enjoy evaluative work that aims to build up knowledge about what works, what does not, for whom, and why, in that particular field.

Maybe an evaluator finds it intriguing to compare what was with what should have been, which would fall under a type of **accountability** evaluation and include the role of a judge. Accountability evaluations look at whether resources are being used efficiently and if the intervention attained its planned results. Evaluators can also work **developmentally,** meaning that in their role they support and work alongside (and are sometimes embedded within) an organization as critical friends—though their work is often more intensive than in improvement evaluations, as their role here is to inform the shape of an innovative intervention as it emerges. It is a role that requires an evaluator to be comfortable with the unknown, and to know what to do when faced with it. Yet perhaps working with extreme flexibility and intense personal engagement is not appealing to you.

Maybe these broad categories are overwhelming, or none attract you. Possibly there is an evaluation niche that excites you, such as statistical analysis, designing web-based surveys, data visualization, or editing and writing evaluation reports. The evaluation field often draws on "knowledgeable others" to fill gaps that are needed on an evaluation team. Selecting a specialty within the evaluation field could be your chosen path. Among other considerations, an evaluator could specialize in different evaluation theories, approaches, and models (in-depth discussions of which are provided in Chapters 14 and 15), which then further defines her role. So what floats your boat?

While the academic books provide nice categorizations (and, as we have seen, different ones) as ways to think through the many roles of evaluation, and what an evaluator does to implement them, the reality is that the lines among categories are often blurred. And within those blurred lines, an evaluator can fill a myriad of roles—but this still does not get to the heart of what an evaluator is. While the intended purpose of the evaluation, or its label, may give some hints at what role an evaluator can play, there are no definitive answers. Some evaluators fill different roles at different points in their careers; various evaluators only fill one or two roles in the course of their working lives; and some evaluators fill an assortment of roles all at once, even if they conduct evaluations for one purpose.

Now that you have learned a bit more about the varying purposes for evaluation, and the many different roles an evaluator can play, let's explore some more considerations through the different positions an evaluator can fill: Do you want to be a sector specialist or an evaluation generalist? Do you want to be an internal or external evaluator? Or do you want to consider some of the more elusive roles that exist in the evaluation field? Let's start our discussion by looking at the distinction between sector specialist and evaluation generalist.

An Evaluator's Role through Self-Identification: Sector Specialist or Evaluation Generalist?

Some say that an evaluator needs to be a **sector specialist** (who is also an evaluator) to understand what is being evaluated. Without subject expertise in education, environment, or health, the evaluator will not know what questions to ask, where to look for data, or how to interpret the data, and will thus be unable to provide solid recommendations. For example, one common argument is that an education program needs an evaluator who is also an education specialist. And in many circumstances, the specialization needs to be even more specific—as the evaluation does not need *just* an education specialist, but a curriculum specialist, a math and science subject specialist, a language education specialist, or a learner assessment specialist.

Then there are those who say that an evaluator should be a **generalist.** They suggest that evaluators need knowledge of various evaluation approaches, theories, and models, and probably (though not always) a broad spectrum of experiences in different thematic areas (e.g., health, education, environment, community development, gender), to strengthen their evaluator capabilities. Not being a specialist suggests that an evaluator does not bring in pre-conceived thinking or assumptions about an intervention, which could influence (positively or negatively) the evaluation approach and its findings. For example, a subject specialist evaluator could assume that she knows something because she has experienced the same intervention in 30 other places thus far, whereas a generalist would be more likely not to make assumptions and rather to ask the "obvious" questions, which can elicit all types of useful data. On the other hand, the sector specialist will have the knowledge to perhaps dig deeper or ask more focused and insightful questions, or to provide stronger analysis based on knowing the content area of the evaluation. Does one of these arguments resonate with you?

Perhaps the idea of working with programs aimed at children, sports, animals, agriculture, or the elderly, and becoming an expert in one of these sectors, appeals to you. Or maybe you want to work in a community setting and address a broader spectrum of interventions; or perhaps you prefer working in pairs or with teammates who bring sector expertise. Considering these arguments and options, would you rather be a specialist or a generalist?

I thought most evaluators worked in teams?

A team approach does often occur in evaluations. Sometimes it is a team of 2, and sometimes a team of 20 or more. A team may consist of someone with evaluation knowledge and skills, a sector specialist with no evaluation knowledge, a community liaison, a translator, a statistician, and a cultural specialist. Here the team members draw on each other's skills. Or there are times when there is one lone evaluator—but do not let that mislead you. For instance, a lone evaluator can draw on knowledgeable others through key informant interviews, or can draw on program staff, to ensure cultural appropriateness and contextual technical expertise.

I am not sure if I want to be a generalist or a specialist. What are some more key points I should consider?

Sometimes it is not a choice; it just happens. For example, a position opens for an education evaluation specialist; you have an education background, and you are hired. You then train as an evaluator, and/or learn on the job, and become an education evaluation specialist. And you love it. Or let's say you work for an organization and have strong research and basic evaluation skills. The organization funds many kinds of community grants. One month they need you to look at a noise pollution intervention; the next month they need you to focus on a community garden project; and the following week an evaluation is needed for a community safety program. And you love it. So there's that. At other times a person will naturally fill the role of a specialist, having trained as an educator, environmentalist, psychologist, nurse, or other specialist, and will then train as an evaluator. I would suggest that if you have a passion about a subject that continually engages your intellect and incites your passion (e.g., children, melting polar ice caps), a specialist role is more likely to be a position that will bring you fulfillment. If you are a person with a shorter attention span, or an insatiable desire to engage in many kinds of activities, a generalist role may be more likely to suit your personal and professional needs. Having said all that, I emphasize that a generalist and a specialist both play important and valuable roles in evaluation.

Can I be both? What if I have specific knowledge about gender issues, but do not want to limit my evaluation work to interventions targeting violence against women, mother–child health, or economic equity? Can I be a specialist and a generalist?

Absolutely. An evaluator can be a specialist in gender issues, as you note, and then also conduct other evaluations as a generalist. I tend to define myself as a generalist. I conduct evaluations in the areas of the environment, education, health, agriculture, youth at risk, community safety, and housing, among others, using a myriad of approaches and evaluation frameworks. I am also a specialist in gender and feminist evaluation, and am sometimes hired to bring my specialist focus to these kinds of evaluations. Here is an example. Last year I was the gender and equity specialist on a large economic trade evaluation, and then, for a different evaluation and drawing on my generalist knowledge, I served as the team leader for a 3-year, four-country education program; my team included education, gender, and system evaluation experts.

AN EVALUATOR'S ROLE THROUGH A FORMAL POSITION: INTERNAL OR EXTERNAL EVALUATOR?

Now let's look at two formal positions that can be filled by an evaluator, and the roles normally associated with those positions. **Internal evaluators** are defined as those who work permanently with an organization. In that role, an evaluator may conduct multiple evaluations for different interventions, or perhaps may only work with a specific program, project, intervention, or policy team. **External evaluators** are those who do not work within an organization as a permanent staff member, but are hired as needed for evaluations. The definitions provided may not work in your context; I get that. In this section, some very general distinctions are made about the roles to make them comparable for the discussion. These differences are drawn from my experience, that of my colleagues, and articles on the topic (Conley-Tyler, 2005; Kennedy, 1983; Kniker, 2011; Minnett, 1999; Volkov, 2011). Although I draw stark contrasts between the two different types of roles, I realize that in real life the distinctions are often fuzzier.

Internal Evaluators

Internal evaluators offer several benefits to an evaluative process. An internal evaluator is very likely to have an insider's knowledge of the intervention, where an external evaluator often needs time to explore and understand the intervention. An internal evaluator is more likely to have appropriate cultural and social understanding, as they are more likely (though not always) to be aware of the politics, power, and culture in which the intervention takes place. Because the person is situated within the organization, they can more easily influence the use of findings and recommendations. These are, of course, the ideal situations. Power, politics, and other contextual challenges may not permit an internal evaluator to fill these roles or bring these benefits to an evaluation.

There are some drawbacks often associated with being an internal evaluator. One example is that a person who works in an organization may be hesitant to critique her peers or colleagues. Another example is that she may feel pressure, real or otherwise, from those who have power over her to provide only positive findings or to bury the negative ones. Unlike an external evaluator, an internal evaluator may have other roles within the organization that do not allow her full attention to be placed on the evaluation. Finally, as noted in Chapter 1, a person may have been assigned to the M&E role with little or no knowledge of evaluation and is now expected to conduct an evaluation (i.e., her specialty is monitoring). These are some challenges that an internal evaluator could face.

Have you ever worked as an internal evaluator? If so, did you like it?

When I worked as an internal evaluator for a nonprofit organization, I enjoyed being a part of the team, providing useful information to my colleagues, being a thinking partner, and slowly informing the theory of change and the program logic (see Chapter 8). I liked providing empirical data and credible evidence that my team could use to continually improve the program and defend it when necessary. I liked the role of being their critical friend. I relished focusing on one organization, knowing it well, and being able to work within the organizational culture—once I figured it out. Also, because I was in a relationship with people, it was often easier to know whom to target with key evaluation messages that were translated into action. At the same time, my evaluation knowledge and skills did not grow past a certain point, and I found myself seeking a wider evaluation experience.

External Evaluators

Some advantages for external evaluators include perceived or real impartiality, and less hesitance than an internal evaluator might feel to criticize an intervention. These factors may lead to an external evaluator's being more likely (or at least being perceived as such) to bring perceived objectivity and therefore greater credibility to the evaluation. (Please consider rereading Chapter 5, which includes a discussion of subjectivity, objectivity, bias, and credibility, before continuing.) Whereas some view in-depth knowledge about a program as an advantage for an internal evaluator, others view not being familiar with the program as encouraging more in-depth questions, a broader search for data, and new perspectives and insights during data analysis. While sometimes external evaluators are viewed as more threatening (because of the perception that "outsiders are here to judge"), they could also be perceived as more trustworthy and neutral, as they are not caught up in office politics. Finally, external evaluators are hired to implement an evaluation, and not to carry out multiple other simultaneous roles. Yet we should note that while an external evaluator may only carry out that one evaluation role for that organization, many external evaluators also conduct more than one evaluation or evaluative process at a time (though not always).

Have you ever been an external evaluator? If so, did you like it?

I am now an external evaluator. I delight in having 7–10 different evaluation processes each year, often in different sectors and different countries. This means that I must draw on, mix, and continually learn (or update my knowledge on) different evaluation approaches and evaluative processes. This keeps me on my toes. I constantly expand my evaluation knowledge and skills, with the bonus of learning about new topics and, at times, new sectors. The challenges include balancing my time among the projects, working with different teams I have never met before, meeting the often-changing demands of so many different clients, and probably never interacting again with the many people I meet through the evaluation process with whom I have formed professional friendships. (There are a few instances in which *not* interacting with someone again may be an advantage, but these are rare.) Being an external evaluator can also look very different from my own approach, such as taking on fewer evaluations, only working in one sector, or balancing teaching at a university with conducting one longer-term evaluation. An external evaluator can have longer-term projects that last for years, or short-term ones that last a day (e.g., a theory-of-change workshop) or a week (e.g., an evaluation that must be brief because of limited funding or is naturally brief due to a small scope).

This discussion provides broad generalizations that offer an inkling of the kinds of factors to be considered, while my personal experiences offer quite particular ones. And I should also note that a person may be a specialist who is an internal evaluator, or a generalist who is an external evaluator; these pairings match rather well. Before we leave the discussion, let's look at some choices that are not as well known.

AN EVALUATOR'S ROLE IN SOME NOT-SO-COMMON POSITIONS

Roles related to evaluation, but not directly to being an evaluator, can strengthen an evaluator's skills and knowledge. Benita Williams, an experienced South African evaluator and former national SAMEA and AFREA board member, talks about roles that are not often associated with being an evaluator, yet have strengthened her as an evaluator. We have met Benita in Chapter 5, where she has provided sage advice on quantitative methods of inquiry. Benita has shared this with me:

> "I find that being in nonevaluation roles related to evaluation has served me quite well as an evaluator. If you sometimes do technical assistance where you help an organization select evaluators by being part of a proposal review committee, you have a better idea how to pitch evaluations. Similarly, if you have been an implementer of an evaluated program, or a beneficiary of an evaluated program, you are likely to better know how to collect data or relate your evaluation approaches or findings. I find that [to be] true of the knowledge management role as well. Being on the other side, so to speak, is a very valuable role, and a way to enhance your skills when you go back to practicing evaluation."

Other experiences in which an evaluator is not actually doing evaluation, yet is strengthening evaluation skills, include being a peer reviewer of evaluation methodologies and evaluation journal articles; a metaevaluator, who conducts a structured review of evaluation reports; an advisor to evaluation processes (e.g., through being part of a steering committee); or the manager of an evaluation. These experiences provide different perspectives for understanding evaluation than an evaluator would otherwise have as an evaluator *doing* evaluation. Thus, though most of these are often opportunities that happen as a person gains evaluation experience, they are evaluation roles that could (and should) be considered as part of an evaluator's pathway, whether they are short term, part time, or even full time. If you are in a more structured monitoring or evaluation role at present, some of these offer ways to expand your horizons, bolster your current work, or redirect your evaluation path.

Thus far in our evaluative journey, we (you and I, remember, we are on this journey together) have covered numerous roles, positions, and identities for an evaluator. All this is a lot to think about. Where you work, what knowledge and skill sets you have, what you like to do, and/or what you are assigned to do will influence the kind of evaluator you are. Yet there is another huge influence that will inform how you identify, or who you are, as an evaluator. Let's talk about that intriguing topic next: an evaluation and an evaluator's role in society.

Exploring Evaluation's and an Evaluator's Roles in Society

Engaging with the question of how you view evaluation's and an evaluator's roles in society will require some deep reflection and heavy thinking. Your answer will influence all kinds of things—from what you perceive to be useful evaluation, to what roles you expect an evaluator to fill, to the kind of evaluation you are comfortable implementing, to (as you have read in earlier sections) how you categorize the purpose of evaluation. So how do you view an evaluator's (and evaluation's) roles in society?

Some people strongly view evaluators as agents of social change. Others, more passive in their views, suggest that evaluators contribute to change in society. In other words, some people think that evaluators should only contribute to social change through providing information or knowledge for *others* to make program or policy decisions that lead to social change, while some believe that evaluators themselves should play a more active role with that knowledge. Some evaluators do not even think that evaluation is necessarily about social change at all. Let's look at all this a bit more concretely.

An evaluator could dedicate her life to conducting evaluative processes and evaluations to directly improve services to the poor, the marginalized, or the silenced. Or an evaluator could play a more removed role and provide information to a large international funder or a national government, thereby informing decision makers through evaluation. Or an evaluator could work for local government and provide small bits of incremental information that slowly, over time, inform decisions that bring about social change in that vicinity. Or an evaluator who does not view evaluation as a vehicle for social change could see the evaluator's role as one that is about accountability, performance management, or assessing an intervention against standards or benchmarks.

A critical part of being an evaluator is deciding how you will (or would like to) position yourself in the field. It is a tough decision, and thus I provide two thought-provoking questions to consider:

1. What role should *evaluation* play in society, if any?

2. Through being an *evaluator*, do you want to play a role in social change? If so, how? If not, what makes you say that?

You may want to keep these questions spinning in your brain until you finish reading this book, or perhaps engage with them now and see if you have the same thinking after you have completed reading the book.

What do you believe about evaluation's role in society?

I believe that evaluation should contribute to a better society, but not all evaluators agree with that sentiment. It is not that I am right and they are wrong. Rather, we just think very differently. And accepting and valuing other ways of thinking constitute an important part of being an evaluator, and are critical to our world. I try to choose evaluations and evaluative processes that enable me to play at least a small part in supporting social change. For instance, I try to select evaluations focusing on interventions that aim to improve or provide new services to the disadvantaged, the voiceless, and the disempowered. However, because my family is dependent on the income I generate through being an evaluator, sometimes I take on evaluations that are not aimed at social change. In these situations, I actively seek ways to educate, facilitate, or bring some value or learning to the people with whom I engage; these could be the people who implement the intervention, their beneficiaries, or even the donors or funders themselves (see my next response). Nonetheless, I conduct evaluation that aims to support social change when I can because of how I view my role as an evaluator and the role of evaluation in society. Thus how you view your role as an evaluator will influence (to the extent it can, in practical terms) the kinds of evaluation in which you choose to be involved.

I like the idea of the social change role for an evaluator. However, I am in a role where I do accountability evaluations on grantees, and then the report goes to my boss and stays there. I want to do more than just report to my boss; I want to ensure that evaluation is useful to people in the intervention. How can I do that?

Process use is an approach to evaluation in which the evaluator uses the evaluation process to bring about learning, change, or some type of benefit to those involved in the process; it encourages evaluative thinking (Amo & Cousins, 2007; Patton, 2008; Podems, 2007; Shaw & Campbell, 2014). By now, you know that evaluation terms have multiple meanings, so it should be no surprise that the word *process* is also used to describe a type of evaluation, **process evaluation,** which essentially means assessing how a program is being implemented and the services it delivers. We'll talk about process evaluation in Chapter 15. For now, let's explore a bit more about process use.

As an evaluator, if you so choose, you can ensure innovatively, thoughtfully, and often at little to no cost to the evaluation (in time or money) that learning takes place during the evaluation. While process use can be planned and budgeted for, I am going to speak about the kinds of process use that are more common: the unplanned and unbudgeted ones.

No matter what role you are currently in, there are ways to ensure process use. For example, take a few minutes to explain and answer questions about an evaluation process for beneficiaries or your colleagues. Discuss alternative evaluation designs with the funder, and demonstrate how different approaches are likely to yield different insights. Think through the theory of change with the implementers and beneficiaries, even when doing so is not a part of the intended (e.g., paid) process. Sometimes the evaluation report will be shelved because it is a check box (tick box) evaluation, meaning that it must be done but few people (if any) are interested in what it says (despite an evaluator's best efforts). It is in these kinds of instances where the *evaluator* benefits the most from process use—knowing that despite the fact that the evaluation is being shelved, the evaluator's time and efforts are benefitting someone, somehow. It is a selfish reason, I know.

> ### BOX 11.2. Check Box/Tick Box Evaluations
>
> "Check box" (in U.S. English) or "tick box" (in U.K. English) is evaluator slang for an evaluation that is *only* being done because someone has required an evaluation. It is evident from the start that the evaluation itself is highly unlikely to be used, despite the best efforts of the evaluator. Rather, a manager or other person in charge can "check off" or "tick off" that an evaluation took place.

How does someone ensure that an evaluator incorporates process use when it is not a formal part of the evaluation?

It is rare that someone will check to see if an evaluator did, or did not, bring process use to bear in an evaluation. In more than 20 years of my doing evaluation and drawing on process use, not one person has ever asked me about it when it was not part of the evaluation design. No one has paid me more during an evaluation for doing it. What then, if anything, should motivate an evaluator to ensure process use? *What do you think?*

An emerging evaluator was one of the reviewers of this book, and when she read this question she responded in the margin:

> I think this speaks a lot to integrity and one's real desire for social change. I often feel that, as an external evaluator, influencing those in charge of programs through the process of the evaluation is the closest I can get to influencing 'real change,' particularly in tick box evaluations.

She then went on to ask, "How does an evaluator know that process use has made a difference? If there is no way of knowing, is process use something that an evaluator does because she hopes in some way something will catch on?"

The examples provided demonstrate immediate observed use, a person's understanding, a dialogue that would have otherwise never taken place, and/or use of the evaluation process to bring together beneficiaries who never or rarely engage. This kind of immediate use, no matter how small, is worth any extra effort to me, even if it does not have (or I cannot prove) lingering effects. It is enough for me to observe immediate effects and hope for the lingering ones. The benefits of process use may be evident when an evaluator is internal to an organization, or is engaged in repeated or longer-term relationships with an intervention or its organization.

Process Use: Making the Process Useful

- **Have a few minutes?** Read J. Bradley Cousins's (2007) editor's notes in "Process Use in Theory, Research, and Practice," in an issue of *New Directions in Evaluation (NDE)*, Volume 2007, Issue 116, pp. 1–4.

- **Have 90 minutes?** Read Jessica Shaw and Rebecca Campbell's 2014 article "The 'Process' of Process Use," in the *American Journal of Evaluation*, Volume 35, Issue 2, pp. 250–260.

- **Have a few hours?** Read the whole *NDE* journal mentioned above, "Process Use in Theory, Research, and Practice," which provides various examples of process use.

Your journey to becoming an accomplished and happy evaluator will probably not start with a clear vision or pathway (though it could). Often it is only through trying out different types of evaluation roles that a person begins to identify what they like to do or do not want to do—and, more importantly, where the person's strengths lie. Even if you cannot change what you do right now, it is a good time to start thinking about questions such as these: What do you want to spend most of your days doing, and what kinds of people do you want to work with? Do you enjoy facilitating processes with community groups? Would you rather spend time designing evaluation instruments or crunching data? Do you have a passion for children's health or perhaps gender issues? Do you delight in working with big data sets, or revel in exploring words and meanings of single cases? Do you like working with government, donors, or foundations, or interacting with smaller nonprofits, or perhaps all of the above? Do you prefer to manage evaluators? Do you like being a part of an organization? Some evaluation roles are likely to resonate more strongly with your values, experiences, and personality. Set your course and begin to navigate your path. You may veer off that path, and this is OK—as it may open a door that you never knew existed and launch you into new adventures, or it may identify what you do not want to do again, ever.

So now that we have learned about the plethora of roles that an evaluator can fill, and are contemplating the role of evaluation and an evaluator in society, let's talk about four ways to get started, or continue, on your evaluation journey.

Listening

Attend an evaluation conference and go to every session on the topics that interest you. Speak to the presenters. If you cannot attend a conference, you have several alternatives. Sometimes conferences are streamed for free or at a greatly reduced price, or segments can be found on You-Tube. Often associations post papers and presentations on their websites after a conference. After listening to some speakers who resonate with you, or who make you think, "Yes, that is the type of evaluation I want to do," or "Wow, I need to learn more about that," watch their presentations online, and/or read their articles and/or books. In the bibliographies of their articles and books, see which writers *they* read, and read those articles. This overlaps with my next suggestion.

Reading

Start reading. There are hundreds of websites, books, blogs, journals, and other written materials available. Each topic discussed in this book has various reading and listening suggestions. One caution: Be wary of what you search for online and which websites you land on. Several websites and books are mentioned in this book, which can get you started.

Formal Learning

Courses are provided online, through universities and evaluation institutes, and often at the beginning or end of an evaluation conference. Courses vary in length from a half day, to several months, to a semester (4–5 months), or more. Universities often have evaluation courses buried within different disciplines, so explore education, psychology, development studies, international studies, social work, and public management as places to start looking within universities for their evaluation courses. Some universities have winter or summer schools that focus on evaluation. Contact a university, or an evaluation society or association, near you and ask. Another alternative is to ask conference presenters where they went to school, where they teach, or what courses or universities they recommend.

Shadowing

Ask a colleague who does this kind of work, or a friend who knows a friend (networking), to identify someone you can shadow through an evaluative process. This may also lead to finding a mentor, which has been an invaluable part of my own growth as an evaluator.

Is there some hard line or distinction between who is, and who is not, an evaluator?

Chapter 2 has provided a long discussion of the differences between an evaluator and a researcher. The question you ask here is slightly different. Discussing who is, and who is not, an evaluator is a contentious conversation. With that caution, let's dive into the murky waters of the skills and knowledge needed to be an evaluator. Many evaluation societies, international organizations, governments, and private companies list what *they* consider to be necessary competencies, knowledge, and/or skill areas for evaluators. These lists often reflect a mixture of a society's or organization's values, culture, power, and politics, and show how evaluation is perceived within that society or organization. Being familiar with the different evaluator competencies can provide useful guidance. Next, I present just a few of those sets.

BOX 11.3. Competency and Competence

The term **competencies** refers to specific knowledge and skills, while **competence** is a person's ability to do what is needed in a situation, skillfully and appropriately (Wilcox & King, 2014).

Who Is Considered an Evaluator, and Who Is Not?

There is no unanimous agreement on who is, and who is not, an evaluator. Where you live, and who you work for, are good places to begin to understand how to answer the question within your context. If you work for a specific agency or organization, investigate if this group has a list of evaluator competencies or other guidance on who is considered an evaluator. Different organizations and different evaluation societies and associations define a competent evaluator differently, and some do not define one at all. Consult your local or national evaluation organization, *and* look at other national and international evaluation societies and associations, for guidance. These evaluation organizations are called **voluntary organizations of professional evaluators** (VOPEs). Different countries and evaluation associations have defined competencies in different ways (and do not always call them *competencies*), and sometimes offer dissimilar guidance. Some of the lists offer nearly identical suggestions on what an evaluator needs to bring to the table, so to speak; some overlap in some ways; and others have very nuanced or explicit differences. What does it all mean? There are various understandings of who is an evaluator, depending on where you live and for whom you work. Understanding these different viewpoints is important, as your own path to being an evaluator may involve different knowledge and skills than someone else's may.

Five evaluation societies that can provide some insights into the skills and knowledge needed to be an evaluator are listed below. There are many more organizations generating competency lists even as I write this book, so consider these five as your jumping-off point.

- **Canadian Evaluation Society** (CES; *https://evaluationcanada.ca*). The CES Credentialed Evaluator (CE) designation is designed to support professionalization efforts by defining, recognizing, and promoting the practice of ethical, high-quality, and competent evaluation in Canada. It is based on a set of competencies developed by Stevahn and colleagues. To view these initial competencies, take a look at the article "Establishing Essential Competencies for Program Evaluators" in the *American Journal of Evaluation* (Stevahn, King, Ghere, & Minnema, 2005).

- **European Evaluation Society** (EES; *www.europeanevaluation.org*). The EES has an Evaluation Capabilities Framework that includes three thematic areas: evaluation knowledge, professional practice, and dispositions and attitudes. To strengthen evaluators, they have piloted what is called Voluntary Evaluator Peer Review (VEPR). They describe VEPR as " . . . professional development and accountability concept based on reflective practice and peer review systems."

- **UK Evaluation Society** (UKES; *www.evaluation.org.uk*). The UKES has an Evaluation Capabilities Framework that includes three thematic areas: evaluation knowledge, professional practice, and qualities and dispositions. UKES is also piloting VEPR, which they describe as a " . . . voluntary structured professional practice review."

- **Aotearoa New Zealand Evaluation Association** (ANZEA; *www.anzea.org.nz*). The ANZEA developed evaluator competencies in 2011 and have since moved forward with professionalization by (1) providing evaluators with a self-review tool and professional development guide; (2) supporting the development of employment criteria for evaluator roles; and (3) providing guidance to evaluation trainers, teachers, and tertiary institutions. Insights from this organization can be summed up in two words: *collaboration* and *culture.*

- **American Evaluation Association** (AEA; *www.eval.org*). The AEA Board approved evaluator competencies in 2018. The association also provides Guiding Principles for Evaluators and a Statement on Cultural Competence in Evaluation.

That is a lot of mixed guidance. I hire evaluators. If someone claims to be an evaluator, how would I know? What questions can I ask that will help me determine if a person is, or is not, an evaluator?

When I meet someone who self-identifies as an evaluator, I ask a few conversational questions. I ask them about their favorite theorists. And I ask them what other theories or approaches they like, and what makes them say that. I ask how they value their findings. I ask them what the difference is between an evaluator and a researcher, and what type of inquiry they most often use. I ask them how they distinguish between an outcome and an impact. I ask them about their last evaluation experience. I ask what evaluation associations or societies they belong to, and/or if they have ever presented at the conferences, or published. I ask them how they view evaluation's role in society, and how they perceive their role as an evaluator. If the person can thoughtfully engage in conversation on these topics (*Note:* I did not say "agree with me on these topics" that ask for an opinion) and explain what is an evaluable and plausible program (which for me is a core competency and covered in Chapters 3–10), then I consider this person an evaluator. But these are just the informal criteria I use.

Can I get a degree in evaluation? And if I can, does that make me an evaluator?

There are many university programs at the graduate level that train evaluators. Because there are no universally agreed-upon competencies for evaluators, the graduate training courses vary around the world. Being an evaluator means more than having theoretical knowledge, though having theoretical knowledge provided by a recognized evaluation program (which may also provide some skills) provides a solid foundation for being an evaluator. In addition to a degree, an evaluator needs to practice evaluation and think like an evaluator, which is a core message in this book. Essentially, though, because there is no definitive answer to the question of who is/is not an evaluator, the jury is still out on your question.

Can I be a professional evaluator?

You can be a professional who practices evaluation. Evaluation is not (yet) a profession, at least not in the sense that one *needs* a license or specific degree to practice it. Evaluation has emerged as a formal field of practice. It has its own books, journals, awards, associations, and conferences. Since the late 1980s, evaluation associations and societies have been exploring ways to enhance professionalism in evaluation through the development of practice standards, ethical guidelines, and (more recently) frameworks to identify the knowledge base, skills, and capabilities required for high-quality evaluation. Globally in the past 60 years, there have been significant changes with regard to demand for evaluation and formal recognition of the field (Donaldson & Lipsey, 2006; Podems & King, 2014; Rugh & Segone, 2013; Wilcox & King, 2014):

- Significant growth in regional, national, and international evaluation associations and societies around the world, suggesting an increase of people interested in program evaluation.
- The International Year of Evaluation in 2015, which celebrated the practice of evaluation globally, and aimed to strengthen the demand for, and use of, evaluation.
- The increase in the published evaluation literature (Picciotto, 2011; Quesnel, 2010).
- The increase in universities offering specialized courses on evaluation (Podems & King, 2014).

Since the 1970s, there have been multiple debates in the evaluation literature about whether evaluation should become more formally professionalized, or indeed whether it is already a profession (Worthen, 1994). Some have argued that evaluation is a professionalized practice (Schwandt, 1997), a discipline (Scriven, 1991), or a field (Podems & King, 2014). These debates continue (Jacob & Boisvert, 2010; King & Stevahn, 2015; Podems & King, 2014), with no consensus on whether evaluation is a profession or, if not, whether it should be.

WRAPPING UP

An evaluation career path can be a bit mind-boggling, with so many evaluation roles to choose from (if, indeed, you have a choice), as well as the lack of clear agreement on who is, and who is not, an evaluator. This chapter has aimed to provide some guidance. In the chapter, we have first looked at a list of roles, and then explored them by evaluation purpose. We have then considered how people may lean more toward one type of evaluation or another, based on what they prefer to do. Then we have had to acknowledge that no matter how hard we try, concretely describing what an evaluator does, and capturing the essence of an evaluator, are slippery tasks. Finally, we have questioned the meaning of evaluation, and that of an evaluator's role, in society. These are questions that you are perhaps still contemplating.

Values seem to bubble to the surface everywhere in this book, and it is no different in this chapter. The next chapter discusses how values influence you, and every part of the evaluations that you conduct. Before you move on to learn more about values, however, come have a conversation with me.

 ### *Our Conversation: Between You and Me*

The chapter provides a wealth of information that can be used for reflection. To better support that reflection process, I ask two questions and suggest two activities that aim to inform your contemplation about the kind of evaluator you want to be.

1. *Question: What kind of evaluator are you—and what kind do you want to be?* Of all the roles suggested in the chapter, which ones resonate with you the most? Which hold no interest for you, and would thus be better filled by a knowledgeable other?

2. *Question: How would you answer the question of what an evaluator does?* If you were sitting next to a person on an airplane or train, or in a coffee shop, and they asked you what you do or what an evaluator does, what would you say? How would you describe the essence of an evaluator? Explaining what an evaluator does, and capturing the heart of what one is, is tougher than it sounds—at least for me.

3. *Action: Find an evaluation association or society.* Research it. Attend a conference. Join the association. Speak to members. Present a paper at their conference. Become active in the association or society by volunteering for committees or task forces. If you already belong to an association or society, consider researching and joining another one, which may bring different networks and perspectives.

4. *Action: Compare yourself against one or more competency sets that resonate with you. Or have a colleague or mentor assess you according to a chosen set of standards and criteria.* Then reflect on your self-assessment or the assessment the other person has completed. Which competencies do you have? Which ones do you wish you had? Which ones do you have, but need to improve? Based on that assessment, develop a plan and choose a path for self-development. For example, select one competency area and endeavor to read one journal article or book chapter a month, and actively seek evaluation opportunities where you can practice.

What about a conversation with me, the nonevaluator who needs to hire evaluators?

I did not mean to leave you out. Sorry. If your organization is looking to hire an evaluator, how do you know if someone is an evaluator? That question is still a bit of a conundrum. Refer back to my answer to your earlier question, where I suggest various things to ask someone to determine if they are an evaluator. I might also ask: Does the person have any formal training in evaluation, and if so, from what institution or VOPE? Does the person belong to an evaluation society or association? (Caution: Being a member of an evaluation society or association does not make someone an evaluator; one can become a member of most of these groups just by paying the annual fee.) If you live in a country that has credentialing (e.g., Canada) or some way to assess evaluators (e.g., Japan), check to see if the person has been through that process. If not, ask: Has the person published in peer-reviewed journals or books? Do they present at conferences? Do they have a track record of implementing evaluations? Ask them how they would establish criteria to value an evaluation. Determining if someone has the skills and knowledge that will result in a credible evaluation, and in some cases whether the evaluator brings appropriate values to the evaluation, is a process that deserves a good discussion—not just a review of someone's curriculum vitae.

CHAPTER 12

Thinking about Values

I have a friend from my university days, Leslie, whose mom passed away. A few weeks after the funeral, she and her siblings went through her mom's household goods to figure out what to keep, what to give to charity, and what to sell. There were many valuable objects (i.e., things that were genuinely worth a lot of money) in the house, and the siblings easily agreed on what to do with them. The only substantive argument arose when they were deciding what to do with an old, beaten-up spatula. They all had a strong attachment to that spatula, as it reminded each of them of their mom when she used to stand at the stove and flip pancakes or other food, which they all loved to watch her do. That spatula was the most valuable (and valued) object in the entire house not because of its monetary worth, but because of the sentimental value placed on it by the siblings.

We all value things in different ways, and what has value for one person (the spatula) may have no value at all to someone else (e.g., the spatula had no value to me). It is no different in evaluation. The values that people bring to the evaluative process—how people see and make sense of the world—are the tinted lenses that influence their views of the entire process. Although values play a major role in that *entire* evaluative process, it is often an implicit one. Nevertheless, values are so significant in the evaluative process that I have given them their own chapter.

Discussing the role of values (our own and others) in any evaluative process is often complicated, befuddling, and uncomfortable. It is awkward. It is knotty. It is sometimes silent. It is full of twists and turns. Your role as an evaluator is to engage, facilitate, and carefully negotiate the values discussion, as it informs everything from how the intervention was designed, to how the evaluation is done to how the intervention is determined to have succeeded or failed. Sometimes values are hidden in an evaluation approach or report, under the phrase *criteria for success*.

What Are Values?

Values are what someone views as important in life. They are contingent on how you were raised, and who raised you, how you were educated and where, and by the multiple influences you experience (such as the workplace, religious organizations, multimedia, and your community, to name a few). The terms *ethics, values,* and *morals* are often used interchangeably, so before moving ahead to focus on values, let's clarify the differences among the three.

Ethics, Values, and Morals: The Practical Differences

Sometimes in an evaluation, the question of **ethics** is discussed in close association with **values,** and this discussion then often raises the topic of **morals.** The term *ethics* describes a generally accepted set of moral principles, so it is broader than *morals*. Morals guide actions, and therefore determine whether actions are right or wrong. Values are what are important to people. Many evaluation associations and societies provide evaluation ethics to guide evaluation work, whereas most evaluation approaches are built on a specific (though sometimes very implicit) set of values. A common evaluation ethic, and one I always try to adhere to, is "I will do no harm." To be honest, I should modify that and say, "I will not knowingly do harm, and I will take it upon myself to be aware of how and to whom the evaluation process and evaluation findings may bring harm, and to minimize that harm to the best of my abilities." I make this modification because sometimes, in the real world, what benefits some may harm someone or something else. Although this chapter mainly focuses on values, I devote a special section to ethics at the end of the chapter.

Exploring Your Values

Given that evaluation is laden with values, it is critical to explore your own. Your values are informed by your parental figures, colleagues, peers, education, religion, experiences, and other factors. Being explicit about your values is critical to any evaluative process, as your values will influence how you act and what you do, and inform the evaluation approaches that you choose to guide you. In some evaluative processes, your values may be your main guide; at other times, you will be guided by the values of others (e.g., evaluation commissioner, evaluation user, beneficiaries), which may be the same or different; and in still other situations, the values used are a convoluted mix of both.

Exploring Your Values

Evaluators need to know what their own values are. If you want to explore your values, check out these two videos to get your thinking started.

- **Have 2 minutes?** Check out the video available at this link (*www.mindtools.com/pages/article/newTED_85.htm*), and if you have more time, read the accompanying short article on identifying your values.

- **Have 6 minutes?** Listen to Jason Howarth's TEDxCPP talk "Adding Value to Your Life" (*www.youtube.com/watch?v=crAtVz0EKmM*).

Considering that values are such a critical part of an evaluative process, I find it a bit odd that I am rarely asked about mine when someone considers hiring me. Because I write on feminist evaluation (among other thematic areas), every once in a blue moon I am hired because of having made these values explicit, and sometimes I am not hired for the very same reason. When I apply for evaluation positions, I am normally asked about my research skills (and sometimes only that; please see Chapter 2 for that discussion), about my past experience, and sometimes about how I would conduct the evaluation with regard to steps or phases. Although these answers might provide some insight into my values, values are not formally or explicitly addressed. Among the first questions that I would ask if I were hiring someone to help improve or judge my intervention would be "What are your values, and how will you establish criteria to value the intervention? For example, what valuing process will you put in place?" Or, if values have already been established for these criteria, I would then ask the evaluator how she would engage with them throughout the evaluative process.

Where to Find Values to Inform the Evaluative Process

Quick, look over your shoulder. All clear? Then keep reading; I have another well-kept trade secret that I want to tell you. Most often, by the time an evaluation begins, many of the values that are needed to evaluate the intervention are determined; they are just "hidden in plain sight." Contrary to popular belief, values are usually not new to the evaluation discussion when the question of how to judge an intervention (i.e., merit, value, or significance) enters the conversation. What do I mean by that, you may ask? While evaluation is value-laden, so are the very interventions being evaluated. Values are infused before an evaluator enters the equation; the decisions even to conduct the intervention, and to provide resources to it, are value-laden.

Thus values are infused in everything relevant to an evaluation. Here are six places to start looking for values that can be used to inform (1) the selection of an evaluation approach, (2) the evaluation design, and (3) the criteria used to value the intervention.

- *The intervention itself.* This includes the decision to conduct the intervention (problem statement), how it was designed, by whom, for whom, where it was implemented, the resources it receives, who has implemented it, and its intended results.
- *The implementer.* The implementation organization's values. Whether it be government departments, foundations, donors, for-profits, or nonprofits, values exist.
- *Beneficiaries and un-beneficiaries.* The beneficiaries (the people who receive the services, or otherwise benefit from the intervention in some way) bring critical values; after all, the intervention is for them. Then the values of the un-beneficiaries (see Chapter 3) must also be considered.
- *The commissioner.* The decision to have an evaluation is laden with values. At the same time, the group funding the evaluation brings a variety of values.
- *Evaluation users.* Often the main evaluation users hold the most critical values for an evaluator to understand and engage with, though not always. Other, secondary users may also have values that influence the evaluation process. (For a broader discussion on stakeholders, see Chapter 3.)
- *The evaluator.* Although an evaluator is neutral (see Chapter 5), he does bring values into the process, which may be reflected in his choices for methods of inquiry, the evaluation approach, methods of data interpretation, means of facilitating the process, persons who are listened to, and recommendations made. If there is an evaluation team, its members present even more values (more people = more values).

Clearly, then, the evaluation's focus, questions, methods of inquiry, and data-gathering techniques, as well as what to look for and where to look, whom to interview or what to observe, how to assess the intervention's merit/worth/significance, how to draw conclusions and make recommendations (and with whom), and how (and with whom) to share the evaluation findings, are not merely technical issues; they are value-laden decisions.

BOX 12.1. Values

Values are often thought about in evaluation with regard to judging an intervention. However, values are present in the entire evaluative process. An evaluator needs to be aware of how, what, and whose values are wrapped up in every part of the evaluative process—from choosing to have an intervention, to choosing to evaluate it, to the evaluation itself, and all the decisions in between.

What happens when values are not explicitly discussed?

In one word? Often frustration, for some or everyone involved. Here's an example. Several years ago, I led a team conducting an evaluation of an economic program that aimed to increase trade in eastern Africa. The program's goal was this: "To improve people's lives through increasing regional trade." We implemented the third evaluation undertaken that year, with all evaluations bringing slightly different foci. Before you ask, I was an external evaluator who was only involved in the third evaluation, and so I do not know why the organization had so many evaluations. My team consisted of economists who crunched numbers and did all sorts of fancy modeling to determine trade deficits/surpluses and economic trends. The economists provided empirical, interesting, and useful information to answer most of the evaluation questions. However, several things were not clear: how the donor's interventions led to or aimed to increase trade, and for whom; how that would be valued beyond its monetary benefit, and by whom; and who or what was likely to be negatively affected, if anyone. In other words, how were people's lives improved?

I raised two thoughts with the evaluation's steering committee at two points in the evaluation process—the beginning (i.e., the design phase) and the end (the findings). The steering committee, which made all the decisions, consisted of six male non-African economists and one female secretary. I now share part of the story, which took place in the design phase.

During this early phase, I suggested that different people value results in different ways, and that the evaluation might provide more useful information if we could further understand who valued what, and how that influenced their lives and their economic situation. Thus I suggested that we look at other ways to determine success, beyond, for example, trade deficits. For instance, how would a woman trader at the border value any changes in her life because of the donor's program; did she benefit in any way? Or, because of the program, who would benefit, and who would be potentially negatively affected? Perhaps increased trade would cause damage to traders in a certain sector, or perhaps the environment would be negatively affected. My suggestion was met with cold, dead stares, and complete silence for what seemed an eternity. I was then lectured on economic modeling and trade, and told that I did not understand the intervention's purpose. Silly me! I had thought that "improving people's lives" was indeed part of the intervention's purpose. Although we did manage to look to some extent at who benefitted, through other parts of the evaluation design, the evaluation's resources did not permit understanding the questions of who valued what from a beneficiary's perspective, and who or what was not benefitting or negatively affected.

This vignette illustrates how a clash of values can lead to different interpretations of an intervention's stated purpose, which can then lead to different interpretations of what should be evaluated. Being aware what values, and whose values, underpin each decision (and knowing whose values trump whose) provides an excellent place to explore how to design and conduct what various users consider a credible evaluation. Read the story in Box 12.2, and explore how values infiltrate the Kingdom of Xanadu's intervention.

BOX 12.2. The Kingdom of Xanadu

In the Kingdom of Xanadu, there are three leaders. Each leader represents a separate constituency, and each has considerable money and power. Together, they rule Xanadu. After a recent board meeting, which focused on how to ensure a happy kingdom, the leaders agreed that resources needed to be invested to improve people's rights.

- The King of Aces decided to fund interventions that would provide the greatest good for the greatest number of people.
- The Queen of Hearts decided to use her resources to fund programs to improve equity, even if that meant supporting unequal distribution of resources, as long as it would help the least well off.
- The Jack of Diamonds decided to fund interventions that supported improving human rights, as long as the interventions did not infringe on other persons' legal, ethical, and moral rights.

Thus, while the three most powerful persons in Xanadu agreed on, and valued, improving people's rights, they each brought different values to realizing and understanding what it would mean to do that. An evaluation that sought to understand how, and to what extent, each leader's program would improve human rights would look for, and value, each intervention and its results differently because each program defined improving people's rights with different value systems. Imagine, however, that an evaluator was only told to assess each program on the basis of its ability to improve people's human rights. From whom would data be collected? What would be the criteria for success (i.e., whose values would be used to make judgments about the program)? Knowing whose values, and what values, have had what influence on the intervention design is critical to informing how an intervention should be judged for both its quality and its value. That is not to say that other values cannot be brought in (and in some cases that might be beneficial, while in other cases it would be perceived as unfair).

Understanding the array of values that influence interventions and evaluations also provides insights into why evaluations can be complicated, stressful, accepted, useful, appreciated, contested, or simply dismissed. In addition, being aware of how extensive the infiltration of values is in the evaluative process will help you to mitigate the inevitable bumps and bruises that often find their way into one. Given the important role that values play in each part of the evaluation process, let's stop and take a closer look at values through a practical activity.

ACTIVITY 12.1. An Exercise on Value and Valuing

Purpose: To demonstrate how we use our values to make a judgment, and how quickly we often make them.

Materials: You will need a picture (printed or drawn on flip chart paper) of a boy running from a shop, with bananas (or any fruit or piece of food) in his hand. You will also need several simple scenarios written on smaller pieces of paper, each explaining a little "story" giving one set of reasons why the boy is stealing the bananas. Here are some examples: he is a well-off kid who enjoys tormenting the immigrant shopkeeper;

he is a boy who is very poor and is trying to get food for his sick sister; he is just having fun; he has been dared to do it by his friends. Each of these pieces of paper can be placed in its own envelope, or each can be folded over and closed with a piece of tape, so the groups cannot see what is written on them.

Time: You will need about 10 minutes for individual group discussion, 5 minutes for initial feedback (assuming that there are three groups of four or five people), and then 10–20 minutes for large-group discussion. Total approximate time: 25–35 minutes.

The activity: Divide the room into groups of four or five people. Show the picture of the boy running from the shop with the bananas in his hand. Then provide a sealed envelope to each group; do not let the group members share what is inside with other groups. After each group opens its envelope and reads the "back story," ask the members to discuss these two questions within their group:

1. Is it OK that this boy is stealing the bananas? (And is stealing ever seen as justified?)

2. If the boy is caught, what should happen to the boy?

Provide these rules: The answer to Question 1 must be "Yes" or "No." The answer to the second question may be a few sentences long, but no longer. The answers are to be written down. Allow for several minutes of small-group discussion. Then have one person from each group share the group's answers to Questions 1 and 2. However, the person *must not* share what was written on the envelope the group was given, or read anything more than what the group has written down as the responses to the two questions. After all groups have given their answers to Questions 1 and 2, *then* allow a member of each group to explain that group's circumstances for the boy and provide the group's reasons. The challenge for you as the facilitator is to help the participants have a discussion without a heated argument, and yet constantly to point out how context and their own personal values influence their understanding of the situation and what they consider fair consequences.

Critical learning points: Values are often buried; they can be hard to bring to the surface and make clear. The aim is for the participants to learn how context matters, how people's interpretations of that context are based on their values, and that an evaluator needs to engage in a process to understand these values. The values and understanding of context are then used to inform an evaluation design and to provide the criteria for valuing the intervention.

THE EVALUATOR'S ROLE IN IDENTIFYING AND APPLYING CRITERIA TO VALUE AN INTERVENTION

An evaluator uses values to inform decisions on how to conduct an evaluation, and to determine an intervention's success. The evaluator can have two roles in the valuing process: He can (1) *apply* criteria to value an intervention, or (2) *facilitate* others in applying criteria to value an intervention. Furthermore, an evaluator can work with two kinds of values. He can apply **organic values,** which are values that stem from the beneficiaries, program implementers, or others involved directly with the program. Or he can apply **external values,** which are values developed by persons or groups external to the intervention. For example, these external values may emanate from global or academic thinking on poverty, education, or the environment; they may be the commissioner's valuing criteria; or they may be the

TABLE 12.1. Valuing an Intervention: Organic versus External Valuing

Evaluator	Organic valuing	External valuing
Facilitation role	Evaluator identifies valuing criteria from beneficiaries or others touched by the program, and facilitates them in valuing the intervention.	Evaluator provides external valuing criteria to beneficiaries or others touched by the program, and facilitates them in valuing the intervention.
Expert role	Evaluator identifies valuing criteria from beneficiaries or others touched by the program, and applies those criteria to value the intervention.	Evaluator uses external valuing criteria to value the intervention.

evaluator's own valuing criteria, grounded in his experience and the relevant literature (e.g., on education, health, community safety, or environment programs). See Table 12.1 for a comparison of organic and external valuing. At times, though more rarely, he may use both.

Organic Values

Let me start this section by noting that organic values may be explicit. Indeed, organizations or beneficiaries may have an overt, clearly stated set of values that are unmistakably used to develop, manage, and assess the intervention. Ask if these exist. In my experience, it is more common that while organic values do exist, they are often implicit. We (you and I, the evaluators) need to make them explicit, as organic values should (though they may not; see the next section on external values and Chapter 13's discussion on politics and power) constitute an invaluable part of the entire evaluative process. How do we make them explicit? Unfortunately, asking a straightforward question such as "So tell me, what do you value?" does not often result in a straightforward answer; it is a complicated question. To unearth values, an evaluator can ask, for example, program managers, implementers, and beneficiaries of the program, the following thematic questions. These thematic questions should be followed up with an ample use of probes (e.g., "Can you tell me more?" or "What makes you say that?") that avoid the use of "why." (See Chapter 3 for an explanation on the challenges of asking "why.")

- Of all the *problems* that could have been addressed, what made [someone] choose this problem? Who sees it as a problem?
- These are the intended *results*. Who identified these results? Is one result more important than the others? To whom? If the intervention achieved only one result, or set of results, which one would you say is most important? Should some results be listed that are not?
- Tell me about the intervention's *design*. Were there other options? What made [someone] choose this design?

- The intervention aims to address these *beneficiaries* [name specific beneficiaries; see Chapter 3]. What made [someone] choose these beneficiaries? Who else, or what else, should benefit? Because these are the beneficiaries, who are possible un-beneficiaries? (*Note:* In some circumstances, the beneficiaries may have self-identified and developed their own intervention.)

- What does *success* look like? For whom?

When time is short, you can ask only the final question (i.e., What does success look like? For whom?), though it will be less illuminating. The decision to use a longer process (i.e., ask all the questions) will inform how the evaluation is done (e.g., how to do fieldwork) *and* how to value the intervention, whereas the shorter one-question approach (with probes) will only provide insight into how to value the intervention.

The work of E. Jane Davidson and her colleagues on **evaluative rubrics** is an inspiring and practical approach to answering the question of what success looks like and for whom. Davidson writes extensively about the rubric approach and demonstrates how, when well facilitated and properly developed, it is an approach that assesses quality by ensuring that the values, criteria, and evaluative reasoning used are explicit. When those criteria are developed with those who are implementing and/or receiving the service, the criteria reflect different people's perspectives about the quality and value of the intervention and its results (Davidson, 2005, 2012, 2014). Davidson (2010) explains:

> A useful tool for generating real evaluative conclusions is an *evaluative rubric*. This is a table describing what different levels of performance, value, or effectiveness 'look like' in terms of the mix of evidence on each criterion. Grading rubrics have been used for many years in student assessment. Evaluative rubrics make transparent how quality and value are defined and applied. I sometimes refer to rubrics as the antidote to both 'Rorschach inkblot' ("You work it out") and 'divine judgment' ("I looked upon it and saw that it was good")-type evaluations.

Davidson goes on to say that a clear understanding of not just *what* evidence to look at, but *how* to look at it, is what leads to strong evaluative conclusions. That is because the values and criteria used to assess the intervention, as well as the evaluative reasoning used to apply those values to the evidence, are made explicit with words that provide meaning, insight, and guidance with regard to what and how to value.

External Values

It is as common for external values to be implicit as they are to be explicit. Implicit values could be when an evaluator or commissioner brings his own values to bear on an evaluative process, yet does not overtly articulate them. Let me be clear: These values need to be clearly articulated for a fair and just evaluative process. At other times, the external values may be explicit, such as when an evaluator is required to use the donor, government, or commissioner's valuing framework. An example of an external valuing framework (also called *evaluation standards and criteria*) used to value interventions in developing countries is described next. These valuing criteria are often familiar to, and accessed by, evaluators all over the world.

The Organisation for Economic Co-operation and Development's (OECD) Development Assistance Committee (DAC) is a forum to discuss donor aid. Simply stated, *donor aid* is the provision of money and other resources by richer countries (also known as *developed countries*) to poorer countries (also known as *developing countries*). The OECD DAC framework for evaluating donor aid includes five standards or criteria for valuing interventions: *relevance, effectiveness, efficiency, impact,* and *sustainability.* Associated with each standard or criterion (value) are more specific criteria. These OECD DAC standards are not to be confused with the OECD DAC Evaluation Quality Standards, which are provided to assess the quality of an evaluation (these are discussed in Chapter 15). An organization that focuses on evaluating humanitarian interventions, called the Active Learning Network for Accountability and Performance (ALNAP), has added three further criteria for its context: *connectedness, coherence,* and *coverage* (see *www.alnap.org*).

In addition to the OECD DAC standards, other organizations, governments, and evaluation associations and societies have accepted standards for assessing the quality of an intervention, program, or policy. These standards are in line with their own inherent values (e.g., those of faith-based donors).

When you are conducting an evaluation, identify whether any of these standards and criteria have been or must be used to value the intervention. If so, interrogate those standards, explore how to apply them in the evaluation, and raise any potential issues with them (either before starting the evaluation, or as soon as they emerge during the evaluation), such as conflicting with the organic valuing framework.

So an evaluator does not necessarily use his own values to establish criteria to value something, and he can draw on other people's values or on valuing criteria developed by a government agency, foundation, or donor, for example. Can he use multiple ways to value in one evaluation?

An evaluator ensures that valuing happens and is explicit, and his intent is that the evaluation will be used. So he will need to consider whether using one set or multiple sets of criteria will lead to a more credible evaluation, and whose set(s) of valuing criteria should be used (to read about evaluation credibility, see Chapter 5). For example, he can apply two different external valuing frameworks (e.g., his own values and those provided by the commissioner), which may (or may not) provide two different perspectives. The evaluation user may find that helpful. Or the evaluator can facilitate the development of organic valuing criteria, and then the evaluator can also apply external criteria. Again, these different strategies are likely to provide very different insights, which may be useful to answer the evaluation questions, and provide a useful evaluation.

I have written this book to be used for guidance, reflection, and mentoring—which means that I need to describe real-world experiences, not write perfect textbook answers. So come just a little bit closer; I need to whisper one of evaluation's best-kept trade secrets in your ear. The power to decide what to value, and how to value it, does not always lie with the evaluator. Sometimes the commissioner assigns the role (e.g., you will use the commissioner's criteria to value that intervention); sometimes the program implementer decides (e.g., you will be told to use certain processes and involve certain people); and sometimes time or budget constraints heavily influence the decision. All this raises these questions: To what extent is it the evaluator's role to ensure that, in the valuing of the intervention, different perspectives are recognized, as needed? What happens when the evaluator is complicit in ignoring the voices of the most vulnerable or enforcing the role of the dominant? There is a lot of responsibility in being an evaluator, and evaluators need to be ready to engage with these situations, address them, and (sigh) sometimes just have the courage to acknowledge it.

Here is an example of a situation in which key stakeholders' values were completely overshadowed by the government's and donor's, which negatively affected the evaluation team's ability to conduct the evaluation. A health evaluation in a recently democratized country aimed to provide health benefits to the most marginalized population. However, the evaluation team was not given permission to visit the most marginalized population (for, as they were informed, reasons of safety). While the evaluation team aimed to understand how the beneficiaries valued the intervention, the team was never allowed to talk to them, and was instead asked to use monitoring data and then apply the external criteria to determine the intervention's success.

You mentioned that my values, as an evaluator, are part of the entire process. I thought I was supposed to be value-free?

An evaluator should be neutral—which means not accepting an evaluation assignment with a selfish reason or a strong opinion that influences their actions; in other words, an evaluator should not enter the evaluation process solely to make a point. An evaluator, however, may very well bring in empathy, which is connected to personal values (see Chapter 5 for more discussion of empathy and neutrality). Indeed, the evaluator's values are infused throughout an entire evaluation process, from deciding to do an evaluation (if it was a choice), to designing the approach and informing the questions, implementing data collection, analyzing data, and providing findings and recommendations and communicating them. The reality, however, is that the weight carried by an evaluator's values will fluctuate according to who holds the most power in the process, and to the evaluator's decision on how much their values should influence the process (which is itself a value).

Here is an example of how an evaluator's values influence the evaluative process. Let's say that an evaluator is asked to determine the effectiveness of an intervention (did it do what it said it would do?) that aims to improve farmworkers' knowledge with regard to safety with pesticides. The evaluator does not have an axe to grind, so to speak, about the intervention or the pesticides; she wants to answer the client's question and determine whether the intervention is achieving what it aimed to achieve. She values hearing underrepresented voices (i.e., the farmworkers) in the agriculture community to answer that question. The commissioner (who has requested and paid for, and will approve, the final report) is not particularly interested in hearing those voices; he wants to hear from the farmers. So the evaluator demonstrates how hearing these other perspectives will provide useful insights into the evaluation questions he posed. The commissioner still says no; he is not interested. The evaluator, at no extra cost to the commissioner, collects some insights from farmworkers regarding how they value the intervention, and what could be improved to make it more beneficial to them. In the formal report, she provides the findings and related recommendations as requested by the commissioner. Through an informal discussion, she illustrates how hearing the farmworkers' voices would have provided a different insight by sharing the additional information she collected. In doing so, she educates the commissioner on how hearing different perspectives could be valuable to his decision-making process in the future. Thus, in the evaluation, the evaluator is neutral—but her values have influenced the process to some extent. See the difference? That is, an evaluator's values may be overpowered in one way, but they can still be infused into the evaluation, as appropriate. (This is then an example of an evaluator's playing the roles of both a facilitator and an educator.)

But wait: What about the evaluation approach? Doesn't that more or less tell the evaluator what values to use?

That an evaluator practices, knows, or suggests certain approaches is likely to suggest her values. The evaluation approach itself may overtly suggest values, though the values are not always explicit. Some evaluation approaches are very "in your face" about values (e.g., feminist evaluation, democratic evaluation, empowerment evaluation), while in other approaches the values are a bit . . . muffled. For example, what values are explicit in Stufflebeam's (2007) context, input, process, product (CIPP) framework? Hmm. (See Chapter 15 for more details on evaluation approaches, models, and frameworks.)

Thus, while evaluation approaches, methods, and frameworks have values embedded in them, it is not always immediately clear what those values are. And even evaluation approaches that do engage explicitly with values do not often provide strategies for (1) how to uncover, understand, and use values that influence the intervention and related decisions; (2) how to engage with the values that come to the surface (or should come to the surface) during the evaluative process; or (3) how to make the criteria that are used to value an intervention explicit.

Yet exploring and engaging with values from different angles is the evaluator's responsibility. The evaluator needs to know whose values trump whose because ultimately a judgment will be made. (See the discussion in Chapter 11 of different kinds of judgment in the context of formative and summative evaluation.)

What challenges, if any, arise when the members of an evaluation team bring different values to the process?

Indeed, challenges can arise when evaluation team members have different values. How differing values are dealt with can either hinder or benefit an evaluation. For instance, arguments that stem from different value systems may arise in every part of the evaluation process. The team members may think they are having a purely logistical argument about visiting beneficiaries, when the underlying discussion involves how different team members value beneficiary perspectives. Or there may be disagreements on what the data mean, how to focus the report, or what recommendations to make, because the team members are viewing the evaluation through different value lenses. Although these disagreements or different viewpoints can hinder an evaluation process, they can also benefit it by bringing in different ways of thinking and alternative perspectives that deepen the analysis, enhance the interpretation of the findings, and strengthen the recommendations.

The leadership style of the evaluation leader (often called the **team leader**; this role is equivalent to the **principal investigator** position in a research project), the budget, logistics, and the time frame are all likely to influence how this process unfolds. While a well-facilitated conversation is likely to benefit the evaluation, at other times there will only be the bone-crushing reality of how values are realized in evaluative work.

VALUING

- **Have a few minutes?** Look at the website of your local or national evaluation association or society, or the organization with which you work. Identify if they have standards and criteria for valuing either an intervention or the evaluation of it.

- **Have 30 minutes?** Listen to a podcast with James Coyle and Kylie Hutchinson, featuring E. Jane Davidson on her evaluative rubric (*www.managingforimpact.org/resource/evaluation-rubrics-e-jane-davidson*).

- **Have an hour?** Take a look at Etienne Wenger, Beverly Traynor, and Maarten de Laat's guidance, "Promoting and Assessing Value Creation in Communities and Networks: A Conceptual Framework" (available at *http://wenger-trayner.com/resources/publications/evaluation-framework*).

- **Have a few hours?** Read the thoughts of Thomaz Chianca, an evaluator from Brazil, on the OECD DAC criteria, his suggested changes, and evaluation criteria in general in the *Journal of MultiDisciplinary Evaluation*, 5(9), 41–51.

- **Have more time?** Check out the extensive list of resources on valuing provided on the Better Evaluation website (*www.betterevaluation.org/en/search/site/evaluation%20criteria*).

EVALUATION ETHICS AND PRINCIPLES

Different organizations, governments, evaluation associations, and societies provide guidance on evaluation ethics and principles. The Australasian Evaluation Society (AES; 2013) guidelines include a useful overview that explains the reason for ethical guidelines: "Ethics refers to right and wrong in conduct. These guidelines for ethical behaviour and decision making in evaluation are intended to foster continuing improvement in the theory, practice and use of evaluation by stimulating awareness and discussion of ethical issues" (p. 2).

If you work with a specific organization or government, or belong to an evaluation association or society, find out what ethical guidelines exist. If you answer to more than one organization and must engage with diverse ethics or principles, engage with your client and the implementation organization (and anyone else that needs to be consulted) to decide which explicit ethical guidelines will be used for the evaluation. That explicit discussion and agreement will help you to facilitate an evaluation process that makes ethical decisions transparent, and one that is more likely to be (and to be viewed by others as) fair and just.

Different evaluation associations have articulated what is expected of members in regard to conducting ethical and high-quality evaluations. The AES (2013) *Guidelines for the Ethical Conduct of Evaluations* is divided into three categories of ethics: (1) commissioning and preparing for an evaluation, (2) conducting an evaluation, and (3) reporting the results of an evaluation. The American Evaluation Association (AEA; 2004) provides five guiding principles, summarized below:

A. *Systematic inquiry:* Evaluators conduct systematic, data-based inquiries.

B. *Competence:* Evaluators provide competent performance to stakeholders.

C. *Integrity/honesty:* Evaluators ensure the honesty and integrity of their own behavior and take responsibility for an ethical process.

D. *Respect for people:* Evaluators respect the security, dignity, and self-worth of all stakeholders with whom they interact.

E. *Responsibilities for general and public welfare:* Evaluators articulate and take into account the diversity of interests and values that may be related to the general and public welfare.

What if an evaluator is told to use certain ethics, and he is uncomfortable with the ethics used in the evaluation?

Although there are multiple options, here are three.

1. *Do not take the work.* If the ethical issues are apparent before the work starts, do not do the work. When I first started working as an evaluator, I was not aware that it was actually professionally acceptable to turn down work for that reason. It is. *It is perfectly acceptable to say no to an evaluation for ethical reasons.* For some evaluators, who are dependent on their evaluation income, this may not always be a feasible or easy choice. If the ethical or value issues becomes apparent after the evaluation has begun, refer to a contract, or discuss the situation with a human resource or contracts person, on how to ethically and legally disengage.

2. *Discuss and document all decisions.* As the evaluator, you can clarify the ethical issues as they arise with whoever needs to know (the issues and the need-to-know personnel will vary by evaluation), so that these issues are transparent to all involved. You should also explicitly describe these discussions in the evaluation report (or in an annex or appendix, though this is less likely to be read), and make it clear how the ethical decision influenced the evaluation. You can then describe other options or decisions that could have been made, and/or were suggested, based on different ethics. Documenting decisions provides needed transparency; it ensures that those who read the report understand how, and who, made ethical (and other) decisions in the evaluation process. My advice here is based on some hard-earned lessons. Sometimes, when I read my reports on evaluations where decisions were out of my control and/or where my ethics were compromised, I think, "If someone else read the evaluation report, how would they know that certain decisions were not mine, and that those are not my ethics?" Learn from my mistakes; make all ethical decisions (and for that matter, all decisions) transparent through conversations and documentation.

3. *Talk about it—ethically.* The third choice can be combined with the second, or this choice can stand alone. After an evaluation is concluded, you can reflect on the process alone or with others, to better understand what (if anything) could be done differently next time. You can use the reflection to inform your own work. You can also use it if you publish an account of the experience (removing any names or links to the actual process so that, ethically, people are protected), to ensure that others learn from the experience.

Although there are more possible choices than these, I hope that these suggestions will help you to brainstorm other ideas appropriate to your context.

What if there are no formal ethics? Are there any generic ethics?

That situation is extremely unlikely, as each evaluation is likely to be guided by the ethical guidelines of the commissioner's organization, the implementing organization, the local or national evaluation association, or others. While ethical guidelines will probably be influenced by contextual factors, below I provide six general guidelines that may be helpful to consider.

1. *Follow the three Belmont Principles.* Informed by monthly discussions that spanned nearly 4 years, as well as an intensive 4 days of deliberation in 1976, the National Commission for the Protection of Human Subjects of Biomedical and Behavioral Research published the Belmont Report, which identifies basic ethical principles and guidelines that address issues arising from the conduct of research with human subjects (see *www.hhs.gov/ohrp/ regulations-and-policy/belmont-report/index.html*). The three Belmont Principles—respect for persons, beneficence, and justice—provide guidance to evaluators. With regard to beneficence, two general rules are often considered: (a) do no harm and (b) maximize possible benefits and minimize possible harms. However, a wide array of procedures and practices support each principle, and evaluators should identify what those are for each context (Medical Advocates for Social Justice, n.d.).

During work in the field, the topic of an informed consent process is often discussed. The process will vary widely, depending on where and for whom you work. The guidelines provided by the Belmont Report for informed consent list three elements of an informed consent process: information, comprehension, and voluntariness (Human Subjects Office/ Institutional Review Board, University of Iowa, n.d.). How the process is carried out, whether or not a consent form needs to be signed, and other decisions will be guided by the context in which you work. It is your responsibility as an evaluator to know what these are and adhere to them.

2. *Respect the team members' safety and the safety of those with whom they engage.* For example, no data are worth obtaining at the risk of the evaluation team, or those engaged in the evaluation, including those from whom they seek information.

3. *Know administrative requirements.* Identify formal permissions that may be needed. For example, engaging with a local school, health clinic, or nature reserve may require national or regional permission.

4. *Give attention to sensitive issues.* Some topics may be extremely sensitive for some people, such as asking questions about sex, addictions, or other topics that are politics- or power-sensitive (e.g., sexual orientation, local political decisions). Think carefully about how to ask these questions, or if they even need to be asked. If they do need to be asked, consider when, where, and how to ask the questions (e.g., in safe spaces, using appropriate language, not linking the person in any way to the data-gathering process).

5. *Avoid causing hardships to participants or the organization.* Be mindful of what is asked of the people who manage or implement the intervention, those who receive services or benefits, or others, in terms of personal time or other costs, because of the evaluation or the evaluation team. If participants need special considerations, ensure that they are provided (e.g., interpreters, wheelchair access, visual aids, audio), and respect participants' time or other constraints, such as if they need to access public transport or have other responsibilities (e.g., school pickups, elderly care).

6. *Be culturally sensitive.* Recognize and honor how people interact, dress, and communicate. Be aware of and sensitive to gender relations, power roles, and other dynamics particular to the culture in which you are working. Some examples would be wearing appropriate clothing, understanding who can be interviewed by whom and where, what permissions are needed, what is off limits, what is offensive, what makes people uncomfortable (and comfortable), and what is expected in terms of an evaluative process. See Chapter 13 for resources on being a culturally responsive evaluator.

What happens if I find out something I did not intend to, and it's pretty sensitive information? What do I do with that "extra-sensitive" information?

A few years ago, I was evaluating a donor's scholarship program. Through this process, I accidentally uncovered information about the program's one and only medical doctor, who provided a negative experience for female candidates that all needed a health clearance from him. Although I did not doubt the few, similar reports I received from the women candidates, I could not interview the male doctor or observe any medical checkups. Plus, this information fell way outside the scope of my evaluation. A tricky situation, indeed. Regardless, I provided feedback to the program manager that some sensitive information had been uncovered (though not fully triangulated), which strongly indicated that offering female students the option to have a medical examination with a woman doctor should be something to strongly consider. The finding that women were being abused by the medical doctor, and the recommendation to suggest an alternative to the women, were in keeping with the well-established evaluation ethic of "do no harm." However, decisions like these are sensitive, ethical decisions that need to be based on *your* ethics and the ethics that you have agreed to abide by.

BIAS AND ETHICS

- **Have 45 minutes?** Look at the guidelines provided by the AEA (*www.eval.org/p/cm/ld/fid=51*) and the AES (*www.aes.asn.au/images/stories/files/membership/AES_Guidelines_web_v2.pdf*).

- **Have a few hours?** Select a few sections of Michael Morris's book *Evaluation Ethics for Best Practice: Cases and Commentaries* (2008).
- **Have a few more hours?** Read E. Jane Davidson's (2010) online article "'Process Values' and 'Deep Values' in Evaluation" (*http://journals.sfu.ca/jmde/index.php/jmde_1/article/view/262*).
- **Have a few days?** Read Ernest House's book *Evaluating: Values, Biases, and Practical Wisdom* (2015).
- **Have a few hours a night over severals weeks?** Read *Ethics in Social Science Research: Becoming Culturally Responsive* by Mariah Lahman (2018).

WRAPPING UP

Values permeate every decision about an intervention, and every step of any evaluative process. Engaging in a valuing discussion is not a process either to avoid or to conduct in haste. Knowing one's own values, and being explicit about them, are necessary prerequisites for any evaluator. Bringing other people's values to the surface, knowing and understanding values from various perspectives, and then participating in and negotiating discussions of those values during an evaluative process can take considerable patience, deep self-awareness, and strong facilitation skills. In any evaluation, how something (or anything) is valued needs to be transparent; yet an evaluator needs to engage with values that are infused throughout the entire process. In situations where external values are used with which to value the intervention, engaging in a values discussion is still necessary, as these values provide insight into, for example, decisions made about the evaluation approach and its criteria for success.

Values are often the translucent (or invisible) elephant in the room, and it is an evaluator's role to make them visible and engage with them throughout the entire evaluative process.

Evaluation societies and other organizations provide ethical guidelines and principles to guide an evaluator through an evaluative process, from informing the evaluator's own behavior to engaging with the behavior of others. It is the evaluator's role to facilitate a fair and just process. *As such, the challenge of how to engage with values and valuing, and to adhere to ethical and principled conduct, is the evaluator's burden.* Before you leave the chapter, come have a conversation with me.

Our Conversation: Between You and Me

Engaging with values can be a challenge to an evaluator and a commissioner of evaluations. Thus here I provide three pieces of advice. The first piece provides the chance to practice engaging in the values discussion; the second one encourages quiet contemplation; and the third one is directed at those who hire evaluators.

Talk to a Practicing Evaluator

Most practicing evaluators will regale you with multiple stories filled with dilemmas over issues related to values (and thus to power, ethics, politics, and language)—issues that influenced their evaluations. Ask them about how they engaged in these situations (or chose not to), and what advice they have for you.

Reflect on Your Values

Take a moment to reflect on your personal values as they might affect your practice of evaluation:

- What if you think that it is better to be kind than to be right? How would this personal value influence your actions as an evaluator? Can someone with these kinds of values be an effective evaluator?

- If someone asked you how your approach to evaluation reflects your values, what would you say? If a client asked you how your values will influence an evaluation, what would you say? How do your values influence the work you do, the methods you choose, or the approaches or processes that you find most useful? What would you do if your values were extremely different from the values of your client?

Ask about Values

When you are hiring an evaluator, talk about values. Describe the power structure, language, culture, and context in which the intervention was designed, and in which it is implemented. Encourage the evaluator to lead you through a process of how she would potentially engage in value discussions. Ask her how and what values, and whose, could influence the evaluation process and the judgment of its results.

CHAPTER 13

Thinking about Power, Politics, Culture, Language, and Context

Evaluation is so much more than methods of inquiry. When the evaluation conversation starts with methods of inquiry, I say, "Whoa. Stop. Hold your horses." While choosing methods of inquiry (and evaluation approaches) are certainly core parts of any evaluation discussion, evaluators also need to engage with other influences, as these can either positively inform the evaluative process or wreak havoc with it.

Psst. Over here. I have a tiny trade secret to share. Selecting appropriate methods of inquiry to answer the evaluation question is one of the easier parts of conducting an evaluation. Choosing an evaluation approach that matches the evaluation's purpose and context becomes a bit more challenging. Choosing a method of inquiry, evaluation approach, and explicit way to value that are technically, culturally, socially, and politically acceptable is even tougher. Paying attention to power and language in that process makes it trickier still. Then ensuring that these choices result in answering evaluation questions, and producing a credible evaluation that is used to inform change? Now things are getting complicated! Let me tell you about all this.

EVALUATION CHOICES: A LITTLE BIT TECHNICAL

Some questions are clearly better answered with qualitative inquiry, others with quantitative inquiry, and some with mixed methods (see Chapter 5 on methods of inquiry). Some evaluation purposes are better served by certain kinds of evaluation models, approaches, or theories (see Chapter 15 on this topic). Ultimately, the decisions made in the process of answering evaluation questions with what evaluation users consider to be credible evidence *and* providing a credible evaluation (credibility is covered in Chapter 5) are always influenced by five factors. Four of these are power, politics, culture, and language—which are all of course connected to and infused with the fifth factor, values. Although an important aspect of designing an evaluation is technical in the sense of choosing a method of inquiry, an equally important aspect is understanding the power, politics, culture, language, and values that influence the evaluation. Therefore, ignoring these powerful influencers in the course of selecting methods of inquiry and an evaluation approach can be a huge detriment to the evaluation process, its product, and the potential evaluation use. Chapter 12 has discussed values in depth—and, just as values are, politics, power, culture, and language are critical to *any* evaluative process that draws on *any* methodological approach.

When my daughter was young, she loved the game of putting her hands over her eyes because she thought that when she did, she was invisible and I could not see her. And she could not see me; therefore, I did not exist either. I used to stand and stare at this little human, hiding in plain sight giggling away, and laugh to myself. That was funny. It is not so funny when evaluators cover their eyes and pretend that power, politics, culture, language, and values do not influence evaluation because they cannot see them. Perhaps they cannot see them because they are choosing not to look. Or, perhaps it is not that evaluators' eyes are covered on purpose, it is just that they do not know how or where to look or what to look for. Hence the chapter's focus.

Evaluators need to be aware of how each of these factors influences all evaluation decisions, and ultimately the acceptance of the evaluation product, its findings, and its recommendations. Normally, when I write a strong statement like that, I change "all" to "almost all" or "most" because that is often appropriate. This time, I have left my original statement alone because I have no doubt that all five factors influence all evaluations in some way. This is why all (note use of "all") evaluators need to pay attention to these factors, have the requisite skill sets to facilitate conversations that make these influencers explicit, and understand what to do with them when their influences are identified. The next sections provide guidance on how to engage with the "fabulous five" plus one (i.e., context is our "plus one," which wraps them all together and includes a bit more).

EVALUATION INFLUENCERS: THE FABULOUS FIVE

Again, there are five key influencers in evaluation: **power, politics, culture, language,** and **values.** Values have just been discussed in Chapter 12, and although they are not reexplored here specifically, keep in mind that values infiltrate all discussions of power, politics, culture, and language. I discuss context separately at the end of the chapter, as its umbrella status makes it difficult to concretely engage with. For instance, its broad label could encompass each of the five listed above, and more; therefore, context needs, and gets, its own clarifying chat. Potential evaluator roles identified in Chapter 11 that are useful for engaging with the fabulous five are the negotiator, facilitator, and educator roles. Let's begin by exploring the influence of power and politics.

Power and Politics (and Values)

Power and politics can be subtle, explicit, nuanced, forceful, helpful, or detrimental, and may be all of the above at different points in the same evaluative process. But there is no doubt about it: Power and politics are always influencing evaluation decisions.

Let me share a thinly veiled trade secret before we talk in more depth about power and politics: Most often key evaluation decisions are made by those in power, and those who hold the most power in the evaluative process are seldom the evaluators. Knowing this, how should you prepare for any evaluation? Enter all evaluation processes with eyes wide open, not with eyes wide shut, which is not so uncommon an occurrence. At a minimum, identify the power and political dynamics, and make them explicit, even when your hands are tied with regard to negating their potential (negative) influence. Power and politics can influence the evaluation at three points in the evaluative process:

- Before it starts (e.g., the reason for the intervention and its intended results, the reason to have an evaluation, whom to hire, the design, the questions).
- During its implementation (e.g., where to gather data, whom to talk to, how to access information).
- After the data gathering (e.g., whom to involve in data analysis and interpretation, how to value findings, or how or with whom to share findings).

In other words, power and politics are factors at every step of the way.

We start by addressing the concept of power because I am writing the book and I have the power to decide that. First, let's look at a practical approach on how to identify power in an evaluative process; then let's look at some real-life experiences. In any evaluation, an evaluator needs to be clear about who is making what final decisions. Consider asking the nine questions presented and discussed below.

The Nine Necessary "Who" Questions: Identifying Who Has the Power in an Evaluative Process

1. Who decides to have the evaluation?

2. Who determines the evaluation budget?

3. Who decides on the evaluation questions?

4. Who approves the inception report or the evaluation design?

5. Who can stop or otherwise block any part of an evaluation process?

6. Who can support or facilitate what parts of the process?

7. Who signs off on (and ultimately approves) the evaluation and its products?

8. Who decides on how (and if) findings are shared and with whom?

9. Who owns the evaluation and its data?

Having clear answers to each of these questions *can* help to implement a useful evaluation process.

When you are asking the nine questions, be careful of accepting answers that are likely to prove useless. Here are some "nonanswers" and some hints for avoiding or mitigating them:

- *The "right" answer.* Sometimes people often like to give what they believe is the "right" answer, which is not to be confused with the real answer. Be sure to check the information elicited for each response, and confirm it from different sources and from different perspectives. (See Chapter 5 for a description of triangulation.)
- *The "suitcase" answer.* Be mindful of answers using suitcase words, such as "the beneficiaries" or even "the donor," unless it is very clear who is specifically referred to. (See Chapter 7 for a discussion of suitcase words and how to unpack them.)
- *The "group" answer.* When the response is that a steering committee or reference group will make the decisions, a little red flag should go up in your brain. Ask specifically about how decisions are made in that group and who communicates that answer to the evaluation team. Be very clear with regard to, within that group, "where the buck stops" or who has the final decision-making authority, and be sure to establish clear lines of communication.

I often find that the answers to these nine questions inform the evaluation design, and help me to negotiate, navigate, and make sense of the evaluation process. Knowing who has the power to make what decisions can prove useful many times over. For example, when an evaluator knows that the donor is making all decisions for an evaluation that is most likely going to be used by the implementer, he can facilitate a process that demonstrates how involving the implementer in decisions will probably lead to a more useful evaluation. At other times, knowing about decision-making power is helpful when the evaluation comes to a grinding halt "for some reason"; the evaluator can then quickly identify what that reason is, and can determine who can help to get the wheels turning again.

However, it would be misleading to suggest that these nine questions alone provide the magic answers to sorting out power issues and guarantee a smooth process. They do not. Let me share some examples where, although I knew who was making all the decisions, it did not change what happened. Knowing why things happened the way they did, however, provided partial relief; it was comforting to know why they happened, even if I could not prevent them from happening. To put this another way, it kept me stable.

- *The evaluator's advice is disregarded.* Sometimes an evaluator can disagree with the approach chosen by the client. Years back, I had a client who had just read Michael Patton's book on developmental evaluation (DE). She hired me to figure out how to evaluate her intervention, and she asked me to use DE. The problem was that her intervention was not a fit for DE, and implementing the approach would not result in what she wanted (e.g., products, such as an M&E plan with indicators). Although I explained this in multiple ways, she insisted on the DE approach, so I used it. While the evaluation was appreciated for its process, in the end the client did not have the final products she wanted, and she was therefore unhappy with the evaluation. The client held power over my livelihood (I needed the work), so I had to do what went against my better judgment. Though I acted ethically by telling the client that DE would not provide what she wanted, or needed, from the evaluation, she insisted.

- *The evaluator is caught in the middle.* An international organization hired me to conduct an evaluation in an African country, and on behalf of an African government. The international organization informed me that the evaluation's primary purpose was to demonstrate to the country's government how evaluation would be useful to inform their policy decisions. Then the international organization proceeded to dictate how and when the evaluation would be done, told me to develop the evaluation questions before I even arrived in the country (through a desk review), approved the final report, and controlled all financial aspects of the evaluation (including my payment). The African government, representatives of which I eventually did meet, had very different expectations and understandings for the process and the final evaluation report. The donor exercised complete power.

- *The evaluator is sidelined.* A European for-profit consulting company implemented a health evaluation in Asia. A board of directors governed the project. The European company hired me as the lead evaluator to design and oversee the evaluation. The board of directors did not like the evaluation findings or the recommendations, and wanted the evaluation changed to what they wanted to hear. I refused to change the findings, though I offered to conduct additional data gathering, analysis, and interpretation. The consulting company, whose staff members were not evaluators or health experts, rewrote the report findings and the recommendations, without ever leaving their European offices. The changed report, which said everything the board wanted to hear, was sent to the board and accepted. I left the project. I was never paid for my work, as my contract clearly stated that if I did not get the report approved, I would not be paid. Was standing up to power worth losing substantial income? Was it more ethical not to tamper with the evaluation findings, or to skip a few monthly health insurance premium payments for my children? Sometimes, when an evaluator chooses to stand up for what is right (according to her own ethics), there can be severe consequences. Speaking truth to power is a nice saying; it can be very hard to do in practice.

In each of the stories shared above, I had answers to every single one of the nine questions. While that knowledge did not change the ultimate results, it did provide transparency and understanding for how decisions were made and who made them. To what benefit? Sometimes it is helpful just to understand what is going on. At the start of this section, I have noted how just knowing what is happening is a relief; indeed, it lowers my frustration levels.

These things happen in the real world, and very few people write about them. What keeps evaluators from writing about these situations more often? Maybe it is too dangerous to speak up (political backlash), or too embarrassing to admit some things ("If I admit to that, I look foolish"). Two things happen when evaluators do not talk and write about these situations, however: (1) evaluators feel isolated when such things occur, and (2) effective ways of engaging with these challenges are not developed.

Not all engagements with power are negative. Evaluation decisions influenced by power may not have *any* detrimental consequences, and can have multiple positive ones. Decisions made by people in positions of power are often necessary (i.e., someone must decide), and their decisions can support and facilitate the evaluation process. Examples include committing more funds to an evaluation, opening "doors" to allow evaluators to explore an organization more deeply, or even calling for an evaluation in the first place. The important things for an evaluator to know are where the power resides, and how what decisions, made by whom, influence all aspects of the evaluation process.

Before we leave our discussion of power, let's look at a particularly powerful role in any evaluative process, that of **gatekeeper.** Gatekeepers are people who can block information and/or access during an evaluation. Here are a few examples of how a gatekeeper can stymie an evaluation process:

- A finance manager compares what was in the evaluation's terms of reference (written 2 years ago by a committee) with what is in the evaluation report (which now reflects the reality in the field and current management needs). The report and terms of reference need to match before funds can be released. Although transparent changes were made during the evaluation process, the evaluation does not meet contractual obligations. Report rejected.

- A foundation wants an evaluation conducted to judge its education program. A letter is needed from the nation's department of education before any schools can be approached for interviews, which are critical to the evaluation approach. The department does not like the evaluation questions or approach, and no letter is granted. Access denied.

- The management office at a health clinic needs to approve all questions before patients can be interviewed. However, the very problem the intervention is intended to solve is poor management that (appears to) lead to poor patient care. No questions are approved. Access denied.

- An evaluation seeks to understand how a recent intervention to involve homeless people in decision making on newly constructed shelters has influenced the local government's decision making. The city management refuses to answer any questions or provide any relevant documents. Information denied.

- A community leader insists on a participatory approach that requires the evaluation team to spend 5 days in the community. The evaluation commissioner will not approve (or provide funds for) an evaluation design that has the evaluation team in any one place for more than 2 days. Request denied.

There are also examples of how power positively influences social change and evaluative processes. For example, the government of the Netherlands is currently investing in a global feminist movement and providing funds to evaluate that effort. That effort garnered notice, and now the Bill and Melinda Gates Foundation has indicated that it will provide additional support. Power . . . and politics . . . and values.

I have begun this discussion of power by providing questions to identify who holds the power in an evaluative process and explaining why it is useful to know this. Then I have offered some examples of how power can challenge an evaluation process in the real world, and have acknowledged that it can also be beneficial to the process. Although knowing who makes decisions does not necessarily promise a smooth evaluation, clarity on this point does help us to understand why things sometimes happen the way they do.

What about Politics?

Let's start with a story and draw out from the story what is meant by politics in evaluation. A national government contracted with an evaluator to identify how well the government's approach to strengthening evaluation in the country was working, and to provide recommendations for moving forward. The government's view was that it was in the country's best interest for the government to keep control over the development of the evaluation profession. The evaluation findings demonstrated something different: They indicated that the government should cede its role to a professional association or to academic universities. The findings were not received well by the government, though it was well received by the professional association. The evaluation findings conflicted with the government's ideology. The government refused to pay for the report until "certain" changes were made, and in the end had the political power to squelch the findings. The "certain changes" included, among others, quantifying qualitative data, changing some of the findings and related recommendations. In other words, the evaluation did not serve the political interests of those who were in power.

Although a government example is provided, it could have easily been an example from a foundation, nonprofit organization, or university. Any organization or group where political ideologies exist can be threatened by evaluation findings that are the opposite of what the power brokers want.

What is being evaluated can provide clues to the likelihood of becoming tangled up with challenging political issues. When there are high stakes (as in the story above, when an evaluation demonstrated a need to shift power from one group to another), or when a policy or program is highly visible to the public, it is more likely to be influenced by politics (Patton, 2008; Weiss, 1987). And let's not forget the example in Chapter 12, where an intervention was put in place not to solve a social problem but to support a political agenda; an evaluation of that intervention proved to be highly political. What gets funded, what gets evaluated, and/or what findings are shared and with whom all have the potential to be influenced by politics.

Certain types of evaluation approaches invite a higher likelihood of political confrontation. Democratic evaluation and feminist evaluation are two such approaches. These evaluation approaches overtly aim to address and confront injustices in society. Thus these approaches are more likely to identify and confront issues that invite not-so-pleasant responses from those in power. For example, let's say that an evaluation finds evidence that women are paid less than men, receive fewer benefits from the intervention, and face more barriers to participation. The evaluators recommend that men and women receive equal pay and equal benefits, and that the barriers to women's access be addressed. These recommendations then challenge cultural and social norms, and, as such, the findings and recommendations politicize the evaluation. In a situation like this, people might go so far as to hide an evaluation and its findings, and even to say when asked about it, "What evaluation?"

It is time to look at some practical strategies for engaging with power *and* politics.

Strategies for Engaging with Power and Politics

- *Be reflective and, in particular, be self-reflective.* Be sensitive to, and aware of, the realities related to power, politics, and values—your own and everyone else's.

- *Be aware of the larger political context.* Understand the intervention in its larger political context, and gain a sense of how likely any evaluation (or a particular evaluation approach) is to encounter various political challenges.

- *Be active, not passive.* Actively seek to understand who affects what, where, when, how, and why, and to determine how all this can influence the evaluation, at what stage, and to what extent. Even if you cannot change these circumstances, being aware of how power and politics influence the evaluative process will help to keep you calm and reflective.

- *Be explicit about potential consequences.* Seek to grasp, and make explicit, the potential consequences of power and politics on the entire evaluative process.

- *Be a good documenter.* Make all decisions transparent, yours and everyone else's. Document all processes, key decisions, and makers of key decisions at every critical step of the evaluative process. These key decisions are likely to include (1) the evaluation purpose and its questions, (2) the evaluation approach, (3) methods of inquiry, (4) criteria with which to value the intervention, (5) the contents and structure of the evaluation report (or any other product), and (6) communication of findings (i.e., how it is done and who is involved).

- *Be true to yourself.* Make decisions that allow you to sleep at night.

Culture and Language (and Values)

Culture and language are heavily intertwined. Although I address culture first and then language, the two factors (and conversations about them) often overlap.

Culture

How an evaluator engages in the evaluative process, and how people engage with the evaluator and her evaluative process, are both influenced by culture. More specifically, how the evaluator conducts the evaluation, what is seen and not seen, how something is interpreted and valued, and how findings are communicated and used are all influenced by culture.

What is meant by the term *culture*? An anthropologist would define it as the "shared set of (implicit and explicit) values, ideas, concepts, and rules of behavior that allow a social group to function" (Hudelson, 2004). According to the *Oxford Living Dictionaries: English* (2018), culture is "the ideas, customs and social behaviour of a particular group or society"; when the term is used with a specific modifier, it also signifies "the attitudes and behaviour characteristic of a particular social group." Trying to define or identify culture in an evaluative process, and then understand how it influences the evaluative process, can be a difficult task.

SenGupta, Hopson, and Thompson-Robinson (2004) state:

> Culture is an undeniably integral part of the diverse contexts of evaluation, and therefore an integral part of evaluation. Culture is present in evaluation not only in the context in which programs are implemented, but also in the designs of these programs, and the approach, stance or method an evaluator chooses to use in their work . . . culture shapes values, beliefs and world-views. . . . (p. 5)

SenGupta and colleagues' views on evaluation and culture are reflected in my own approach to demystifying evaluation in this book. This demystification has not begun with a focus on methods, but with a focus on language (Chapter 1) and an intervention. Chapters 3–10 provide an explicit process for detangling the intervention, which then prepares the evaluator to explore further how culture (and language and power and politics and values) have influenced the intervention's shape. This understanding can then be used to guide every aspect of the evaluation process, and at times simply to understand it. One metaphor for viewing something in a specific way is using a particular *lens*.

So, in other words, the process laid out in Chapters 3–10 allows an evaluator to apply different lenses. Just as putting on glasses that have red lenses, or ones with dark green lenses, shows you a different view of the world, so do these different conceptual lenses. However, looking at a mess (i.e., a tangled intervention) through lenses of any color still shows us a mess; it's just a mess of a different color. To make culture more tangible, let's read a story about how it influences a situation. Then let's discuss how to engage practically with culture in an evaluation.

When I was teaching a class on program evaluation, I asked students to think about how culture influences an evaluative process. For example, how does culture influence the ways an evaluator gathers or interprets data? One of my Alaskan students shared the following story:

"I think of a story my father tells. Years ago, there was a Russian Orthodox priest out in western Alaska, way out in the middle of nowhere (or the center of the universe, depending on your viewpoint), who married a Yupik woman. One holiday season, they went to Anchorage to see friends and family, and went to dinner one night at a friend's house. They finished dinner and were sitting around chatting after the meal, as old friends tend to do, when the priest said, 'Well, it looks like we should head out soon.' Upon hearing this, his wife promptly got up, put on her coat, and went out to the car without saying a word.

"Now one might think she was being rude, especially coming from a Western perspective. A declaration like what the husband said might mean, in a Western context, sitting and talking for a bit longer, slowly getting up still chatting, cleaning up, visiting some more, getting to the door and putting on coats and shoes still talking, and finally heading out to the porch for the final visiting session of the night before waving as one drives away. All in all, this could be upwards of an hour before guests actually leave. From the Yupik perspective, one only speaks when they have something to say, and it is literal, no added fluff. In this particular situation, the end of the night had been announced, so the night was over, and the wife left. In her mind, she did the politest thing possible, and showed respect to all involved and took the initiative to move first (showing leadership). Same story, two different perspectives."

When my student shared that story, she also provided me with a link to a YouTube video featuring one of the people central to the story, the Russian Orthodox priest. Father Michael Oleksa is an adjunct professor of Alaska studies at Alaska Pacific University, and he provides practical insight into culture for a practicing evaluator. He explains that culture is (1) the way someone sees the world; (2) the game of life, as a person understands and plays it; and (3) the story into which a person is born. Watch his video (*www.youtube.com/ watch?v=GjPxu5wCJ14*). His practical explanation of culture is useful; it cuts right to the chase, so to speak, of how to consider culture in any evaluative process.

Father Oleksa's practical advice is useful because engaging with culture in an evaluation can be overwhelming, and much of the literature surrounding culture can be quite theoretical. Keep these explanations of culture in mind when considering four broad categories that have the potential to influence the evaluation.

- *The evaluator, and her organization and/or team.* Within the evaluation organization (e.g., a private consulting company), there may be multiple cultures—for example, within different departments, or among different staff members. An evaluator may work independently, and therefore may only need to consider her own culture. If there is a team of evaluators, however, the team members' cultures need to be considered.

- *The commissioner.* The commissioner's organizational culture may be the dominant culture for the evaluation. Then within the commissioner's organization, there are individuals whose own cultures may influence the evaluation. And if there is one person in charge, his culture may dominate.

- *The implementer.* The organization that implements the intervention possesses its own culture. Depending on the size of the organization (local, national, global), multiple cultures may exist. Then individuals within the organization or department have their own cultures.

- *The place.* The beneficiaries receiving the services are likely to share a common culture, though not always, and while a culture may be shared, other existing cultures may also influence beneficiaries who live in one place (e.g., religious, academic). If the intervention is implemented in multiple places, there are likely to be additional cultural considerations.

These are a lot of cultural considerations. All these cultures may be subtle or overt, or docile or dominant, and may conflict with or complement each other.

To explore and understand culture, an evaluator needs to be self-reflective and aware: aware of her own culture, of other people's cultures, and of how all these cultures play out in the evaluation process. Hazel Symonette (2004) writes about self-reflection and awareness, suggesting that an evaluator needs to engage in "ongoing personal homework" to be culturally sensitive (p. 97). Specifically, she suggests that the evaluator needs to be (1) aware of how what differences in people influence "access, process, and success"; (2) aware of power, privilege, and other social structures; and (3) self-aware, constantly reflecting on how she sees what she sees, what she does not see, and why that is.

And I cannot write a section on culture in evaluation without reflecting on *culturally responsive evaluation,* an evaluation approach that encompasses race, ethnicity, and language (Hood, Hopson, & Frierson, 2015). As we have learned through this book, almost a prerequisite for an evaluation term to be invited into the evaluation "club" is that it must have multiple associated concepts, definitions, meanings, and labels, and it is no different here. Other terms associated with culturally responsive evaluation are *cultural competence, cultural humility, multicultural evaluation, cross-cultural evaluation,* and *cultural responsibility.* Although it is not clear how these differ, or if they do (Bledsoe & Donaldson, 2015; Chouinard & Cousins, 2009), what each offers is insight, guidance, and thoughtful thinking about what role(s) culture plays in an evaluation, and how an evaluator can and should engage in a thoughtful discussion on it.

Understanding how culture influences an evaluative process provides insight into how to design an evaluation that (1) gathers data in an appropriate manner; (2) has fewer potential bumps and barriers, and when they do occur, enables them to be understood and mitigated; (3) results in an evaluative process and findings that are credible to evaluation users; and (4) does no (or the least possible amount of) harm to all involved.

Language

Now let's shift the discussion and tackle the topic of language. *Tackle?* What an odd choice of words. A commonly used term in sports, it means to stop your opponent. The term also means to address something head on, instead of avoiding it. Some of you reading the book may be thinking, "Awesome! A direct discussion on language that does not mince words." To others of you, that word choice of *tackle* may seem too aggressive, too sports-centric, or perhaps even patriarchal, and for these reasons may be offensive. For that matter, the word *awesome* may be deemed inappropriate for a book on evaluation. In fact, you may no longer be interested in what I am going to say about language because the word *tackle* is bouncing around in your brain and the word *awesome* has lowered my credibility. I may have lost you right at the beginning of my explanation. Wait! Come back! I promise to be more careful with my word choice.

BOX 13.1. The English Language

My mother tongue is English; American English to be exact. I grew up in the United States (I am a Jersey girl, though I lost that accent long ago). I now live in South Africa. My children were born in South Africa and South African English is their mother tongue. When my mom (whom my kids call Gogo) visits us, I spend time translating between American English and South African English. "Do not ask Gogo for a plaster; ask her for a Band-Aid." "Mom, don't ask the kids for a Kleenex; ask for a tissue." "Kids, don't ask Gogo to bring you a rubber; she will have a heart attack." (Note that *rubber* means *eraser* in South Africa, and in American English, it means condom, and my children are 9 and 12 years old at this writing.) And similar things happen at work. When I first arrived in South Africa, I asked for a document from my South African colleague. He said he would give it to me "now," so I waited at his desk. And waited. However, what he meant by "now" would be translated into American English as "in a few minutes" or "a bit later." So that was a bit awkward. Then I asked for directions to the closest supermarket. He told me to go out the front of the building and then turn left at the first robot. I thought, "How cool are South Africans? They have robots in the street!" I left the building looking for something like R2D2 from *Star Wars*. It turned out that traffic lights are called *robots* in South Africa.

And how we communicate is cultural. In this book, most of my stories are personal ones, and those reading them may have very different reactions to them. A South African friend once described to me her version of a typical first meeting between a South African and a North American. She said that when a North American meets a new person, the American talks about themselves with the intent to show friendliness—and then waits for the South African to talk. But the South African does not share personal information; they wait to be asked questions so that they can answer them. However, when the South African does not readily share information, the American is hesitant to ask questions because that would seem to be prying; the American is thinking that the South African would share information if they wanted to. Although this awkward pattern may not be a universal one, my friend's description certainly made me rethink my interactions. Imagine how these kinds of cultural differences influence any evaluative process.

The discussion that follows assumes (assumptions are dangerous, I know) that the language spoken during the evaluation is a primary or native language (also known as the mother tongue), or a language in which people are comfortable listening and speaking. The discussion does not cover how to work with translators or in second languages (which both need their own guidance). With that understanding, the next discussion focuses on how to use language effectively in an evaluation process.

Here are four practical thematic considerations with regard to language in any evaluative process.

1. *Word choice for gathering data.* When an evaluator is gathering data, questions should be phrased so that they are understandable to those who need to answer the question. Specifically, when designing a data-capturing tool or questions to ask a respondent (i.e., the evaluator is the tool), an evaluator needs to be aware of to whom she is speaking, to ensure that her word choice and the phrasing of the question are appropriate. At the same time, when listening, an evaluator needs to know who is saying a word or phrase, for what purpose, and in what context, to fully grasp what the person intends by the word or phrase (see examples on pages 4–5 in Chapter 1). Evaluation tools (e.g., questionnaires, focus group guides) are often "pilot-tested" to check that words and phrasing are understandable. When qualitative evaluators collect data with open-ended questions, there is additional pressure; these evaluators need to be even more familiar with how their respondents use language, as much of their inquiry is developed as needed, in the moment. Designing evaluation questions should not be driven by the need to produce the most perfect, nicely worded question in formal, academic language. Although that might be the most appropriate approach in some cases, in general the focus should be on writing clear, concise questions with appropriate words and phrases that will be understood *by the respondents.*

2. *Word choice for managing the evaluation and providing feedback.* Throughout the evaluation's management and decision-making process, and in the feedback of evaluative findings, words and phrases should be used that invite people into the conversation, not exclude them through word choice. While word choice and language are critical in the collection and interpretation of data, they are equally important for engaging with others in every other aspect of the evaluative process. (Read Chapter 1 for an in-depth discussion of evaluation words.) When you are managing an evaluation or providing feedback, carefully consider *how* a word or phrase is spoken or written, as well as *what* is spoken or written. Let's first look at an emphasis on *how* something is said. How a sentence is phrased, with what words, matters. The word *but* is a good example. An evaluator can provide eight positive findings; however, if *but* is used as a connector in the sentence before negative evaluation findings are shared, everything up to the word *but* will likely be forgotten. Try to use the word *and* if you must use a connector—or, even better, just start a new sentence. Now let's briefly look at *what* is said, keeping in mind that no one (that I know of) likes to receive criticism. Use word choice carefully. For instance, switching "It is a problem" to "It is a challenge," or "It failed" to "It did not work as planned," provides words and phrases that are likely more encouraging and likely to invite engagement with the finding. To bring back in the link to culture, different cultures are likely to engage with words and the phrasing of them differently.

3. *Body language.* Throughout the evaluative process, be aware of what signals are sent with nonverbal cues. Body language is influenced by culture. It influences how people engage with the evaluator throughout the entire evaluation process, from data gathering to a feedback session on the evaluation's results. When I am interviewing someone, or listening to someone at a conference, I unwittingly find myself bobbing my head up and down. While subconsciously I mean this as "Yes, please continue, I am listening," it can also be interpreted as "The evaluator asked me something, and I am saying the right thing." As a result, the data obtained may be biased. A respondent sitting with arms crossed may send a signal that she is angry, closed off, or not listening. In some cultures, direct eye contact is necessary; in others, it is not necessary or may even be inappropriate. Julien S. Bourrelle tells a rather rambling and interesting story that includes how body language and other cultural differences influence how people understand (perceive) a situation. Check out his video (*www.youtube.com/watch?v=l-Yy6poJ2zs*).

4. *Tone.* It is sometimes not what is said, but sometimes the inflection—vehemence or calmness, for example—of what is said that matters. Reading someone else's typed interview notes may be misleading because the interviewee's expression, or the way a word or phrase was said, is not apparent. For instance, if someone says, with vehemence and forcefulness, "Great. That is just great!", this is different from hearing someone say, in a very pleasant tone, "Great. That is just great." And both, of course, are different from a very sarcastic "Great. That . . . is . . . just . . . great." Therefore, it is important to note not just that the phrase was said, but the tone in which it was conveyed. So what about when an evaluator is verbally administering closed-ended surveys? Suppose a question calls for a choice between 1 and 5, and a person says, "Um, well, hmm, I don't know, OK . . . well, just circle 4 . . . no, circle 3 . . . um, I really don't know, maybe 2 . . . oh, never mind, let's go with 4." Is this eventually stated "4" different from an adamant "4"? What do you think?

Designing a Language- and Culture-Appropriate Data Collection Process and Tool: A Four-Step Strategy

A facilitated, intentional planning session can generate needed information for designing a culturally and socially appropriate data-gathering process. Here I describe a four-step process that supports developing and implementing such a process; the resulting data-gathering tools are more likely to be clear, understandable, useful, and nonoffensive to respondents. When given proper time and attention, the session can provide not only useful insights about ways to gather data sensitively, but clues for interpreting the data with regard to cultural, power, and political realities. Here are the four steps for the planning session:

- *Step 1: Identify culturally knowledgeable people to attend a group meeting.* Although the ideal number is three to eight people, it can vary, depending on need and availability. The implementing organization can often identify at least one or two people from inside the organization, who can then often identify others within the broader community. The selection criteria are that (1) the people chosen should be likely to provide credible insight into language and culture, and (2) they should be comfortable doing so. A group meeting is more beneficial than meeting people individually. If individuals provide conflicting advice at separate points in time, the evaluator is left to try to reconcile it. When people within a group setting provide different advice (or advice perceived to be different), the evaluator can facilitate a decision on what to do.

- *Step 2: Introduce the broad purpose.* Begin the group meeting by identifying how much time is available for the meeting, and thanking people for bringing their knowledge and insights to share. Then introduce the purpose. For example, you might say, "I was asked to conduct an evaluation on an intervention designed to assist immigrants who are new to the community in the last several years. Each of you brings insights that are needed to help me conduct an evaluation that is culturally sensitive and language-appropriate. In other words, I need your help to make sure that I ask questions in an understandable and nonoffensive way." Then introduce the specific questions that need to be answered, and describe how the information will be used and by whom.

- *Step 3: Engage the group in a discussion of word use and phrasing of questions.* There are two options.

  - *Option 1:* Provide a draft of the questions, and ask the group to reflect on them.
  - *Option 2:* Provide a theme or topic, and ask the group members how they would phrase a question, what words should be used, and what words should not.

Some typical responses when facilitating a group may be someone saying, "No, you cannot ask that because it would be heard as being rude," and someone else stating, "If you use that word, then it means this, not that . . . ," and a third person noting that "I would be scared to answer a question about . . ."

- *Step 4: Engage the group in a discussion of how to administer the questions.* Once word use and phrasing is clear, I then ask questions about how to conduct the interview. Examples of such questions include ones about time ("Should I show up on time, early, or a few minutes late?"); body language ("Do I look someone in the eye?"); gender ("Can a male interview a female? Can females be interviewed alone?"); politeness ("Do I need to make small talk, or should I just launch into an interview?"); power ("Do I need to speak with a certain person or group first?"); and other social norms ("What is the appropriate dress code?" or for surveys, "How do we ensure a high response rate?"). And one of the best-ever evaluation questions to ask is this: "What should I know that I have not asked you?" It is a great question because there have been times when I have made mistakes after I have conducted this process, and when I ask why no one told me not to say this, or do that, the response is, "Because you didn't ask us that question." (*Note:* I often use that as one of my last questions when interviewing respondents during an evaluation process, for the same reason.)

While the process described above informs how to gather data and provides clues about how to interpret data, a similar process can be used for the actual interpretation of data. After data are gathered, cleaned, and made anonymous, facilitating the same or a similar group to interpret those data often provides useful insights.

Language AND *Culture*

Culture matters: Explicit culture and hidden culture; your culture and someone else's. Language matters. Words matter. Who says them, who does not say them, how they are said, and how people interpret them all matter. As evaluators, we must carefully consider the language we use, the language others use to communicate with us, and the ways cultural norms can influence the evaluation process.

Let's explore an evaluation example from southern Africa that depicts how language and culture are intertwined. A women's group in a southern African country supported health clinics that catered to sex workers in urban areas. The evaluation aimed to explore the kinds of support that all sex workers (including men who had sex with men) sought from the clinic, and their experience of the services. Pilot-testing the evaluation tool identified several challenges in the section that asked for demographic information. First, the term *female* was offensive because in this location *female* is only used for animals. *Female* was replaced with *woman*. Second, the identification of men who have sex with men—a population that did exist and did access the clinic—was removed from the questionnaire. Because homosexuality is illegal in this location, answering that question (or, for that matter, even asking it) could have had dire consequences for the interviewers *and* the respondents. The example demonstrates the importance of being aware of how language usage intertwines with culture and how both of these are linked with power and politics. This leads me to one more point, which I discuss next.

 ### *Who Asks What*

How a question is asked is as important as what question is asked, and who asks it.

Language and Culture and Power and Politics (and Values)

Power and politics have roles to play in language and cultural discussions. For example, choosing to conduct an interview in English with a group who speaks a different mother tongue, or only writing a report in French about a population who does not speak French, sends a message about politics, power, and culture by not paying attention to, or purposely ignoring, language. An evaluator who uses overly complicated, technical words in speaking or writing sends a message about power and culture (the evaluator's). It is often challenging to disentangle values, politics, power, language, and culture in any evaluation, and then also to engage with every aspect of these; nevertheless, it is an evaluator's role to recognize the critical influence each of these has on every part of the evaluation process, and to enter the process with eyes wide open.

I have a question I am a little nervous to ask. Sometimes when I ask people why something happened, or to explain a finding, people answer with "It is my culture." But, honestly, I am not sure what to do with that answer.

"It is my culture" can contain a gold mine of information; however, if this response is followed up incorrectly, it can quickly dissolve any trust between the evaluator and the person with whom she is talking. Let's start with the positive experience. When someone uses "It is my culture" as an explanation, ask them to tell you a bit more. Most people like talking about their culture and explaining it to others. You could add that you are not familiar with the culture (if you are not), or if you are, you could ask to hear about the culture from their perspective to get a better understanding of what they mean. These open-ended questions can lead to all sorts of insights and rich data.

On the other hand, a probe such as "What do you mean when you say your culture?" can quickly bubble into a disaster. For instance, asking about the culture may suggest that you do not understand the culture in which you are working, and therefore may give some people the impression that you should not be working in that location. Or perhaps the answer is given as a comfortable, generic response, and the respondent is not sure what it means either. Or maybe the respondent intends the answer to flummox the evaluator and does not expect to be questioned on it—and the respondent sees the inquiry about what it means as an attack.

If the initial response to "Please tell me what you mean by that" seems tense, try discussing the "It is my culture" response with other members who understand or are part of the same culture who are more likely to be receptive to follow-up questions. For example, you could ask another person, "When I interviewed some community members [remember, maintain their confidentiality], they explained the reason as 'It is the culture.' Could you help me understand what they *may* have meant by that?" Again, triangulation is key to that exploration.

POLITICS, POWER, LANGUAGE, AND CULTURE IN EVALUATION

- **Have 2 minutes?** Check out an AEA365 blog post on cultural humility (*http://aea365. org/blog/tag/cultural-humility*). The free AEA365 blog offers quick tips on various evaluation topics. Sign up and get one tip a day emailed to you.

- **Have 5 minutes?** Take a spin through the Center for Culturally Responsive Evaluation and Assessment (CREA) website (*https://crea.education.illinois.edu*).

- **Have 7 minutes?** Check out Eric Liu's TED Talk on what power is and how to understand it (*www.ted.com/talks/eric_liu_how_to_understand_power*).

- **Have 17 minutes?** Check out Steven Pinker's TED Talk on how language emerges and what our language usage reveals (*www.ted.com/talks/steven_pinker_on_language_and_ thought*).

- **Have 20 minutes?** Check out Chimamanda Ngozi Adichie's TED Talk "The Danger of the Single Story" (*www.ted.com/talks/chimamanda_adichie_the_danger_of_a_single_ story?language=en*).

- **Have 60–90 minutes?** Read an article by Bowman and Dodge-Francis (2018) in *New Directions in Evaluation*, "Culturally Responsive Indigenous Evaluation and Tribal Governments: Understanding the Relationship."

- **Have a few hours a day?** Check out Ernest House's fun and interesting book *Regression to the Mean: A Novel of Evaluation Politics* (2007); as one reviewer noted, this is a book that anyone considering becoming an evaluator should read.

- **Have a few hours?** Read "Evaluation, Language, and Untranslatables" by Peter Dahler-Larsen and colleagues (2017) in the *American Journal of Evaluation*. The article talks about the challenges of using evaluation in languages other than English.

- **Have a few hours a night?** Choose a few chapters from an edited book by Stafford Hood, Rodney Hopson, and Henry Frierson, *Continuing the Journey to Reposition Culture and Cultural Context in Evaluation Theory and Practice* (2015).

- **Have some more time?** Do online searches of these evaluation authors, who speak and write on a broad range of topics concerning culture, mostly from a Western perspective: Karen Kirkhart, Stafford Hood, Hazel Symonette, and Rodney Hopson. Check out Nicole Bowman on sovereignty (tribal government policy) and traditional indigenous knowledge and culture. A New Zealand cultural perspective is provided by Fiona Cram, Nan Wehipeihana, and Kate McKegg. Read some or all of these authors, and then look to see which other authors they cite, to broaden your knowledge on culture and evaluation.

Evaluation Context: Broadest of Them All

A well-worn term in any evaluation process, and for a good reason, is **context.** What is meant by the term? In the *Oxford Living Dictionaries: English* (2018), *context* is defined as "the circumstances that form the setting for an event, statement, or idea, and in terms of which it can be fully understood." Most people thoughtfully, yet lazily, use the term because it covers so much (and I am guilty of that as well). In fact, everything discussed in this chapter could be subsumed under context—but don't!

On a practical level, when you are thinking about context, just remember that *everything matters.* Imagine all the factors that affect the intervention, the evaluator, the evaluation process, its findings, and how those findings are received. Some examples include the environment (e.g., rainy weather), the political system (e.g., is it a democracy or an oligarchy?), political strife (e.g., a coup), the economy (e.g., a recession or lack of jobs), the demographics (e.g., people's age or religion), or simply the physical space in which an intervention takes place.

All of the examples of contextual factors we have discussed (and many more) then inform the intervention, and shape people's expectations and perceptions of the intervention, its results, and the evaluation. It is unlikely that every aspect of the context that has potentially influenced the intervention or evaluation can be identified, explored, and articulated. Two evaluation approaches that aim to focus the evaluator on issues of context are Daniel Stufflebeam's (Stufflebeam & Zhang, 2017) context, input, process, product (CIPP) approach, and Pawson and Tilly's (1997) realist evaluation—an approach that looks at the context (circumstances), mechanism (what brought about change), and outcome (results) to describe and explain an intervention's achievement or lack thereof. Specifically, Pawson and Tilly's approach explores what works for whom and why (and in what context). Let's look at context in evaluation from a different perspective.

Kerstin Rausch Waddell, a colleague of mine who was an evaluator, trained as a psychologist, and is now a personal life coach, provides these next insights. She says that we all decide meanings socially—through what we say and do together during social interactions such as conversations and community rituals; through the production of research literature and other media; and through the various systems, organizations, and groups of people with whom we affiliate ourselves. She draws on Hedtke and Winslade (2017) and Miehls (2011), among others, to explain that in this way we form what she calls "social agreements" about what we think is important and true in relation to how we see the world and ourselves. We also form social agreements about what we think is not important—through what we do not say or do together, such as when we silence certain conversations, assume that everyone has the same understandings, leave out certain practices, or just do not think of venturing into certain territories because it simply never occurred to us (Hedtke & Winslade, 2017; Miehls, 2011). In this way, among others, context influences what and how we think, what we see and do not see, and what we question. In other words, it affects how we evaluate and ultimately value an intervention.

A common concept in evaluation is the *socioeconomic* context, which is an impressive term for the ways in which social factors and economic factors, when combined, influence a situation. One example of exploring socioeconomic context would be to explore how a person is viewed (social status) in society is based on how much money they make (economic). The reality is that not all contextual elements can be accounted for in most evaluations. Should you want to explore context in an evaluation, I leave you in the capable hands of Pawson and Tilly, Stufflebeam, and Greene to get you started (see the end of the section).

Practical Advice for Exploring Context

- *Questions can be broad to start with, yet they need to be narrowed down and made more specific.* For example, a recent policy change, or a shift in school governance, or even a drought can serve as a place for an evaluator to begin exploring how that factor influenced the intervention and its results, and in what way.

- *Answers can also be broad to begin with, but need to be narrowed down and made more specific.* Answers cannot be suitcase words (see Chapter 7 on the havoc caused by these words). For instance, a question "What contextual factors influenced the intervention?" and the response "The political economy influenced it" are not helpful enough. The evaluator will need to unpack the suitcase term *political economy* to make the response specific enough to be useful.

- *Questions or answers that are too narrow may also be detrimental.* While narrowing down the contextual factors is useful, starting out being too focused (for a question or an answer) may cause the evaluator to miss out on other useful influences, or the necessary broader understanding.

Context

- **Have half an hour?** An evaluation approach that addresses context overtly is the CIPP approach, developed by Daniel Stufflebeam. It is one of the earliest evaluation approaches to explicitly consider context. To learn more about the approach, look at a detailed checklist developed by Stufflebeam in 2007 (*www.wmich.edu/sites/default/files/attachments/u350/2014/cippchecklist_mar07.pdf*).

- **Have a few months?** Read a recent book by Daniel Stufflebeam and Guili Zhang, *The CIPP Evaluation Model* (2017), published by Guilford Press.

- **Have a few hours a night?** Read a special issue of *New Directions for Evaluation*, titled *Context: A Framework for Its Influence on Evaluation Practice* (Volume 2012, Issue 135).

- **Have some time for an online search?** In the evaluation field, a few theorists who provide further insight into how context matters are Karen Kirkhart (United States),

Jennifer Greene (United States), and Peter Dahler-Larson (Denmark). Search each of their names with the word *context*.

- **Feel adventurous?** Community psychology, sociology, and anthropology are a few fields that offer a wide range of literature on understanding context. As a start, try searching for Clifford Geertz, an interpretive anthropologist. He explains how cultures can be understood by studying what people think about, their ideas, and the meanings that are important to them.

WRAPPING UP

Understanding the intervention and the reason for it, and discussing evaluation questions and methods of inquiry, are important factors in any evaluation—yet there is so much more. This chapter has focused on how, and whose, power, politics, culture, and language (which are infiltrated by values and could be subsumed under context) influence an intervention, its results (or lack thereof), and the entire evaluative process. Through engaging with each, I laid the foundation to encourage reflective practice. Each of the "fabulous five, plus one" (the "plus one" being context) affects every aspect of the intervention and the evaluation. Yet evaluation is still *more* than even this; for example, every evaluation needs to be guided by an evaluation theory, approach, or model, as discussed in the next two chapters. Chapter 14 first introduces the scholarly side of being an evaluator and talks about evaluation theories, approaches, and models, while a more pragmatic side to evaluation is discussed in Chapter 15. Before you leave our discussion of the fab five plus one, join me in a conversation.

Our Conversation: Between You and Me

This chapter provides a wealth of information that can be used to inform any evaluation process. I would like you to apply what we have just discussed, and ask you a few questions about power, politics, language, and culture.

1. **Consider this evaluation question for people who live within a 5-mile radius of your home, "Tell me how safe you feel in your community":** How would you rephrase that question, if at all, for an 11-year-old child, a teenager, a university student, a retired person, and a young single parent? What different probes might you use with different people? Does gender make a difference? What other differences would make a difference? What makes you say that?

2. **Reflect on your cultural competence.** If someone asked you how culturally competent you were in terms of designing and conducting an evaluation, how would you respond?

CHAPTER 14

The Scholarly Side of Being an Evaluator

The more that you read, the more things you will know.
The more that you learn, the more places you'll go.
—Dr. Seuss, *I Can Read With My Eyes Shut!*

We have talked about the different roles an evaluator can play, and some important factors (values, politics, power, culture, language, and context) that influence an evaluator's choices and, ultimately, the evaluation. Regardless of the type of evaluator you are or want to be, learning a bit about the evaluation literature is fundamental to being an evaluator; you cannot know who you are as an evaluator unless you delve into it. An evaluator cannot design, manage, or implement a credible evaluation without knowledge of the academic side, just as she cannot do any of this without experience on the practical side. How deep that dive into the academic side should go is less certain, as the literature about evaluation can be overwhelming; a person can get lost in the vast amounts of literature and never emerge. On the other hand, labeling yourself an evaluator and not knowing at least something about evaluation theory seems a bit . . . unfathomable. This chapter helps to guide you through how to engage with, and learn about and from, the evaluation literature.

KNOWING THE EVALUATION LITERATURE: IT MATTERS

William Shadish (1998), a past president of the American Evaluation Association (AEA) and an evaluation theorist, takes a very strong position regarding evaluators' knowing evaluation theory. He clearly states that evaluation theory is the substance of who evaluators are, and what they do; I could not agree more about the importance of learning evaluation theory. Evaluation is more than just methods of inquiry. I suggest five reasons to read some evaluation literature if you are going to be an evaluator. Some reasons are a tad academic and suggest how reading or otherwise learning the literature (such as by listening to a lecture or podcast) will influence you in more abstract ways; others are just downright practical.

1. *It is about guiding an evaluator's career.* To begin with, evaluation literature provides an understanding of how the field has evolved, and provides a window into the drastically diverse ways of thinking about evaluation and its changing role in a changing society. Understanding evaluation's history, and how its published thinkers think, influences a person's understanding of evaluation, shapes one's views of evaluation and its role in society, and inspires the type of evaluator one wishes to be.

2. *It is about credibility.* Imagine meeting a psychiatrist who was not familiar with the influential work of Sigmund Freud, who introduced the now familiar concepts of ego, id, superego, and libido. Or what if you met an anthropologist who has never read Margaret Mead, one of the field's foremost thinkers and writers. Or what would your reaction be if you met a human rights activist who could not discuss Nelson Mandela or the philosophy of Gandhi? What would you think if these "professionals" had never heard of these leading figures in their fields? Would you have confidence in them? Or would you wonder, "Are these persons who they think they are, or claim to be?"

3. *An evaluator who draws on the literature shows that he is well read, knowledgeable, and prepared; he is a confident evaluator.* Knowing the literature demonstrates that the evaluator has read, researched, and carefully thought about the ways he is engaging in evaluation. Furthermore, it allows for a nonpersonal discussion. Here's an example. When I lecture or present a paper on feminist evaluation, I am often attacked both personally and professionally. I find it a huge benefit to draw on the literature. Primarily, it separates out the personal "I think; therefore it is" from describing or drawing on peer-reviewed approaches, theories, and frameworks. Rather than simply relying on personal opinions, in other words, an evaluator who is well read can talk about various authors, theorists, and their examples which can then be discussed in a more neutral and thoughtful way. Disagreeing with one person's opinions is different from disagreeing with years of research and various peer-reviewed published papers. Furthermore, reading the literature can give evaluators a better appreciation of opposing views; this allows an evaluator to be prepared for discussions, and sometimes even changes her viewpoints.

4. *Knowing how and when to mix and match approaches prepares you to be an evaluator in the real world.* Reading the literature guides you in the many ways of how to think about and do evaluation—the potential pitfalls, the practicalities, the facilitators, and other considerations. It is only with a breadth of evaluation knowledge that we can be prepared to make sound technical evaluation decisions, and be aware of the many nontechnical ones. In my 20-plus years of doing evaluation, I have never implemented a pure theory or approach; I have always mixed, matched, and adapted.

5. *It is a key aspect of what separates us from researchers.* Need I say more? If so, read Chapter 2.

I hope that at least one of these reasons resonates with you. Perhaps you have a reason you want to add?

WAYS TO START ENGAGING WITH THE LITERATURE

OK, I am convinced. Is there a basic list of people whose works I should read?

Before I answer that, there are several ways to learn about evaluation theories, approaches, and methods. One way is to choose one thematic area that resonates with you—for example, approaches that focus on use. Then begin your reading list by focusing on these kinds of approaches. The other way is to read works by particular people, who will refer you to more works by different people (i.e., the thinkers they talk about and cite), and so on. Table 14.1 is my own laundry list based on evaluators who publish in English, and who have taught me at least one important idea or concept that I continually use in nearly all my evaluation work. This is not a list of the all-time greats (though for me they are great), or necessarily the iconic writers or theorists of evaluation. It is obviously very biased. Yet, when I think about how different theorists influenced how I do evaluation in the field, it is this list that I want to share. The list gives you a bit of insight into my own evaluation journey, and suggests how reading different theorists influenced how I think about evaluation. At the end of this answer, I provide a box that names some of the more prominent names in evaluation (those whose works are often covered in evaluation foundation courses and key evaluation textbooks).

As I have said, Table 14.1 and Box 14.1 are very biased and very short lists. Ask your colleagues, your friends, and other evaluators this question: If they had a dinner party and could invite five evaluation theorists or writers, who would they invite, and why? Here are some more ideas for choosing thinkers/authors to read (or listen to podcasts or online presentations) to inform your role as an evaluator:

- Choose a few of your favorite evaluation articles (or just one) and look at their reference lists or bibliographies. A reference list is a list of works cited in a paper; a bibliography may list just the works cited, or may list all the works that were read for the paper (not all of which may be cited in it).
- Choose an evaluation approach (see Chapter 15) that interests you and see who writes about it and who critiques it, and read them.
- Take an evaluation course at a university, which then provides a reading list. The AEA (*www.eval.org*) has a webpage dedicated to universities that offer program evaluation courses all over the world. Look also at the websites of universities that offer evaluation courses; sometimes they provide their syllabi online, which offers detailed reading lists.

TABLE 14.1. Evaluation Theorists or Practitioners Who Have Influenced Me

Evaluation theorist(s) or practitioner(s)	Biggest "aha" moment that I have used in my everyday work after I read their work[a]
Maria Bustelo	Maria's ways of thinking about feminist and gender concepts continually inspire my own writing on these topics.
Fiona Cram and Nicky Bowman	Fiona and Nicky's practical, grounded, and thoughtful examples keep me reading, and both bring a passion to their work that has opened my eyes to what it really means to be culturally sensitive.
E. Jane Davidson and Nan Wehipeihana	Jane's rubrics work and Nan's practical examples have transformed how I think about and design processes for valuing an intervention. Jane's practical advice is just never-ending.
Jennifer Greene	Jennifer's writings on participation, democratic evaluation, and voice have encouraged a wide range of thinking from the start of my career. Her insights have influenced how I design evaluations to engage those for whom the services are intended, and have made me think about how their perspectives and voices should be acknowledged in the evaluation's purpose, process, and valuing of findings.
Melvin Hall	Melvin has taught me how to think about the complexities of race and culture, and what these mean in an evaluation setting.
Rodney Hopson	Rodney's writing on culture, values, and ethics are inspiring to me.
Ernest House	Ernie has influenced me in many ways; one of his greatest contributions is his description of advocating for the disempowered through using empirical data. His writing has made me rethink evaluation's role in a democratic society and my own role in it, and has encouraged me to pay careful attention to gathering empirical data. He has taught me that empirical evidence is one of the best gifts I can offer to those who do not have a voice.
Beverly Parsons	Beverly's explanation of systems thinking has changed how I think about complexity, and has enabled me to engage with the systems literature and implement systems evaluation approaches.
Michael Patton	Michael has inspired me to be my own kind of evaluator. His writing brings much-needed practicality to my approaches, and his influence is seen in my adherence to always asking who is going to use something, and how. I draw on his ideas about reality checks all the time. His work on process use and developmental evaluation has influenced much of my later work, and his more recent work on principles-focused evaluation is inspirational.
Patricia Rogers	Patricia's explanation of randomized controlled trials (RCTs) and their practicalities, and her description of what she calls "randomization fairies" (among other logical arguments concerning methodology), always stick in my head. Her practical, intelligent, writing inspires me in how to engage with clients on complex topics.
Michael Scriven and Thomas Schwandt	These two authors do not necessarily bring the same ideologies to evaluation. Reading one, then the other, then the first one again, and so on has taught me how to think with different kinds of academic reasoning; this has greatly benefitted my practical evaluation work.
Hazel Symonette	Hazel's work in diversity and culturally responsive evaluation helps me to see the world in different ways; her writing provides thoughtful insights that help me to reflect on my evaluation work.
Robert Stake	I had a big "aha" moment when I read Robert's assertion that an evaluation approach can provide more of a way of thinking than a step-by-step approach. As I became a more experienced evaluator, this advice allowed me to start thinking more, and stop seeking step-by-step approaches that needed to be methodically applied.

[a]Although other authors may have said something or made a point first, this author or authors put it in a way that influenced me.

> **BOX 14.1. Mystery Box**
>
> So let's play a game. Having a long list of evaluators, and their chosen areas of study, would be one way to list potential authors to read. There are three reasons why I do not do that. First, that seems kind of boring. Second, a long list of authors and readings is not in line with the culture, context, politics, and power of this book. Third, if you have an area of interest, you may only read authors in that subject area while neglecting unlikely choices, who may end up providing useful insights. Reading someone who thinks like you is calming, while reading someone who does not think like you can be invigorating.
>
> So, rather than my telling you what these authors write about, here's what I suggest: Close your eyes (no cheating), and point at one of the names listed below. If your finger ends up in the margin or on a blank space between names, try again. Then visit a library, or do a web search on this evaluator. Your mystery box awaits!
>
> Peter Dahler-Larsen, Katrina Bledsoe, Denise Seigart, Kate McKegg, Robert Chambers, Thomas Cook, Nan Wehipeihana, Lee J. Cronbach, Jess Dart, Stuart Donaldson, Irene Guijt, Joseph Wholey, Stafford Hood, Robert Picciotto, Karen Kirkhart, Saville Kushner, John Mayne, Robin Miller, Katherine Newcomer, Gary Henry, Zenda Ofir, Eleanor Chelimsky, Ray Pawson, Peter Rossi, Donna Mertens, Michael Scriven, Robert Stake, Rick Davies, Daniel Stufflebeam, Fiona Cram, and Donald Campbell.

Human beings are theoretical; we use theory to inform and shape everything we do. Evaluation theory (as well as its various frameworks, approaches, and models) informs how and why an evaluator does what he does, which then allows him to provide explicit reasoning for his evaluation decisions. The more you read, chill out to a podcast, or listen to speakers at evaluation conferences, the more nuggets you will find that influence and support ways of thinking about evaluation.

THEORIES, APPROACHES, AND METHODS

- **Have an hour?** Sometimes it can be fun to watch great evaluation theorists debate. Let's choose Michael Patton and Michael Scriven, two evaluators with fundamentally different ideas about evaluation. Watch a video of one of their famous debates, held at the Claremont Graduate School (*http://ccdl.libraries.claremont.edu/cdm/singleitem/ collection/lap/id/70*). Like what you see? Click on a few more links on that Claremont page (perhaps the one with Fetterman, Patton, and Scriven).

- **Have a few days?** Read Marvin C. Alkin's (2013) *Evaluation Roots: A Wider Perspective of Theorists' Views and Influences.* This North America–focused book centers around the idea that evaluation has three roots: methods, use, and valuing. Mertens and Wilson (2012) also discuss methods, use, and values (which they call *branches*) in their textbook, and they have added a social justice branch. Each branch contributes to the field in different ways. Mertens and Wilson then introduce different authors according to which branch they represent.

- **Have some time to follow up?** Carden and Alkin supplement Alkin's book with a 2012 article, "Evaluation Roots: An International Perspective," published in the online free-access *Journal for MultiDisciplinary Evaluation*. This article offers a wider perspective on critical influencers in the evaluation field.

- **Enjoy heavy theory?** For those who enjoy heavier theory, read William Shadish, Thomas D. Cook, and Laura C. Leviton's (1991) *Foundations of Program Evaluation*, which formed the basis for my own entry into the field of evaluation. I suggest forming a study group to read sections of this book together and discuss their meaning; it's dense. Parts of this book provide some heavy theory. This is a book that I still occasionally pick up and reread a few pages at a time, and then contemplate. As several evaluator colleagues have told me, "This is the text that made me an evaluator."

- **Want to explore some critiques of evaluation theory?** Read Daniel Stufflebeam and Chris Coryn's (2014) *Evaluation Theory, Models, and Applications*.

- **Want to have some fun?** Select any two evaluation books. Choose a topic (e.g., participation, values, outcomes), and go to the subject index in these books. Find the subject you have chosen in each book, and write down the numbers of the relevant page(s) in each book. Then look at those pages and compare what each author says, who they cite, or note which authors do not even mention that topic. This is a quick way to begin to understand the diverse plethora of information out there.

WRAPPING UP

The thinkers and writers whose work you read or listen to, and the persons and organizations you work with and for, will subtly (or not so subtly) influence your thinking about evaluation. Every field has its early influencers, and evaluation is no different. Grounding your understanding of evaluation in works by some of the people who helped build the foundations of modern program evaluation (though as we note in Chapter 1, evaluation extends beyond just programs), and reading the works of those who continue to contribute to this emerging field, will enable you to provide more thoughtful evaluation. Thoughtful evaluation is likely to be better evaluation, which is then likely to be more useful evaluation, which is then likely to result in better interventions that have a higher likelihood of benefitting the people they aim to serve. Phew—now that is a results chain of note! (See Chapters 3–8, particularly Chapter 7, for more on that topic.) With some academic literature on specific theorists to orient you in the field of evaluation, the next chapter explores evaluation more deeply, discussing topics such as common evaluation labels, evaluation theory, approaches and methods, designing an evaluation, and evaluating the evaluation. Before you leave this chapter, however, please come have a chat with me.

Our Conversation: Between You and Me

Sometimes efforts to get focused on what to read can be overwhelming. It is sometimes helpful to pick a topic (say, process use or culturally appropriate evaluations) and then read a wide assortment of authors on these topics. Here are some more ideas to guide you in delving deeper into the literature.

- *Which person in evaluation do you admire, or what themes excite you?* Who does the type of evaluation work that you want to do? Who does the type of evaluation work that inspires you? My evaluation work was greatly influenced by my experience of poverty—first in the Peace Corps, later with AmeriCorps, and then while living in a developing country. I saw evaluation as one way that I could positively influence people's lives and promote social justice. I sought out approaches and articles on evaluation and social justice, and evaluation and use; these readings led me to study under Michael Patton (use) and Jennifer Greene (social justice). *What about you?*

- *Take a certificate course, or get a degree.* Sometimes it is nice to have someone else set up a guided tour of the literature. There is no better way to get that guidance than to pursue a degree or certificate in evaluation. Many universities on several continents offer individual courses, certificates, master's degrees, and doctorates in evaluation, with some courses even available online (*www.eval.org* provides a list, though at my last glance it was not complete). Choose one that interests you and fits your budget. If there are barriers to full-time study, look for short courses at institutes, universities, or courses held in conjunction with conferences. Look for free public seminars and online seminars provided by institutes and evaluation associations and societies.

- *Attend an evaluation conference.* Once you arrive at the conference, chose themes or topics that interest you. Often speakers will mention theorists or new ideas that you can then research at a later date. If a speaker piques your interest, approach the speaker at the conference and ask them for recommendations on who to read; or, better yet, ask the speaker some questions that have been swimming in your head.

CHAPTER 15

Navigating the Maze of Evaluation Choices

Look for choices, pick the best one, and then go with it.
—PAT RILEY, American professional basketball
coach and player

We have talked about the different roles and actions associated with being an evaluator (Chapter 11); the values that influence an evaluator and evaluation (Chapter 12); other influences on an evaluator and evaluation (Chapter 13); and being inspired by evaluation theorists through the literature and the scholarly side of being an evaluator (Chapter 14). This chapter begins by looking at how people often request evaluation (the names they use), and takes a "nutshell" approach to exploring a few different evaluation approaches, theories, and models. The chapter then wraps up with a focus on evaluation designs, reports, and evaluating the evaluation. Let's first clarify some common terms often associated with evaluation.

WHEN SOMEONE WANTS AN EVALUATION: THE NAMES THEY USE

Requests for evaluations come with many names, and for many reasons. Some of the more familiar names are *midterm*, *final*, *summative*, and *formative*. Sometimes a client will request a particular approach, such as a *utilization-focused* approach or a *participatory* approach. There are an endless number of reasons to request an evaluation, some of which are political (to showcase an intervention, or to get rid of it), bureaucratic (to check/tick off boxes on a form), and even practical (to answer questions raised by monitoring data). When people request an evaluation by name, or by approach, the reason for the evaluation is not always clear in that request, and it often needs to be expounded upon. Only once a clear reason or purpose for the evaluation is determined can an approach to evaluation can be selected. Clarifying that initial request is covered in these first few pages of the chapter, followed by brief descriptions of different approaches.

Hi. My clients are asking me to do a midterm evaluation this year and a final evaluation next year. What are they asking for? Are these the same as a formative and a summative evaluation, respectively?

All that is clear from those labels is that the client is asking for evaluations at certain times. I understand the connection you make; an assumption could be made that a midterm evaluation aims to inform the intervention (formative), and that a final one aims to sum it up and judge its merit, worth, and significance (summative). However, guesses are always dangerous. That a person is requesting, and planning for evaluation, is excellent. To encourage that, seek clarity with these two questions:

- *Who wants the evaluation?* Answers to this question will give some insight into the evaluation's reason and purpose, as well as hint at the potential power and political issues that you may well need to be engaged with during the evaluation.
- *What information is needed, by whom, when, to do what?* Answers to this quesion provide insight into what specific person needs what specific information to make what decisions. This further clarifies the evaluation purpose, and *also* hints at the power and politics in the evaluation process.

These questions are thus likely to provide answers that lead to more thoughtful questions—the answers to which further clarify not only the purpose, but the key questions, potential methods of inquiry, possible evaluation approaches, the most likely valuing process, and probable ways to communicate the findings. A third question always in the back of my head, yet one I am constantly aware of, is this: Who can get hurt by the evaluation, and who stands to benefit from the evaluation (Patton, 2008)? Let's continue to look at other ways in which clients request evaluations.

IMPLEMENTATION, OUTCOME, AND IMPACT LABELS

Other common ways in which people often request evaluations, or label them, are with these three words: **implementation, outcome,** and **impact.** When someone uses one of these labels, or asks for one of these types of evaluation, it provides a vague idea of what kind of information they seek. *Never* assume, however, that whoever requested that evaluation has the same understanding or expectations for the same term as you do. For example, Part I of this book (specifically, see Chapters 6 and 7) explains, in detail, how someone's outcome can be another person's impact. Go back to those chapters and review those discussions, and then draw on that understanding to walk forward into the evaluation discussion.

Before exploring implementation, outcome, and impact evaluations, the advice provided in the section above is repeated. *An evaluator needs to clarify who has what purpose for the evaluation before engaging further.* Just as the terms *midterm* and *final* evaluation provide an idea of the evaluation's timing, and *formative* and *summative* offer a vague idea of its intended use, the request for an *implementation, outcome,* or *impact* evaluation offers some foggy clarity around what results to evaluate. We need to defog, however.

Implementation Evaluation: The "What Is Done" and Sometimes "How and What" Conversation

Implementation evaluation looks at how an intervention is . . . implemented. Implementation evaluations can be conducted at any time during an intervention's life, though it is often better to conduct an implementation evaluation early in its life. How early? Early enough so that if challenges or problems are identified, or changes are otherwise needed, the modifications can be made so that the intervention is more likely to achieve its intended results. Sometimes an implementation evaluation is conducted as part of an outcome or impact evaluation (see the next section for a discussion of these); it then provides insight into the intervention results, or lack thereof.

My client asked for a process evaluation; is that the same thing as an implementation evaluation?

It could be. Some people interchange the words *process* and *implementation* evaluation, while others use them quite differently. Drawing from Patton (2008), Mertens and Wilson (2012), and Rossi, Lipsey, and Freeman (2004) and from my own field experience, I explain the distinction this way: Process evaluation focuses on *how* an intervention is done, and implementation evaluation focuses on *what* is done. An implementation evaluation explores the extent to which the intervention was implemented as designed, to see if the intervention is moving toward achieving its intended results. A process evaluation also explores to see if an intervention is moving toward its intended results; however, the process evaluation focuses more on, for example, the participants' experience of the intervention, and seeks to understand how and why something is happening. Just to note, a few people do talk about implementation evaluation as a type of process research. Sigh. If someone asks for an implementation evaluation, a process evaluation, or process research, clarify if they are interested in what is done, how something is done, or both. Then delve into the reasons for the request, again using the two questions listed and discussed on the previous page:

- Who wants the evaluation?
- What information is needed, by whom, when, to do what?

Use the answers to these questions and conversations to inform the evaluation's design. Do not let anyone (including yourself) use a label until it is clear what is expected from the evaluation.

> ### BOX 15.1. Implementation Evaluation
>
> Michael Patton (2002) describes implementation evaluations as evaluations that "tell decision makers what is going on in the program, how the program has developed, and how and why programs deviate from initial plans and expectations" (p. 161). He goes on to say that if there are limited funds for evaluation and one must choose between an implementation or outcome evaluation, it is often better to choose the implementation evaluation. "Unless one knows that a program is operating according to design, there may be little reason to expect it to produce the desired outcomes. Where outcomes are evaluated without knowledge of implementation, the results seldom provide a direction for action because the decision makers lack the information about what produces the observed outcome (or lack of outcome)" (Patton, 2002, p. 161).

My client asked for an implementation evaluation that looks at accountability; is that even possible?

Evaluation, to be useful, needs to meet a client's needs, and thus many terms and their definitions can be flexible. It is also what creates a bit of mayhem (see Chapter 1 for more on evaluation language). Patton (2008) writes that an implementation evaluation can be done for several reasons. One is for *accountability*. For example, in a school system, there could be a standard that all children in Grade 1 are tested for scoliosis. So an implementation evaluation focused on accountability would assess the extent to which that standard is being met. Patton and others (Mertens & Wilson, 2012), note that implementation evaluation can also be done for program *improvement*. In this case, the focus is on what is working well and what is not, so that program implementers can make changes as needed. So, rather than assessing the scoliosis testing program against a standard, the evaluator would assess what was working well (e.g., testing children during physical education classes works well for the boys) and what is not working well (e.g., it does not work well for girls).

Patton then describes a few more types of implementation evaluation. One is implementation evaluation with a *learning* focus. Here, what is learned is intended to inform other programs or the general literature, so the purpose is to use the findings more broadly, with a summative focus. What? Yes, that is right, summative; the focus is on learning more about the intervention by assessing it against what was supposed to happen (i.e., the standard) and to understand what has emerged that is different with regard to its implementation, and in doing so, to judge its merit and worth. The key point to remember is that, regardless of the type of implementation evaluation, it is all about implementation.

Goodness. That is a lot of labels. Can I just stick to calling it implementation evaluation?

In evaluation, there are a lot of useful labels that come with distinct meanings, which support an evaluator in producing an evaluation that meets a client's needs. However, if the labels get in the way and muddle up what you as an evaluator need to do, my advice is not to use the labels. My further advice is to stick with the two questions suggested on page 286: Seek to understand who needs what information to make what decisions, and by when. Once the answers to the two questions are very clear, then apply a label if you want to, or if you must.

What are some questions that are often part of an implementation evaluation?

The guiding, or overarching, question is this: What happens during implementation of the intervention, as compared to what was supposed to happen? Here are some specific questions that are often part of an implementation evaluation (*www.betterevaluation.org*; Mertens & Wilson, 2012; Patton, 2008). The different kinds of implementation evaluation will entail their own distinct and narrowed questions; however, each question will still focus on implementation.

- What is working well? What is not?
- What does the program consist of?
- What are the key characteristics?
- What do staff members do?
- Who are the intended beneficiaries?
- Does the theory of change appear to be working, and is it likely that the outcomes will be achieved?
- What needs to be done to strengthen the program and to overcome blockages?

My client wants an implementation evaluation to learn about what is working well and what is not, and what can be improved, for a rather large project. I'm kind of overwhelmed in deciding where to start the data collection. Do you have any suggestions?

For *any* evaluation, seek to understand what *credible* evidence exists (if any) that can be used to answer or inform evaluation questions. (To revisit the difference among credible data, credible evidence, and credible evaluation, see Chapter 5.) These two thematic areas can guide you:

- *Previous evaluations.* Previous evaluations can be useful in several ways. These evaluations can have credible data, identify data sources, and provide other hints on how to focus the data collection. The evaluation may also provide overt or covert clues to the power, politics, language, and cultural considerations (e.g., read an earlier report's limitations section). Finally, find out how the evaluation was used (and if not, why not), and use that information to guide the design of your evaluation.
- *Monitoring data.* Explore those data: Are they accessible? Are they accurate? Do

they raise questions or answer them? Sometimes several evaluation questions (or even parts of them) can be answered with the monitoring data. Even if a question is answered with monitoring data, though, it may still be an area to explore, perhaps from different perspectives or with different kinds of data.

Wait a second. I was asked to do an implementation evaluation, and what was supposed to happen during the intervention is all a bit unclear. How can I evaluate what was supposed to happen if it isn't clear to begin with?

Actually, these situations are among the reasons I enjoy being an evaluator. Sometimes I am asked to evaluate a model, or a specific design, but then there is no written documentation or any explanation of what the actual model or design is. Then part of the evaluation (or sometimes the entire evaluation) involves documenting and explaining the model/design. In these situations, I drop the label and revert to the two questions discussed on page 286 (i.e., who needs to know what, by when, to do what). Perhaps the donor or government manager needs the evaluation because they are unclear about what is supposed to happen and/or what is actually happening. The evaluation would still focus on exploring how things are being done, so technically it would be labeled an implementation evaluation. Things can get a bit messy out there in the real world, however, so do not get too hooked on labels; as always, seek explanation and understanding.

I think I get it. So an implementation evaluation focuses on what happens, and does not focus on results.

That is correct. An implementation evaluation does *not* focus on the results. Two of the more common types of evaluation that focus on results are called *outcome* and *impact* evaluations. Let's talk about those next.

Outcome and Impact Evaluations: The Results Conversations

Outcome and impact evaluations focus on understanding whether (and, if so, to what extent) results happened (and consider yet go beyond output results; see Chapters 6–8 for further explanation), *and* on exploring how those results are connected to the intervention. These results can be intended, meaning those that the intervention planned to achieve, or unintended, meaning those that the intervention did not set out to achieve, but happened anyway. Unintended results can be negative (e.g., a wetland environment is destroyed to build a school) or positive (e.g., a new school built to improve access to education for preschoolers also provides a safe space for a fathers' peer-to-peer meeting that aims to improve girls' access to education). Some people would specifically define an impact evaluation as one that focuses on accountability (i.e., by determining whether the intervention has brought about the results intended) and learning (i.e., by creating an evidence base of what interventions work) (White & Raitzer, 2017).

Outcome. Impact. People never seem to agree which is what. Chapters 6 and 7 have showed me how to engage in the results label discussion when clarifying the intervention, and Chapter 8 has helped too. Should that same discussion be held here?

Absolutely. When a client or colleague uses the term *outcome* or *impact* with no clear definitions, stop the conversation immediately, *remove the label from the conversation,* and ask the following two (now very familiar) questions:

- Who wants the evaluation?
- What information is needed, by whom, when, to do what?

Furthermore, as you mentioned, it would be useful to support that discussion with a conversation like those that we had in Chapters 6 and 7. Again, too, do not let anyone (including yourself) use a label before its time. After it is clear what the key evaluation questions are, and who will use the findings to do what, go ahead and apply any relevant label you like.

In general, what are outcome and impact evaluations mainly focused on? Is it just whether the intervention has achieved its intended results?

Essentially, outcome and impact evaluations are mainly focusing on effectiveness: Has the intervention achieved what it set out to achieve? Some people define outcome evaluation as looking for lower-level effectiveness results, while they view impact evaluations as searching for higher-level (often societal-level) changes. Regardless of whether it is labeled an outcome or impact evaluation, the evaluation needs to show *some* link between what the intervention did and what results were achieved (intended or unintended). How that link is determined causes (pun intended) intense conversations in the field. The issue of causal inference is a critical one that evaluators should be comfortable explaining.

OK, so you said outcome and impact evaluation are about effectiveness. The other day someone told me that there is effectiveness and this other term, efficacy. Then there is also efficiency. What is the difference among the three terms?

I am going to provide an answer given two decades ago by Brian Haynes, who in turn drew his explanation from Archie Cochrane. Haynes (1999, p. 652) stated, "Efficacy is the extent to which an intervention does more good than harm under ideal circumstances ('Can it work?'). Effectiveness assesses whether an intervention does more good than harm when provided under usual circumstances . . . ('Does it work in practice?'). Efficiency measures the effect of an intervention in relation to the resources it consumes ('Is it worth it?')."

When someone says they want an outcome or impact evaluation, what are they most likely looking to evaluate?

In a nutshell, they probably want to know if the intervention worked. Outcome (and, for some, impact) evaluations typically look at changes in knowledge, skills, attitudes, and the intention to act (i.e., do something), though not the actual act. The next level of focus (which some evaluators would still place under outcome evaluation, while others would shift to calling it impact evaluation) then involves looking at actual behavior change—a person actually doing something, or something else happening as a result of shifts in knowledge, skills, or attitudes. Here is another way of putting it. An outcome evaluation explores whether people's knowledge has changed, and an impact evaluation then looks to see if, because of that knowledge change, actual behavior has changed. In an impact evaluation, some would look for changes at a societal level. Many interventions that I evaluate make assumptions (as shown through a theory of change) that when an intervention shifts people's knowledge and attitudes, it then follows that behavior changes. That is a big assumption (which is why it is evaluated).

What I have just described, however, is *my understanding* of outcome and impact evaluation. When you are working with a client who requests an outcome or impact evaluation, clarify the *client's* understanding of outcome or impact—or, better yet, focus on understanding the client's purpose for the evaluation, and who needs to know what, to do what, by when.

Can you just clarify, briefly, why someone would want to do an outcome or impact evaluation?

There can be many reasons someone asks for an outcome or impact evaluation. Usually, a person is interested in identifying what worked to produce what result, and what did not work.

Wait! A bit earlier in the section, you mentioned causality and causal inference. Please, can you go back to that discussion?

OK. As I have noted in earlier chapters, E. Jane Davidson is a well-known evaluation theorist who has written several books and shares a blog called Genuine Evaluation (*www. genuineevaluation.com*) with Patricia Rogers, another well-known evaluation theorist who is also one of the masterminds behind the website Better Evaluation (*www.betterevaluation. org*). In a 2010 post on Genuine Evaluation, Rogers and Davidson engage in a very straightforward discussion of causality (*http://genuineevaluation.com/causal-inference-for-program-theory-evaluation*). I have drawn on that dialogue here.

At the start of that conversation, Rogers provides a concrete definition and explanation for the term *causal inference*. She notes that "By causal inference we mean both causal attribution (working out what was THE cause) and causal contribution (identifying what was one or more of the causes that together produced the outcomes and impacts)."

Thus Rogers explains the three critical terms in the causality conversation: **causal inference, attribution,** and **contribution.** I cannot emphasize enough the importance of knowing and understanding these terms, particularly when having any discussion of outcome and impact evaluation. As Rogers notes, *causal inference* can refer to either attribution or contribution. She then clarifies that an evaluation question can seek to understand either the cause of the result (*attribution*) or what contributed to the result (*contribution*). These are different questions that necessitate different evaluation designs.

When a client, commissioner, or colleague requests a design that shows attribution, reframe that conversation as one about causal inference. Often people are not aware that there are two options for exploring the "what caused that" question. A straightforward question to ask is this: "Do you want to know if your intervention caused the result [attribution] or helped to cause the result [contribution]?"

If a person says that they need to know if their intervention caused the result, ask, "What makes you say that?" If they provide reasons, such as that the donor or government mandates this level of understanding, then the evaluation design needs to address attribution. If a client does not have a clear reason, discuss the likely usefulness of contribution. Because many factors often contribute to an intervention's results, the concept of contribution is a practical concept in the real world of evaluation.

A book that provides a deeper understanding of contribution is Earl, Carden, and Smutylo's *Outcome Mapping: Building Learning and Reflection into Development Programs* (2001). In this book, the authors talk in depth about the concept of contribution and reasons to consider it.

John Mayne's (2012) description of contribution analysis is worth knowing. *Contribution analysis* is a theory-oriented approach that enables an evaluator to confirm whether an intervention is a contributory cause of an outcome or impact. Mayne explains that the evaluator is aiming to identify if and how the intervention has contributed to identified outcomes or impacts. He then notes that often interventions are implemented in a context where there are many influencing factors, not just the intervention being evaluated. Thus contribution analysis is an approach to determining how the intervention, among these other factors, has contributed to (i.e., is a contributory cause of) identified results.

Attribution and contribution can both play a vital role in evaluation. Sometimes in one evaluation, some questions may lend themselves to attribution, while others are more appropriately explored through contribution. (For a longer explanation, read through the logic explained in Chapters 3–7.) Here is an example. An evaluator assesses an intervention to determine the extent of improvement in math scores for boys between the ages of 11 and 13 who live in inner cities with high levels of school absenteeism. Data show that within 2 years of implementation, the targeted boys have improved their math scores by an average of 20%, which the evaluation shows as *attributable* to the math intervention. The results are highly valued by the boys, their parents, and the school administration. Another question, in the same evaluation, asks about the influence of the intervention on the school attendance of the targeted boys. The answer to this question is that the intervention has *contributed* to improved attendance, a result valued by the school's teachers and administration. In other words, the intervention has been one of reasons why the boys' attendance has improved—along with many other factors, such as an improved sports program, free breakfast, and the adoption and enforcement of an anti-bullying policy.

What strategies should I learn about to engage with causal inference?

In the blog post cited on page 292, Rogers and Davidson (*http://genuineevaluation.com/causal-inference-for-program-theory-evaluation*) talk about useful strategies to engage with causal inference. They describe three groups of methods for answering causal questions:

- Comparing results to a *counterfactual*—an estimate of what would have happened in the absence of the program or policy.
- Checking that the results match the program theory.
- Identifying and ruling out alternative explanations.

The sample questions provided on page 289 for implementation evaluations are useful. Can you provide some sample questions for outcome and impact evaluations as well?

I am glad to. The overarching question for an outcome or impact evaluation is to determine the extent to which the intervention has achieved what it set out to achieve, and/or how it has influenced or created change. In general, when someone is referring to an outcome or impact evaluation, they are asking these kinds of questions (*www.betterevaluation.org*; Patton, 2008):

- How effective was the program? (Has the intervention achieved what it set out to achieve?)
- What are the unintended effects, if any?
- Can the changes in outcomes be explained by the program, or are they the result of some other factors occurring simultaneously?
- Should an intervention be continued or replicated?
- Do results vary across different groups of intended beneficiaries (e.g., males vs. females), in different areas, over different time periods?
- How effective is the program in comparison with alternative interventions?

My parting words on outcome and impact evaluations are words of caution. The debate still rages over what is an outcome evaluation and what is an impact evaluation, or even whether such a thing as an impact evaluation exists. *Do not engage in this debate* (unless you so choose in an academic or other learning setting, where it can be invigorating). Rather, if someone asks for an outcome or impact evaluation, delve into the reasons for the request (the evaluation's purpose), the questions that need to be answered, how the findings will be used, when, and by whom—*and then* agree on the evaluation label (if a label is needed). Again, define first and label later. I am sure that the advice sounds familiar by now.

A Few Other Purposes for Evaluations

The chapter so far has covered the labels most commonly used when a person requests an evaluation. Because those in the field of evaluation appear to like labels and categories, and because nuanced differences abound among those labels and concepts, there are a few more types of evaluation that suggest a specific purpose. These include *economic* evaluation, *cost–benefit* evaluation, *sustainability* evaluation, and *design* evaluation, to name a few. While their names provide clues to their intended purposes, how people define the terms may vary—and if these variations are not clarified, this can cause all kinds of havoc for an evaluator. At the same time, when definitions are clear, the surplus of choices for evaluation purposes can be just what is needed. Evaluators need to be able to engage others in a discussion that makes an evaluation's purpose (and whose purpose) clear, and have the knowledge and skills to clarify the evaluation labels (see Chapter 1).

BOX 15.2. Adding to the List: Focusing an Evaluation by Label

Patton's (2012) book, *Essentials of Utilization-Focused Evaluation,* offers more than 70 ways to focus an evaluation. I encourage having a look at the plethora of terms that you may encounter. I have randomly selected three as examples (pp. 182–188):

- *Compliance-focused:* Are rules and regulations being followed?
- *Equity-focused:* Are participants treated fairly and justly?
- *Quality assurance:* Are minimum and accepted standards of care being routinely and systematically provided to participants and clients?

Two other terms that suggest a specific purpose for an evaluation are *value for money* (VFM) and *social return on investment* (SROI), both of which take a stand on how to value findings. Can you guess one of those determining values? (Hint: $!)

At the end of the day, it is fundamental to any evaluation process for an evaluator to be clear about (1) what the evaluation's purpose (not the label) is, (2) whose purpose it is, and

(3) how an evaluation will support (4) whom in making or informing (5) what decisions or areas of knowledge. Negotiating the evaluation's purpose may be part of an evaluator's role, or it may be a foregone conclusion before the evaluator is invited to the party—I mean, into the process.

Is there a difference among the many purposes of evaluation in terms of cost?

There is no way to determine the cost of an evaluation by its stated purpose. The resources and time needed for any evaluation will vary according to the number of evaluation questions, the size of the intervention, the availability of credible data, the logistics of collecting data, and multiple other factors. The very popular answer to the question "How long is a piece of string?" (i.e., "It depends") is also a good response to the question of how much an evaluation will cost.

Once an evaluator has established a clear evaluation purpose, understands who is going to use the data to inform what decisions, and has finalized the key evaluation questions with all relevant parties, she begins to think about how to approach the evaluation. It is now time for a discussion of evaluation approaches, theories, and models. Some evaluation purposes and evaluation approaches are perfect matches, while others are like oil and water (they do not mix). Evaluators need to choose an approach, or otherwise modify or mix parts of several approaches, that guides them to create an appropriate, useful, feasible, accountable, accurate, and altogether credible evaluation that meets the evaluation's purpose (or objective) and answers the evaluation questions.

APPROACHES TO EVALUATION

Evaluation approaches, theories, and models abound (hereafter usually called just *approaches*), and each brings unique benefits and challenges to the evaluation process. Different approaches offer a plethora of ways to engage (or not) with values as well as cultural, political, language, power, and other contextual issues. An evaluator needs to be familiar with the multiple ways that diverse approaches can provide guidance for designing and implementing an evaluation, and to be aware that these approaches can result in different answers to the same evaluation question. Thus knowing a range of evaluation approaches is a benefit to any evaluator and her client. This section provides a smorgasbord of appetizers to whet your appetite for evaluation approaches, and then refers you to some experts who offer full meals.

As noted earlier, the words *approach*, *theory*, and *model* are often used interchangeably in both the evaluation literature and the practice of evaluation. If I were asked, I would say that a theory explains why you do something; an approach, model, or framework is something that builds on a theory, is more concrete, and is prescriptive about how to implement the evaluation. However, this is not always how the evaluation world unfolds and engages with these terms. For the purposes of our discussion, I have chosen the term *approach* to mean something that offers guidance to an evaluator; it describes her role in the evaluation and informs decision making during the evaluation process. Many, many different evaluation approaches are described in the evaluation literature; some are quite distinct, while others are slight variations of each other. And then there is the complication that what people publish as an example of an approach does not actually exemplify the approach as described by its original theorist. Miller and Campbell (2006) studied 53 evaluations labeled as *empowerment evaluation*. This was what they found:

> [The] 47 case examples examined in this review were remarkably different in their approaches to empowerment evaluation and degree of adherence to its espoused principles of practice . . . although many evaluation projects get labeled (and relabeled) as empowerment evaluations, frequently, these evaluations do not embody the core principles that are supposed to undergird empowerment evaluation practice. (pp. 313–314)

Although being an evaluator involves so much more than knowing an approach (as this book has demonstrated), one cannot be an evaluator without them. Choosing which approach (or whose version of an approach) to read about and learn can be a huge decision—one that is often only guided by implementing an evaluation and experiencing a huge learning curve. At the same time, Miller (2010) notes:

> In the real world of practice, evaluators may not use any theory as more than a vague map to facilitate and guide their action. Evaluators may also use combinations of theories rather than apply any theory in pure fashion. And, the demands of the particular evaluation situation may predominate over theoretical prescriptions, preferences, and training. (p. 397)

This section of this chapter only touches the tip of the iceberg on what approaches can guide an evaluator. The section's purposes are to raise your awareness of the many choices that exist; to inspire you to learn more about each one; and to encourage you to read more about the others not mentioned here, though identified throughout the book (e.g., developmental evaluation, culturally responsive evaluation, empowerment evaluation).

After a nutshell description of each type, I provide resources to place you in the hands of experts who provide in-depth explanations. Luckily, an amazing range of books, blogs, journal articles, and other resources that delve specifically into various approaches, theories, and models is available. To apply a metaphor from the medical field, I am a general practitioner who will explain the basics, and then send you to a podiatrist, cardiologist, orthopedic surgeon, or pediatrician for detailed, specific advice.

> **BOX 15.3. An Evaluator's Approach to Using Theories, Models, and Approaches**
>
> Most evaluators draw on multiple theories, models, and approaches, and then add a dash of experience, a pinch of common sense, and touch of luck.

Wait! I have a burning question that I need to ask before you start. I have heard some people argue that evaluation theory is not a theory.

I think I know where that statement comes from. Social science theories aim to predict or explain behavior; in other words, they are generalizable statements that aim to predict or explain something. While evaluation theories do not predict behavior or attempt to explain it, there are evaluation approaches that make claims about what will happen if an evaluator uses them. For example, using empowerment evaluation will empower staff, or using participatory approaches will lead to evaluation use. An evaluation theory serves as a guide for an evaluator and provides the philosophical justification for making decisions.

With that understanding, let's explore some evaluation approaches. The website Better Evaluation (*www.betterevaluation.org*) offers a plethora of approaches and themes for guiding an evaluation, and suggests that an evaluation approach is something that offers an "integrated set of options used to do some or all of the tasks involved in evaluation." Using that broad guidance, I have selected the 10 approaches I believe are most likely to offer a wide introduction to what is out there.

The descriptions of some approaches begin with mentions of their creators or principal theorists; at other times, a type of approach is described first and then some theorists are mentioned. There is no rhyme or reason for doing this, other than that I often encounter such variations in my reading and my work. Some approaches seem to be strongly attached to one person, while other approaches are associated with multiple authors, theorists, and practitioners. I have not written this section so that you will be able to use these approaches based on the small snippets of information I provide, or even know all their key aspects. Rather, as noted on the previous page, the section exposes you to a tiny sample that provides an idea of how different approaches offer contrasting ways to inform evaluations and their design.

Utilization-Focused Evaluation

If you find yourself wondering how to implement an evaluation process, and have a core value that evaluations are meant to be used, *utilization-focused evaluation* (UFE) is an approach to consider. Michael Patton is the creator and principal theorist of UFE. His approach is attentive to process use *and* use of the findings. He provides clear guidance on how to manage and implement an evaluation so that it will be used by what he calls its *intended users*. Patton's approach provides clear guidance for how the evaluator can encourage use by being attentive to every step in an evaluation. The UFE framework has evolved over the years; it first provided 5 steps, then expanded these to 17, and now has 21 steps to guide the evaluator through each part of an evaluative process (Podems, 2014b). Patton places the evaluator in the role of a facilitator, negotiator, and educator. UFE provides a process for choosing an appropriate method, theory, or approach to be used with UFE, or simply asking UFE questions can be an approach on its own. If you wish to focus on evaluation use, you like having structured guidance (with ample flexibility within that guidance) for the entire evaluative process, and you appreciate a plethora of supportive material, then UFE is a good evaluation theory to consider.

UTILIZATION-FOCUSED EVALUATION

- **Have a few minutes?** Look at the Better Evaluation website's page on UFE (*www.betterevaluation.org/en/plan/approach/utilization_focused_evaluation*).

- **Have an hour?** Take a look at this UFE checklist (*www.wmich.edu/sites/default/files/attachments/u350/2014/UFE_checklist_2013.pdf*).

- **Plan on implementing the approach?** There are two books, both Patton's: *Utilization-Focused Evaluation* (2008) and *Essentials of Utilization-Focused Evaluation* (2012). If you plan on implementing UFE, I would recommend reading (or owning) both books. Even if you decide that UFE is not an approach you want to try, I encourage reading either book (though if you are completely new to evaluation, I would recommend the 2008 book). Patton is a master storyteller and engages the reader in learning about evaluation more broadly, introducing all sorts of evaluation approaches, techniques, methods, stories, examples, ideas, and references to other material.

While this is a section on evaluation approaches, UFE cannot be discussed without touching on what is meant by *use*. Here are some types of use to consider:

- *Instrumental use.* Instrumental use occurs when someone uses the evaluation findings and recommendations to make changes to the intervention.

- *Conceptual use.* Conceptual use occurs when evaluation results (and often the synthesis of multiple evaluations) provide new information or bring about new ideas and concepts.

- *Process use.* If you have read this book straight through from Chapter 1, by now you are aware that one of my favorite types of uses is process use. Process use refers to learning or other kinds of use happening during the life of the evaluation. Process use can bring about personal or organizational changes and can add value in a multitude of other ways. (See Chapter 11.)

- *Legitimizing use.* This is one to be very careful with: Legitimizing use occurs when the evaluation legitimizes existing thinking. These can also quickly become *pork-barrel* evaluations, or ones that are done to keep powerful individuals or groups in power.

- *Symbolic use.* Symbolic use involves what I have called *check box* or *tick box* evaluations, discussed in Chapter 10. These evaluations are implemented just so someone can say that an evaluation was completed.

- *Misuse.* I would be dishonest to not mention that in the real world, one type of use is misuse. As evaluators, we need to do our best to ensure that this does not happen, and engaging in discussions of power, politics, culture, and language is one way to prevent misuse (see Chapter 13).

- *Non-use.* Sometimes non-use is mentioned as an alternative form of use. Yet for me, there is always some use. Even a check box/tick box evaluation has a use: It often results in meeting some requirement for the intervention to continue. The same can be said for monitoring data: Although a program implementer may not use the data that are required to be collected to inform the intervention, those data are probably used to meet an accountability need, which may influence whether or not the intervention continues to be funded (Alkin & King, 2017; Patton, 2008, 2012; Weiss, 1998).

Democratic Evaluation

If democracy, power, transparency, and/or public accountability are themes that are important to the evaluation users, *democratic evaluation* is an approach to consider. At its core, democratic evaluation encourages evaluative thinking in various spheres of society to bring about social change. Democratic evaluation suggests that evaluation processes and the information generated should support public decision making, and in this way support the attainment of social justice (Greene, 2007; House & Howe, 1999, 2000; MacDonald, 1987; Patton, 2002; Ryan, 2005).

British evaluator Barry MacDonald was the first known theorist to publish on the democratic evaluation concept, which he did in the 1970s. MacDonald (1987) explains that democratic evaluation is guided by the ethic that the public has a right to have enough information with which to engage meaningfully and thoughtfully on an issue. Kushner (2016) adds that particular emphasis should be placed on the need to involve marginalized populations in the evaluation process. House and Howe (1999, 2000) introduce *deliberative democratic evaluation,* an approach that supports a deliberative democracy, which is a form of democracy in which deliberation is inclusive and a part of any process that is central to decision making.

Democratic evaluation commits the evaluator to strive for meaningful social change (Podems, 2017). While it does not provide a step-by-step guided process, it does introduce a way of thinking and concepts that support the development of an evaluation design. It is an approach that can use qualitative, quantitative, or mixed methods of inquiry.

Democratic Evaluation

- **Have a minute?** Check out the Better Evaluation website's page on democratic evaluation (*www.betterevaluation.org/en/plan/approach/democratic_evaluation*).

- **Have 30 minutes?** Look at this checklist on deliberative democratic evaluation (*https://wmich.edu/sites/default/files/attachments/u58/2014/deliberative-democratic-evaluation-checklist.pdf*).

- **Have a few hours?** Read House and Howe's (2000) article, "Deliberative Democratic Evaluation," in *New Directions for Evaluation, 2000, 3–12*.

- **Have some more time?** Look at an edited book, *Democratic Evaluation and Democracy: Exploring the Reality* (Podems, 2017). This volume shows the application of democratic evaluation in South Africa and elsewhere in southern Africa, and provides a concise chapter that explains various understandings of democratic evaluation.

Feminist Evaluation

If the evaluation purpose is to explore how differences in structural power and politics influence interventions and its results, *feminist evaluation* (FE) is an approach to consider using. Normally associated with evaluating interventions focused on women, FE is an approach to consider for evaluating interventions that aim to benefit, or involve, any marginalized or disempowered group. Contrary to popular belief, a person does not need to be a feminist to implement FE, and an evaluator does not need to use FE only with women's organizations. The approach emphasizes the importance of reflecting on how an evaluator's own values and perspectives influence the evaluation, and gives guidance on how to engage in an equitable way with people during the evaluation process. At its core, it aims to promote social equity (Podems, 2010, 2014a; Sielbeck-Bowen, Brisolara, Seigart, Tischler, & Whitmore, 2002). FE can use qualitative, quantitative, or mixed methods of inquiry.

Feminist Evaluation

- **Have a minute?** Check out the Better Evaluation website's page on FE (*www.betterevaluation.org/en/themes/feminist_evaluation*).

- **Have 20 minutes?** Check out a slide presentation by Rob Milne that highlights the key aspect of FE and provides some case studies (*https://prezi.com/akfei9qmpxf2/feminist-evaluation*).

- **Have an hour?** Read the article "Feminist Evaluation and Gender Approaches: There's a Difference?" (Podems, 2010), in the *Journal of MultiDisciplinary Evaluation, 6*(14), 1–17.

- **Have a few hours?** Read some selected chapters in an edited volume by Brisolara, Seigart, and SenGupta (2014), *Feminist Evaluation and Research: Theory and Practice*.

Responsive Evaluation

If the evaluation purpose is to explore quality, and focus on how different people and groups experience, understand, and value a program and its activities, then *responsive evaluation* is an approach to consider. While the approach does not necessarily provide steps, responsive evaluation does provide clear guidance on how to implement an evaluation. Basically, the evaluator searches for and documents program quality, with specific attention to key issues or problems, particularly those recognized by people who are directly involved with the intervention. The evaluation design is then focused on those identified issues. Using that design as guidance, the evaluator collects data, and then values those findings by using the value criteria of multiple individuals or groups to determine the program's worth.

Responsive evaluation is not an approach that should be used when core evaluation questions are focused on a program's theory of change, logic model, or stated goals. Rather, it aims to be responsive to "stakeholder concerns" (Stake, 2003), and thus those concerns become the evaluation's core focus. Commonly associated with qualitative methods of inquiry, the approach can also draw on quantitative or mixed methods designs (Stake, 2003).

RESPONSIVE EVALUATION

- **Have a few hours?** Read Tineke Abma's (2005) article in *Evaluation and Program Planning,* which demonstrates an evaluation that uses responsive evaluation, and also offers a nice summary of responsive evaluation in the introduction. Find it at *www. sciencedirect.com/science/article/pii/S0149718905000297.*
- **Have a few hours a night?** Read Robert Stake's (2004) book, *Standards-Based and Responsive Evaluation.*

Theory-Driven Evaluation

If an evaluation's purpose is to explicate an intervention's theory of change, and/or investigate how programs cause intended or observed outcomes, then *theory-driven evaluation* (TDE) is likely a good approach to guide you. Huey Chen is the thinker most commonly associated with this approach, though many other authors publish on it (see the resources provided on the next page). Coryn, Noakes, Westine, and Schroter (2011) provide a nice nutshell description of TDE: "any evaluation strategy or approach that explicitly integrates and uses stakeholder, social science, some combination of, or other types of theories in conceptualizing, designing, conducting, interpreting, and applying an evaluation" (p. 201).

Depending on the author, the ways TDE is applied in practice vary. The good news is that if TDE appeals to you, there is a wide range of choices. I go back to Coryn and colleagues, who provide a succinct summary of how different theorists engage with theory in a TDE approach:

Donaldson . . . has described four potential sources of program theory. These include prior theory and research, implicit theories of those close to the program, observations of the program in operation, and exploratory research to test critical assumptions in regard to a presumed program theory. Patton . . . favors either deductive (i.e., scholarly theories), inductive (i.e., theories grounded in observation of the program), or user-oriented (i.e., stakeholder-derived theories) approaches to developing program theory for evaluation use. Chen . . . , however, has principally advocated a stakeholder-oriented approach to program theory formulation, with the evaluator playing the role of facilitator. (2011, p. 203)

Depending on whose work you are reading (e.g., Patton's, Chen's, or Donaldson's), a different approach would be used to implement TDE, including how to identify and engage with theory. Furthermore (and we know now that this is common in evaluation), other names exist for a theory-oriented approach, including *theory-based evaluation* and *program theory evaluation*. The approach can draw on quantitative, qualitative, or mixed methods designs.

THEORY-DRIVEN EVALUATION

- **Have an hour?** Read Weiss's (2003) article, "On Theory-Based Evaluation: Winning Friends and Influencing People," in *The Evaluation Exchange, 9*(4), 1–5.

- **Have another hour?** Read Rogers's (2007) article, "Theory-Based Evaluations: Reflections Ten Years On," in *New Directions for Evaluation, 2007*(114), 63–67.

- **Have a few hours?** Read Chen's (1994) "Theory-Driven Evaluations: Need, Difficulties and Options," in *Evaluation Practice, 15*(1), 79–82, or Weiss's (2000) "Which Links in Which Theories Shall We Evaluate?" in *New Directions for Evaluation, 2000*(87), 35–45.

- **Have a few days?** Read Chen's book, *Theory-Driven Evaluations* (1990).

Realist Evaluation

If the evaluation purpose is to explore what works for whom, in what respects, to what extent, in what context, and how, then *realist evaluation* is a likely choice to guide that evaluation. Realist evaluation is a form of TDE. Pawson and Tilley (1997) developed the first realist evaluation approach. Essentially, the approach suggests that if evaluation is to be useful to decision makers, then evaluators need to answer how the intervention (for which the term *generative mechanism* is used) caused the outcomes and what role context played in that process (Westhorp, 2014). The concept associated with realist evaluation is context–mechanism–outcome. The approach can draw on qualitative, quantitative, or mixed methods data inquiry.

REALIST EVALUATION

- **Have a few minutes?** Take a spin through Better Evaluation's page on realist evaluation (*www.betterevaluation.org/en/approach/realist_evaluation*).

- **Have a few hours or more?** Read Gill Westhorp's (2014) paper "Realist Impact Evaluation: An Introduction," published online by the Overseas Development Institute's Methods Lab (*www.odi.org/publications/8716-realist-impact-evaluation-introduction*). The paper provides guidance on whether or not to use realist evaluation; if you decide to do one, it then provides concrete steps.

- **Have a few weeks?** Read the original book by Pawson and Tilley, *Realistic Evaluation* (1997).

Context, Input, Process, Product Model

Sometimes explicit steps are helpful. If the evaluation is focusing on accountability or improvement, then consider something like the *context, input, process, product* (CIPP) evaluation model. Daniel Stufflebeam first developed the CIPP evaluation model in the 1960s, and recently coauthored a book on the updated model (Stufflebeam & Zhang, 2017). Through the four stages of context, input, process, and product, this approach investigates an intervention by asking four basic questions: What needs to be done? How should it be done? Is it being done? Did it succeed?

According to Stufflebeam (2007), the CIPP model provides a comprehensive framework that can be used to inform an evaluation for any type of evaluand. The model has a checklist that provides specific details on how to implement the approach, and drills down into each of the four categories. In the CIPP checklist, Stufflebeam takes the overarching question "Did it succeed?" and, step by step, explores specific categories, subcategories, and related questions. While the approach aims to answer questions about merit, worth, and significance, Stufflebeam emphasizes that the evaluation should provide lessons learned. As Stufflebeam says, "The model's main theme is that *evaluation's most important purpose is not to prove, but to improve*" (p. 2; original emphasis). The approach can draw on quantitative, qualitative, or mixed methods designs.

CIPP MODEL

- **Have about 30 minutes?** Take a spin through the 2007 version of Stufflebeam's CIPP checklist (*www.wmich.edu/sites/default/files/attachments/u350/2014/cippchecklist_mar07. pdf*). Then check out the many other checklists provided on the main website.

- **Have a few hours or more?** Read an insightful article by Zhang and colleagues (2011), "Using the Context, Input, Process, and Product Evaluation Model (CIPP) as a

Comprehensive Framework to Guide the Planning, Implementation, and Assessment of Service-Learning Programs," in the *Journal of Higher Education Outreach and Engagement, 15*(4), 57–83 (*http://openjournals.libs.uga.edu/index.php/jheoe/article/view/628*).

- **Plan on implementing the approach?** Read the book by Stufflebeam and Zhang, *The CIPP Evaluation Model: How to Evaluate for Improvement and Accountability* (2017).

Appreciative Inquiry

Appreciative inquiry (abbreviated here as AI, but not to be confused with artificial intelligence) should be considered if the evaluation needs to bring in thinking that encourages a focus on what is working well, and likely a focus on organization improvement. According to Shadish, Cook, and Leviton's (1991) criteria, AI is one of the approaches that would not make the grade in terms of being an evaluation theory; it is what they term an *organization development* approach. Yet it is an approach that evaluators can use to guide their thinking in an evaluation, often in combination with another evaluation approach. AI requires strong facilitation skills, as it relies on group process to identify and address what is not working in an organization in a way "that builds on the successful, effective and energizing experiences of its members" (Preskill & Catsambas, 2006, p. 2). Its basic assumption is that every organization has something that works well. The approach is useful for combating either strong negativity or the opposite, in work with organizations that thrive on positive interaction. The approach provides detailed guidance, such as what questions to ask and what processes to follow. Although it is aimed at assessing an organization, the ideas and concepts can be applied to evaluating a program or intervention.

APPRECIATIVE INQUIRY

- **Have just under 4 minutes?** Take a spin through Jon Townsin's video on AI (*https://appreciativeinquiry.champlain.edu/learn/appreciative-inquiry-introduction*). If you have more time, look at the longer explanation and additional resources.
- **Have a few hours or more a night?** Read the Preskill and Catsambas (2006) book, *Reframing Evaluation through Appreciative Inquiry.*

Principles-Focused Evaluation

As the world continues to change, and as the evaluation field continues to grow with it, new theories and approaches are developed. The newest kid on the block is *principles-focused evaluation* (PFE). If you find yourself in a complex, dynamic situation in which social movements or innovations need to be evaluated, PFE is an approach to consider. Another creation of Michael Patton, PFE engages with these contexts and is based on complexity theory and systems thinking. The approach is premised on the idea that principles can, and should, be evaluated. Patton, through his PFE approach, recognizes that innovation and social movements are guided by principles. These principles need to be clearly articulated, evaluable, and evaluated, to understand what principles lead to what results and how. In other words, how does a principle guide action, and what happens because of that action? PFE provides processes to clarify and articulate a principle so that it is evaluable. It then provides a framework to evaluate the principle, called GUIDE (an acronym for <u>G</u>uiding, <u>U</u>seful, <u>I</u>nspiring, <u>D</u>evelopmental, and <u>E</u>valuable). Patton notes that an evaluation approach needs to match its user; this builds on his earlier thinking, which drove the development of his UFE approach. Patton states that the PFE approach is best matched with principles-driven people doing principles-based initiatives, in innovative and complex situations. The approach can use qualitative, quantitative, or mixed methods of inquiry.

Principles-Focused Evaluation

- **Have 92 minutes?** Listen to Patton describing PFE on his podcast (*www.youtube.com/watch?time_continue=73&v=q4kGbivAAO8*).

- **Have some more time?** Read a new book by Patton, *Principles-Focused Evaluation: The Guide* (2018b).

Randomized Controlled Trials

Donald Campbell (1969) launched the concept of a randomized controlled trial (RCT) as a "truly experimental approach to social reform" (p. 409) in "efforts to extend the logic of laboratory experimentation into the field" (p. 410). Thus an RCT is rooted in the idea of a social experiment (i.e., it is an experimental design). Today some clients request an RCT, not realizing that it is not an approach to evaluation, but a method. Some people approach evaluation through the method, however. A methods-driven approach involves making the method the top criterion for how to do the evaluation. To add a bit more confusion to the mix, an RCT is indeed referred to by some as *randomized evaluation* (White & Raitzer, 2017).

   White and Raitzer (2017, pp. 48–49, 54) describe RCTs as experimental designs in which participants are assigned by chance to separate groups. There are different kinds of RCT designs. The differences relate to (1) the levels of assignment, (2) different approaches to random assignment, and (3) the types of treatment combinations assessed. An RCT needs to be planned before wide-field implementation of an intervention; it cannot be undertaken retrospectively. Another approach, often mentioned in the same breath as an RCT, is a non-experimental design that uses quasi-experimental methods. Here statistical methods replace random assignment (White & Raitzer, 2017).

RANDOMIZED CONTROLLED TRIALS

- **Have 2 minutes?** Watch this World Bank video on RCTs (*https://vimeo.com/92748374*). Note that the World Bank calls an RCT a *randomized impact evaluation.*
- **Have a few hours or more?** Read White and Raitzer's (2017) *Impact Evaluation of Development Interventions,* published by the Asian Development Bank. The resource provides an approximately 150-page guide on RCTs.
- **Have lots of time?** Read a research book recommended at the end of the section on quantitative inquiry in Chapter 5 (Creswell & Creswell, 2018).

An RCT is a quantitative design that is often labeled as an evaluation approach. This reminds me of the so-called "gold standard" debate. Can you talk a bit about that? Is there a gold standard in terms of methodological approaches or approaches for specific purposes?

Some would say, "Yes, there is a gold standard," and some would say, "No! Are you nuts?" Let's look at the debate a bit more closely. Think about the ways people view the world—commonly known in research as *paradigms,* or collections of theories or patterns that are used to make sense of the world. Different people view the world differently, and thus have different opinions on how the world works and how to assess it. At the heart of that debate is the question of what are viewed as credible data. Qualitative and quantitative inquiry are different ways of thinking about, and answering, this question (see Chapter 5).

During the 1990s, there was a heated debate regarding qualitative and quantitative inquiry. That debate has ended in most places, as people often agree that certain questions are better answered by one method of inquiry or the other, or a mix of both, depending on the evaluation purpose, context, and resource considerations in which the evaluation is conducted. However, while the academic debate in the field of evaluation does not rage as it did several years back, practicing evaluators will likely find strong proponents for one type of data collection over the other.

What does remain more in the public eye is the debate regarding what method of inquiry, if any, is best to answer questions on causality (see the discussion of causality earlier in this chapter); this debate is often linked to a discussion on conducting impact evaluations. Here some people suggest that experimental designs are superior to any other method, and thus that an experimental design constitutes the "gold standard."

In a nutshell, people who support the gold standard suggest that there is a "best" way (i.e., experimental designs) to conduct evaluations that seek to understand causality. Those who *do not* support such an idea suggest the importance of choosing a methodology that is appropriate to the purpose of the evaluation, the questions being asked, the budget, time frame, and other contextual factors, and it is only in understanding these factors, that one or several approaches would be considered "fit for purpose."

The Gold Standard Debate

- **Have 5 minutes?** Read a blog post by Duncan Green, who is an advisor for Oxfam Great Britain (*https://oxfamblogs.org/fp2p/randomized-controlled-trials-panacea-or-mirage*).
- **Have 45 minutes?** Read an online article by Florent Bédécarrats, Isabelle Guérin, and François Roubaud (2017), "All That Glitters Is Not Gold: The Political Economy of Randomized Evaluations in Development" (*http://onlinelibrary.wiley.com/doi/10.1111/dech.12378/full*).

The variation among the different approaches stems from how different theorists view evaluation's role in society, their experiences in evaluation, and the paradigms (their worldviews) that guide them. Some approaches provide direct steps and guidance, such as UFE, PFE, and the CIPP model. Others offer formulas, such as realist evaluation and responsive evaluation, and still others offer ways of thinking about evaluation, such as feminist evaluation and democratic evaluation. Then a few sneak in that are immensely useful but do not strictly qualify as evaluation approaches, such as appreciative inquiry and randomized controlled trials.

Each model, approach, and theory has its advantages and disadvantages, and its critics and supporters. Knowing various approaches, theories, or models enables an evaluator to take a little bit from this approach and add a little bit from that one, add a pinch of common sense and a touch of luck, resulting in an evaluation design that is best suited for a particular intervention, in a particular context, at a particular time, with specific resources, for a particular client.

If that is the tip of the iceberg, how deep does that iceberg go? How many methods, approaches, and theories are there?

Heaps. And it depends on how you define a theory, method, or approach. Let's just say there are numerous strategies and guidance on how to design an evaluation. Here are a few more to search, in alphabetical order, that would qualify as evaluation theories according to the Shadish and colleagues (1991) criteria: developmental evaluation, empowerment evaluation, goal-free evaluation, and participatory evaluation. I suggest checking out the *www.betterevaluation.org* homepage and looking under the Themes and Approaches tabs for more ideas and guidance on how to design an evaluation.

How many theories, models, or approaches should I learn?

So many theories, models, and approaches, so little time! Reading about one approach in its entirety, including its supporters, critics, and evaluation examples (being aware of the challenges, as noted by Miller [2010] at the end of this chapter), is of course the best place to start. There are several reasons why evaluators should be familiar with more than one approach, even if they continually evaluate the same type of program, in the same context. Every time I read about a new theory, or a critique of an old approach, or an innovative way to implement one that I have used multiple times before, it influences my next evaluation. The more approaches (and critiques of them) you are familiar with, the more likely it is that you will develop a strong (meaning relevant, feasible, and credible) evaluation design; you can adapt *your* evaluation approach as needed. The same point, made in a slightly different way, is that an evaluator needs to know what exists in order to make the best possible choice in that moment, for that client, for those questions, and in that context. An evaluator should be able to explain to his clients (and colleagues) what options exist, and how different approaches involve different processes and therefore may provide different findings (nuanced or otherwise) and recommendations.

As you read more and more, some approaches will begin to resonate more strongly with your values, your view of evaluation's role in society, and your view of what is appropriate for use in your context. Although you may not be able to apply an approach as it is described in textbooks (and, honestly, I never have), or maybe you do not (at least not right now) have a use for it, having a broad understanding of the many approaches out there is likely to support your journey as an evaluator. Even reading approaches that do not resonate with your values or your context is important; the reflection as to why they do not resonate with you will influence how you choose to do what you do, with sound and explicit reasoning. I am going with the fact that once you read something, you cannot unread it; everything you read will influence you in some way. Even this book.

I am wary of persons only knowing one approach; surely one approach cannot be the most feasible and appropriate approach for every single evaluation situation? So my very long-winded answer to your question is that you should *definitely* know more than one approach; however, there is no magic number for how many you should learn. Sara Vaca summarizes various evaluation choices with amazing visual graphics at her website (*www.saravaca.com*). Look at her Evaluation Periodic Table, for example.

How do you know when to apply only one approach and when to mix and match?

Most evaluators would answer this question with a very common response in evaluation: "It depends." An evaluator needs to provide findings that answer particular questions, for a particular group of people, in a particular context, with a specific amount of resources, all while recognizing the influence of values, power, politics, culture, and language. His approach needs to provide credible data, credible evidence, and credible findings (see Chapter 5). If one approach will provide that, then one approach should be applied (note that applying one approach does not mean only knowing one approach). Otherwise, the evaluator should mix approaches as needed.

Does the evaluator always choose the evaluation approach(es)?

The evaluation approach is sometimes chosen by the evaluator; sometimes it is selected by the commissioner or the client; and sometimes it is a collaborative decision. Nonetheless, how we evaluators *want* to conduct an evaluation, and how we *do* conduct an evaluation, are not always the same thing in the real world. Here are two common reasons:

- *Clients or other decision makers insist on a certain approach.* I have had clients insist on evaluation approaches that I knew were not the most appropriate or even relevant; clients who wanted me to quantify my qualitative data; and clients who wanted me to write limitations to my study that did not actually exist. I could go on, but I am getting off track. (For a longer discussion, jump to Chapter 17.)
- *Resources.* Often my clients are informed, thoughtful collaborators, and we know what we want; we just do not have the resources to do it. To return to a previous question and answer, this is a situation where it helps to know many approaches, so that we can construct a "good enough" approach that meets the clients' needs within resource limitations.

And it is important to mention that many clients are not aware that there even is something called an evaluation approach. In such a case, the evaluator will probably need to educate the client on different evaluation approaches that are likely to be useful. See this chapter and also Chapter 2 to inform a longer discussion.

THE EVALUATION DESIGN

Thinking about how to design an evaluation encompasses everything discussed so far in this book, starting with Chapter 1 and going right through to the point we have reached in this chapter. And it is only with all that information, and all of those thought processes churning, that an evaluation can be thoughtfully designed. An evaluation design, and the level of detail it entails, varies according to the evaluator, the organization, the intervention, and the evaluation approach chosen.

If you are feeling a bit lost on how to design an evaluation, and need some guidance, here are four suggestions. First, find an experienced evaluator and work with that person. The old saying "Two heads are better than one" is very true, especially if one head brings seasoned experience. Second, choose an evaluation approach that provides well-thought-out guidance and steps. Third, consider using a checklist or a framework (see Box 15.4). Fourth, review several evaluation designs and evaluation reports already conducted by, or for, the organization for which you are designing the evaluation.

> **BOX 15.4. Guidance on How to Manage and Design an Evaluation**
>
> - The most recent version of UFE provides 21 steps (*Essentials of Utilitzation-Focused Evaluation*; Patton, 2012), along with facilitation suggestions for each step. *Note:* An earlier version of UFE only has 17 steps, and still earlier versions even fewer. The UFE checklist at the Western Michigan University Evaluation Center (see below) gives the 17-step version.
> - The Better Evaluation website (*www.betterevaluation.org*) offers a 9-step Rainbow Guide to planning and managing an evaluation, along with a whole section connected to numerous web-based resources.
> - The Evaluation Center at Western Michigan University (*https://wmich.edu/evaluation/checklists*) has checklists for the following approaches: deliberative democratic evaluation, empowerment evaluation, UFE, constructivist (fourth-generation) evaluation, and the CIPP model, as well as checklists for many other components of an evaluation process.

I know that this chapter has not focused on teaching us how to design an evaluation per se; rather, it provides the processes, thinking, and tools to design one. But I must confess that I am still not clear about what is in an evaluation design. Can you just list the key components?

An evaluation design is simply a plan for obtaining and processing the information that is required to answer the evaluation questions. Here are some generic elements found in most evaluation designs: (1) evaluation purpose, (2) guiding questions, (3) evaluation method or approach, (4) methods of inquiry and related tools, (5) sampling decisions and framework, (6) data analysis plan, (7) valuing framework, (8) communication plan, and (9) clarification of any logistical or contextual influences. An evaluation design can also include more elements (or fewer), depending on the client. Some clients also want logistics and fieldwork planning, for example, included in the design.

THE EVALUATION REPORT AND OTHER WAYS TO COMMUNICATE

An evaluation report is the primary approach used to communicate with the evaluation's users, so a general rule of thumb is to write an evaluation report that the reader wants to . . . read. Here is a link that provides one perspective on how to write an evaluation report (*https://knowhownonprofit.org/how-to/how-to-write-an-evaluation-report*), and here is another from Western Michigan University (*https://wmich.edu/sites/default/files/attachments/u350/2017/eval-report-content-checklist_0.pdf*).

While these websites provide useful guidance and suggested outlines, I recommend asking the person or group of people who will use the report (e.g., the key evaluation users) and those who will approve the report (e.g., the key evaluation users and/or perhaps the commissioner) what they want in the report and how they want it organized. Start by asking if the organization has a standard, mandatory reporting format. If not, consider asking the clients a few questions: Do they have a page limit or minimum? Do they want a full methodology section in the report or in an annex? Do they want one executive summary, or multiple ones for different potential user groups (e.g., a one-page policy document, a community handout)? Ask to review an evaluation report (or any report) that they have found useful and easy to read.

If they are unsure what they want in the report and there is no mandatory outline, then use the information gathered to develop a detailed report outline. Provide that outline to the client for their reaction. You may need to simply share the outline, or you may need to facilitate a discussion and/or negotiate an agreement. Then, when the users (and the commissioner or whoever needs to sign off on the report) are in agreement, get physical sign-off on the outline (this kind of advice is provided in several sections of the book) before starting the evaluation. What sometimes "pops" out of the conversation on approving a report outline is greater clarity on what people expect from the evaluation. Here are six pieces of advice.

Write Clearly and Appropriately for the Audience

Write in clear, concise sentences. Consider how to write a report that is culturally sensitive, politically sensitive, and nonoffensive. Write a report that the main audience *wants* to read, not what everyone else wants to read. A challenge may arise here, for example, when a commissioner has final approval on a report and expects academic-like writing, but the users are a nonprofit organization and its beneficiaries, who are not likely to engage as well with a report that is so formal. An option is to write two reports, or perhaps two different executive summaries.

Clearly Link Findings to the Evaluation Evidence

Ensure that the readers can clearly see how the evaluative evidence links to the finding(s). While you may develop your own personal style, and while how this is done will vary with qualitative versus quantitative data, ensure that the links are clearly understood and can easily be seen by the readers.

Clearly Link Findings to the Evaluation Questions

The primary reason a person is reading the report is to find answers to his questions; he should not have to hunt through a long report to find answers. Make it easy for the reader. Explicitly link the evaluation findings to the evaluation questions. One way to do this is to use the evaluation questions as headings, or subheadings, in the report. Another suggestion is to state each finding and *then* provide the supporting evidence, rather than having the reader wade through all the evidence and only stumble onto the findings afterward.

Present Visually Enticing Reports

Consider how information (e.g., key messages) is presented. Consider how to make the report engaging and explore the use of data visualization techniques such as infographics. The inclusion of pictures from site visits will likely influence the report's user-friendliness (make sure you have the appropriate permissions). Do not forget the simpler things, such as the font and its size or the amount of white space on a page. Consider the readers' particular needs as well. If the report is meant for visually impaired persons, use larger fonts. If any of the users are color-blind, do not rely on color-coded pie charts. And so on. See data visualization resources on page 309 in this chapter and page 99 in Chapter 5.

Use Active Voice

Passive voice is confusing with regard to who is doing what to whom. Consider reading the following sentence in an evaluation report: "It was then implemented." Who implemented it? Now read this: "The Department of Labor implemented the intervention." Ah, now we know who did what, and it provides a nice segue for the next sentence. Avoid passive voice whenever possible.

Consider Other Ways to Present Findings and Recommendations

There are multiple ways to present evaluation findings and recommendations that are not reports. Consider the audience: Who needs to engage with the findings and recommendations? Would a presentation by beneficiaries, a play by community members, a poem, or a PowerPoint presentation be most effective? Or perhaps something more interactive, such as a workshop where key findings and their recommendations are presented on flip chart paper, and people move around the room and discuss them? Get creative. Or maybe the findings need to be more widely disseminated; social media can be valuable tools for this. Remember, the idea is to have the findings and recommendations used. Having said that, I must add that some organizations require a report, which is judged on its "thunk" factor: The louder the sound the report makes when it hits the desk, the "better" the report. Know your evaluation users.

BOX 15.5. Examples of Evaluation Reports

Wondering what an evaluation report looks like? Here are some examples:

The United States Agency for International Development (USAID) publishes its evaluations from around the world in its Development Experience Clearinghouse (DEC; *https://dec.usaid.gov/dec/home/Default.aspx*).

The United Kingdom Department for International Development (DFID) publishes its evaluation report and related in its Collection of Evaluation Reports (*www.gov. uk/government/collections/evaluation-reports*).

EVALUATING THE EVALUATION

Regardless of the purpose or the approach chosen, there should be an accepted and transparent approach to and criteria for judging an evaluation's quality and accuracy (in addition to the above-mentioned thunk factor). First, I briefly describe a formal approach, metaevaluation. Then I discuss what often happens at the end of an evaluation when a client is provided with an evaluation product, which is most often a report.

Metaevaluation

Metaevaluation is what takes place when a person or team external to the evaluation (i.e., a team that would provide an independent review) is selected to use explicit standards and principles to assess the evaluation's quality and accuracy. These standards and principles can be provided by the local or national evaluation association, although an organization or a government can have its own. For example, the Organisation for Economic Co-operation and Development's Development Assistance Committee (OECD DAC) has its Evaluation Quality Standards for Development Evaluation (*www.oecd.org/development/evaluation/ qualitystandards.pdf*), with four thematic areas (all with their own criteria): (1) overarching considerations; (2) purpose, planning, and design; (3) implementation and reporting; and (4) follow-up use and learning. Another set is the Program Evaluation Standards (Yarbrough, Shulha, Hopson, & Caruthers, 2011):

- Utility (the evaluation meets the needs of its users)
- Feasibility (it is effective and efficient)
- Propriety (it is proper, fair, legal, and just)
- Accurate (it is dependable and truthful)
- Accountability (it focuses on process and product)

An external metaevaluation team will apply these standards and identify the strengths and weaknesses of the evaluation. These reviews rarely result in evaluators' needing to make changes to their reports; the process is more of a way to judge an evaluation report once it is completed. One challenge with metaevaluation is that the assessors do not always know the real-life complications that influenced the quality of the evaluation, which cannot be listed in the limitations section of the report. For example, several years ago I was the team leader on a large impact evaluation. Before we could begin the evaluation, the evaluation design needed approval by an external committee. Over the course of 9 months, I was required to make numerous changes; these resulted in a design that the committee wanted, but one that I was dubious about. The evaluation was implemented, and then a metaevaluation took place. The lead metaevaluator said to me, "I would not have designed the evaluation in this way." So I truthfully said, "Me either."

Discussion between the Evaluator and the Client

While metaevaluations are useful in some circumstances, the discussion of a report's quality and accuracy more often takes place between an individual client and his evaluator.

Here is another trade secret: In an evaluation process, it is not always explicit how the evaluation will be valued and judged. It is for this reason that I place the responsibility on the evaluator to *ask* for clear criteria, and to find out what transparent process will be used to assess the evaluation, before commencing the evaluation. If no clear criteria or process are provided, an evaluator can provide standard criteria (such as the sets discussed on the previous page in the section on metaevaluation), or can provide his own. Here is one strategy with several steps to support an evaluator in his efforts to ensure that the way his (or his team's) evaluation will be judged is transparent.

1. A clear evaluation design is agreed upon before the evaluation begins. All changes that happen during the evaluation are discussed with the client and documented.

2. A report outline details exactly what will be provided. Any changes to the report are clearly documented.

3. The evaluator discusses with the client how the evaluation's quality and accuracy of the evaluation will be judged, and by whom. The agreed-upon criteria are attached to the evaluation design.

4. The evaluator conducts a transparent, credible process, and produces a report that meets agreed-upon quality standards.

Following the four steps will result in a report (or other product) that is accepted and used by the client. Oh. Wait. That is not true. Sometimes there are surprises; personal issues, politics, miscommunications, different subjective understandings of the criteria, or other factors may influence whether (1) the report is accepted, (2) the evaluator is asked to make further changes, or (3) the report is flat-out rejected.

It is not uncommon for an evaluator to produce what he and his team consider a good report that addresses the evaluation questions and follows the evaluation design, and for the client to disagree. One strategy, more fully discussed in Chapter 17, is for the evaluator and the client to agree that one or more external peer reviewers will review the report. A second strategy, or perhaps more of a recognition, is that there are always two sides to a story. An interesting presentation of two different perspectives can be found in an article on the Better Evaluation website, literally titled "Two Sides of the Evaluation Coin" (Cranston, Beynon, & Rowley, 2013). The article details the evaluator's and the client's perception of the same evaluation process.

WRAPPING UP

This chapter began by looking at how people often request evaluation (the names they use) and looked at various ways that evaluations are often requested, such as asking for formative or summative evaluations or outcome and impact. We then took a closer look at implementation, outcome, and impact evaluations, delving into a deeper discussion on the differences among them. The chapter introduced 10 evaluation approaches, theories, and models (where I snuck in two that do not really qualify as such), and then left you in the capable hands of the experts to learn further about each approach. We touched on the gold standard debate, and we looked at useful questions to guide an evaluator to understand her clients' evaluation needs and inform her initial design of an evaluation. We talked about evaluation reports and the need for evaluators to establish how those reports will be judged and by whom. An evaluator needs to take responsibility for identifying (to the best of her ability) how her evaluation will be judged, with what criteria, through what process, and by whom.

As Miller (2010) has shared with us in this chapter, it is extremely rare (if it ever happens) that a practitioner will use a theory, approach, or model in its purest textbook form, thus supporting the idea that an evaluator needs to know more than one evaluation approach. Before you leave this chapter, I invite you to have a short conversation with me.

Our Conversation: Between You and Me

Here, I offer two situations that you may encounter with regard to making design decisions and engaging in how to assess an evaluation. Practicing with these situations will support you when encountering these and similar kinds of situations in the real world.

1. Chatting about RCTs. In this chapter, we have briefly talked about randomized controlled trials (RCTs.) When I am presenting at conferences, engaging with clients, and even doing fieldwork, I find it tremendously helpful to be able to talk about all kinds of designs, particularly RCTs and the gold standard debate. If someone asked you, "What is an RCT, and what are some of the key advantages and challenges associated with RCTs?", *what would you say?* How would you describe the gold standard debate? On which side of the fence do you sit? Straddling the fence is *not* allowed (at least for our discussion purposes).

2. Although being an evaluator involves so much more than knowing an approach, model, or theory (as this book has illustrated), one cannot be an evaluator without them. I have made that very strong statement in this chapter, and it is a sentiment often espoused by academics and evaluation theorists, such as Will Shadish (1998). However, I am not an academic. I am a practitioner. I think that one cannot be an evaluator without practice *and* theory. *Do you agree with me? If not, why not?*

CHAPTER 16

The World of Recommendations (and the Underworld of Critical Feedback)

> One can't prescribe books, even the best books, to people unless one knows a good deal about each individual person.
> —RUDYARD KIPLING, *A Book of Words: Selections from Speeches and Addresses Delivered between 1906 and 1927*

Values have been given their own chapter in this book because of their integral importance to the entire evaluative process. Recommendations also deserve their own space in the book (and get nearly a whole chapter), though for a different reason. Recommendations are often, though not always, provided at the end of an evaluative process and are intended to inform decision making in some way. Although recommendations thus play a critical role in the evaluative process, this role is rarely explicitly discussed in the literature. This chapter, then, is *mostly* about the recommendations. Recommendations often (though not always) derive from findings that are critical of the intervention. Thus, how to provide critical feedback slips in and shares the recommendations chapter.

A RECOMMENDATION: WHAT IS IT?

So what is a **recommendation**? According to the *Oxford Living Dictionaries: English* (2018), a recommendation is "a suggestion or proposal as to the best course of action, especially one put forward by an authoritative body." Quite simply a recommendation is an actionable, informed opinion that provides advice on how to change something. In evaluation, a good recommendation needs to be (1) linked to the evaluation findings, (2) which are connected to the evaluation questions, (3) grounded in local contextual knowledge, social science theory, and/or expert knowledge, and (4) actionable.

In Part I of this book, we have thoroughly explored a girls' education program, from its problem statement through to its results. Let's now assume that the intervention has been implemented, and that the program implementers have decided to have an evaluation process that includes recommendations.

I have a question. What is the purpose of the evaluation?

The purpose is to understand how the intervention is being implemented, what is happening on the ground, and the effectiveness of that implementation. The focus is on the peer-to-peer component of the intervention. (See Chapter 15.)

I have a question too. What are the evaluation questions?

Most of the questions focus on how the peer-to-peer activities have been implemented and the results of that. Some of the questions include: What is working well? What is not? What do staff members do? And to what extent did fathers change their knowledge and perceptions on the importance of sending their daughters to school? (See Chapter 15.)

Me too. Me too. Who are the main users?

The program implementer and his staff.

I also want to know: What is the evaluation approach (or approaches)?

UFE and FE will guide the evaluation. (See Chapter 15.)

Wait, I have another one. What methods of inquiry are used?

Mixed methods. (See Chapter 5.)

One more question: How are the findings valued?

Organic values will be used. (See Chapter 12.)

Wait. This is the last one, I promise. What standards are used to judge the evaluation?

The donor organization has provided clear standards for judging the evaluation. (See Chapter 15.)

Great questions, it's amazing how much you have all learned. So, anyway, let's assume that the evaluation has taken place and provided the following finding and recommendation.

The evaluation data show that while the peer-to-peer intervention for fathers is useful to some extent, it is not shifting the fathers' attitudes and perceptions to the degree that fathers are likely to permit their daughters to attend school. Some data gathered during the interview process suggests that educators are extremely influential in the community. This is further demonstrated by the role educators have recently played in convincing the local government to build a playground, and in convincing parents—particularly fathers—to agree to maintain the equipment. Therefore, it is recommended that educators become involved in the fathers' peer-to-peer intervention on a monthly basis.

Recommendations can be one sentence long, or several paragraphs. A recommendation can be directly linked, in the same paragraph, to its evidence (as shown above). Or it can be provided later in a report, referencing the evidence on which it was based. For example, at the end of the evaluation report, an evaluator can write: "Here is the challenge we identified; here is the evidence that suggested that challenge; and here is the recommendation, which is based on social science theory and technical expertise brought by the evaluation team [or however it has been formulated, which is discussed later in the chapter]."

Who Are the Recommendations For?

It is important to know for whom the recommendations are intended, and how this person or group wants to use the recommendations. In some instances, it may be quite clear who will use the recommendations and how they will be used—but these are not always simple or straightforward matters. Svetlana Negrustuyeva, an international evaluator, shares her experience:

"Sometimes when I conduct an evaluation, it is not always clear who the recommendation is intended for, or who gets to see what. Is it just the implementing organization and their internal team, or is it their donor's management team that has direct oversight over the project? It could be one or the other, or it could be both. If it is both, there are likely to be sets of very different recommendations. Then, if there are two sets of recommendations, does the implementer get to see the set of recommendations that go to the donor? Does the donor see the recommendations that are purely meant for the eyes of the implementer? It is best to clarify these kinds of decisions during the evaluation's design phase, before the evaluation is implemented."

Are there any other real-life experiences to share about recommendations?

Sometimes the evaluation is implemented, and when the assignment is being wrapped up in a final meeting, the client says, "So what do you really think? What would you recommend, beyond the officially presented recommendations?" This conversation needs to be handled carefully. There may be reasons why it is better to provide recommendations orally (e.g., they may be politically sensitive) that did not appear in the report, and so the opportunity to share them in an informal setting is useful. However, it may be the case that the evaluator does not have enough informed experience to answer that question and feels pressured, on the spot, to come up with some. My advice would be to ignore this pressure. Explain that recommendations are not just opinions, but well-thought-out, informed pieces of advice that are clearly linked to the evaluation evidence and, as such, you (the evaluator) need more time to engage with the client's request.

THE EVALUATOR'S ROLE IN RECOMMENDATIONS

There are those who think recommendations are outside the purview of an evaluator. These people think that an evaluation is only intended to provide empirical feedback on, and valuing of, an intervention. Others view recommendations as the critical part of an evaluation, and believe that without recommendations, an evaluation loses its potential usefulness. Prior to starting any evaluation, the evaluator needs to determine if recommendations are required. Having said that, I must add that I have rarely been part of an evaluation process that did *not* require recommendations.

Let's assume for the moment that recommendations are required. How, then, are they to be produced? An evaluator who is a subject expert (e.g., an early childhood development expert, an environmental specialist) can likely offer informed advice based on the evidence gathered and her expertise, experience, and knowledge. An evaluator who is not a subject expert may need to draw on knowledgeable others (see Chapter 1) or follow other processes to develop recommendations. Let's look at some ways to generate meaningful recommendations.

STRATEGIES FOR DEVELOPING MEANINGFUL RECOMMENDATIONS

A recommendation is not a random opinion. A recommendation is also not an informed expert opinion that has no relevance to the evaluation evidence and its findings (for a discussion of what an opinion is, see Chapter 4). So where do recommendations come from? Although recommendations need to have clear links to the evidence, they can be elicited from one or several places. Here are three nonexclusive strategies for developing meaningful recommendations.

1. *The evaluator presents the evaluation question, analyzed data, the key findings, and then facilitates a discussion to develop recommendations with one or all of the following:*

- Key subject experts.
- The intervention's implementation team.
- Beneficiaries.
- The client(s).
- Other relevant stakeholders (see Chapter 3 for a list of potential stakeholders).
- Other members of the evaluation team, who bring different perspectives.

The main potential challenge with this strategy is keeping participants focused on using the evidence to inform recommendations (and not just an uninformed or preformed opinion). A practical suggestion is to begin with a short discussion on the differences among facts, evidence, assumptions, and opinions (see Chapters 1 and 4). Then, present the evaluation finding and its supporting evidence. Do not overwhelm participants with information; rather, break the discussion down into themes or by evaluation questions. Another suggestion is to invite specific groups to address specific themes that are directly relevant to them (i.e., do not present everything to everybody).

2. *The evaluator solicits recommendations as part of an interview strategy.* At the end of each interview, ask the respondent for recommendations. The main potential challenge is that the evaluator needs to be mindful that those recommendations are linked back to, and are supported by, the evidence.

3. *The evaluator writes his own recommendations.* Working with credible evidence, an evaluator can use his own subject expertise, can use evaluation team members' expertise, and/or can draw from the relevant social science theory. The main potential challenge is that, particularly when the evaluator is external to the intervention, the recommendation may not be contextually grounded. While a recommendation can look well written and substantiated ("Great idea! . . ."), it may not be a feasible recommendation for that particular context (" . . . but we cannot do that"). However, clients may value the external insights, as these recommendations can be modified by the program manager or program implementation team or may spur further internal thinking.

STRATEGIES FOR PRESENTING ACCEPTABLE RECOMMENDATIONS

A recommendation that is linked to an evaluation question, finding, and related evidence, and is extremely relevant and actionable, may not be used if it is poorly presented. Here are four pieces of advice for presenting useful recommendations.

Limit the Recommendations

Be realistic: Even if there are 100 substantiated, actionable recommendations, the sheer number is likely to overwhelm any person or organization. We are all only human. Choose a few recommendations that are key to helping the organization improve, and are likely to be addressed. If you must, for some reason, provide all 100 recommendations, identify the key ones, place them in the report, and relegate the remainder to an appendix. Or consider the next piece of advice.

Logically Group and Organize the Recommendations

There are several ways of logically organizing evaluation recommendations. You should consult with your clients to determine if they have a preference, but here are some of the most useful approaches:

- *From easiest to most challenging.* Order them by the easiest to address to the hardest. For example, updating website links is likely to be easier than updating an organizational strategy.
- *By time sensitivity.* List the recommendations in order of their time sensitivity. Which recommendations need to happen now? Which can (or even need to) wait 6 months?
- *By theme.* Thematic categories will vary by evaluation. An example would be to categorize them by content, or by evaluation question, or from their origin (e.g., recommendations made by the evaluator, the subject expert, and the beneficiaries).
- *By the group or individuals responsible.* Consider listing the recommendations by the persons or group that can address them. For example, some recommendations may be directed to those in charge of finances or budgeting, some to project staff at field sites, some to the funder, and some to the management team at the home office.

Provide the Recommendation in Each Relevant Section

Place the relevant recommendation directly at the end of each specific section of the report that has the relevant evidence. In this way, the link is clear between the evidence, the finding, and the recommendation. All recommendations spread throughout the report can be then be collected (i.e., copied and pasted) into the recommendations section at the end of the report, or can be placed in an appendix, with a link (hyperlink or page number) back to the page where each recommendation was initially stated.

Consider Who Presents the Recommendations

What person or group is most credible to the evaluation users? To present the recommendations, consider using a subject expert, a community leader, an evaluator with a well-known name, a professor, or some other person the group will find credible. The presenter, however, must be intimately familiar with the evaluation findings and supportive of the recommendations.

What do I do if the recommendations are rejected?

If the recommendations are rejected, identify what made someone reject them. Here are some reasons why recommendations might be rejected, and suggestions for what to do when that happens.

- *A recommendation is not linked to the evidence.* Remove the recommendation.
- *The recommendation is not clear to the user.* Rewrite the recommendation.
- *The recommendation is not actionable.* Rewrite the recommendation to make it actionable.
- *The recommendation is not feasible.* There are several options, and the choice of one depends on why it is not feasible. Here are three examples: Remove the recommendation if it is not feasible for cultural reasons. Engage with the user if the recommendation needs to be tweaked to make it feasible. Note that although the recommendation is not feasible now (e.g., not enough funding), it may be feasible at a later date.
- *The recommendation is just not liked, and no reason is given.* This is the toughest situation. Either remove the recommendation or facilitate a discussion with those that do not like the recommendation to identify their reasons. For example, one reason may be that the finding (to which the recommendation is linked) was not accepted or well received. The discussion would then need to focus on the finding, not the recommendation. Another reason could be that if the client accepts the recommendation, she also needs to accept responsibility to address the recommendation, which she finds overwhelming. These are just a few of many potential reasons that need to be considered.

How do I write a good recommendation?

A "good" recommendation is based on the evaluation questions, evidence, and findings and is useful, feasible, actionable, informed, and well written. Over the years, the most common challenge I have seen with recommendations is that they are not actionable. Be specific and clear about the action that is being recommended. For example, the recommendation "More thought should be given to how to implement the fathers' peer-to-peer program" is not likely to be useful. However, consider this recommendation: "The program implementer responsible for the fathers' peer-to-peer intervention should consider involving local male educators in this intervention monthly." This version is clear, specific, and actionable. The person reading the recommendation should immediately know how to move forward with the next steps to implement the recommendation.

How do I ensure that good recommendations are used?

The question assumes that it *is* the evaluator's responsibility to ensure that recommendations are used. Some evaluators take the position that it is the evaluator's responsibility to provide clear, actionable recommendations, but that it is the program manager's responsibility to implement them or ensure that they are implemented. Some evaluators do, however, play a more active role. An external evaluator and an internal evaluator (see Chapter 11) would probably engage with this issue differently. Internal evaluators are more likely to have access to those who need to implement the recommendations over a longer period, and can thus support the implementation of the recommendations. External evaluators often (though not always) provide the recommendations and then leave. Regardless, here are two strategies that can be used by either internal or external evaluators.

First, consider presenting recommendations at a workshop. Sometimes hearing recommendations and discussing feasible ways to engage with them leads to higher levels of use. Second, sit down (literally) with whoever needs to engage with the recommendation, and walk the person through the relevant recommendation. For example, one recommendation might be specifically for the administrative department, one for the field workers, and four for the management staff. Meet with members of each group individually, and only talk about the recommendations that are specifically relevant to them. (Note that these strategies assume that people are interested in working with the evaluator, and that this assumption does not always hold true.)

A CHANGING WORLD: SHIFTING FROM RECOMMENDATIONS AT THE END TO LEARNING THROUGHOUT

In recent years, a focus on learning throughout an evaluation has sometimes come to replace recommendations at the end. Organizations and projects that work in partnership with their evaluators sometimes prefer to learn as the evaluative process takes place, rather than waiting until the end of the process to get feedback and recommendations. Learning processes are more compatible with certain kinds of evaluative purposes and evaluation approaches. For example, some participatory evaluation approaches and developmental evaluation lend themselves to learning during the evaluative process and not waiting until the end to suggest recommendations.

Consider this example: An evaluator identifies that something is not working during Month 2 of a 6-month evaluation. He can then use the information identified at Month 2 to engage with the management team. He can facilitate a discussion with all relevant parties to interpret these data, understand the data's meaning or usefulness, generate thinking and ideas based on the data, and then use these thoughts and ideas to inform further decisions immediately.

Closely related to the conversation on recommendations and supporting learning throughout an evaluative process is one on providing feedback that is, well, not so nice to hear. While an evaluator may provide a recommendation when something is working well (e.g., expand the intervention), she is more likely to provide a recommendation in relation to a finding that in some way critizes the intervention. Thus the chapter concludes with a discussion on how to best provide feedback that may be difficult for the client or evaluation user to hear.

Providing Feedback

This section is near and dear to my heart—mostly, I think, because I have a very thin skin. This is not so great for an evaluator, or anyone who writes or works in the public eye. Knowing how to provide feedback is a critical skill that everyone (evaluators and clients alike) involved in the evaluation process should learn, in the interests of communication, improving the evaluation use, and being nice.

Starting a conversation (or even ending one) with "Your intervention is a total dud" is not the best way to provide that feedback, even if it is true. In most evaluations, there is often a balance of good and bad news: There are often things that are going well, some things that can be slightly improved, some components that are just not doing as well as they should, and perhaps a disaster or two. Next, I provide six pieces of advice to help you provide feedback to a client or evaluation user that may be difficult for them to hear.

Provide the Credible Evidence and Logical Reasoning That Support Each Finding and Recommendation

A report should provide information in a logical flow: question, description, analysis, interpretation, finding, recommendation. By presenting the information in this logical flow, the evaluator connects the dots for the reader; I advise sticking to that outline when the need arises to provide feedback that is critical of the intervention. Do not provide the feedback that is critical as the very first statement in a report, or in an oral presentation. If people are sensitive to these kinds of feedback (no matter how carefully worded), they can immediately shut down at that point and not hear the reasoning that supports that criticism. Laying the logical foundation at the start enables the person to follow the logic that has led to that finding. Be ready to answer questions on your method of inquiry, or any other questions on how you identified that finding. Here are some finer points to consider in providing feedback that is critical of the intervention.

Hey, wait a minute. I thought with reports we were supposed to provide the finding first so a reader can find it, then provide all the details. But here you are saying the opposite.

This book aims to provide multiple strategies for various situations. Sometimes your best judgment will tell you that you need to lay the groundwork before presenting a finding that is critical of the intervention. However, even in these cases, the basic advice holds true: The reader should still be able to "find" the finding quickly (i.e., he should not be confused or bored out of his mind by the time he locates the answer). By the time he reads the critical finding, though, he should be ready to read it. Below are some more hints on how to present negative findings.

Choose Your Words and Phrases Carefully

The power of language has been discussed in Chapter 1 and Chapter 13. Nowhere is it more important than when providing feedback. Write clear, direct, specific sentences. Choose words that are not aimed to offend or be taken personally. Do not use overly technical words where they are not necessary, words that can easily be misinterpreted, or words that are phantasmagorical (I'm just making my point with this word). Write, "There were four challenges in the implementation. These challenges were . . ." as opposed to "There were a lot of really devastating problems." Ensure that your chosen words and phrasing are culturally and politically sensitive.

Sandwich the Critical Feedback between Parts of the Positive Feedback

Consider presenting a sequence of positive, then critical, then positive findings. Placing the feedback that is critical of the intervention between parts of the positive feedback often comes across as less threatening, and thus makes the feedback more likely to be heard and accepted.

Link Findings Critical of the Intervention to Actionable Recommendations

Not all findings require recommendations. Findings that provide criticism of the intervention likely need to have them. Do not leave your evaluation user hanging with the message of "It is not working, so you might as well pack up and go home." (In the rare case that is the clear finding, the feedback should be considered and thoughtful.) Rather, focus attention on how the intervention can be improved or changed by suggesting clear, actionable recommendations.

Do Not Shame; Do Not Blame

The report may be a public report, or the findings are likely to be shared in a setting that has more than one person. Do not name names, or link findings that are critical of the intervention to one person or even several people. If you have sensitive information, consider how to provide that information in a manner that respects confidences and shows respect. Do not hide information; rather, share the information so that informed, appropriate management decisions can be made. Avoid sentences that point a finger, such as sentences that include "you" or "your." Instead, replace "you" with "we" where it works, or with the name of the intervention being evaluated.

Read the Report As If You Were the One Receiving the Criticism

Does the report or the oral presentation come across as being given by a critical friend, or a mortal enemy? Remember that, as evaluators, we are aiming to be critical friends.

WRAPPING UP

Recommendations, while not *always* included in an evaluation process, are *often* included. Yet very little about how to write them is available in the evaluation literature. This chapter has aimed to help fill that gap by discussing what is a good recommendation, thinking about an evaluator's role in developing them, identifying where recommendations can come from, and describing how to write and present them. The chapter has then moved from how to make recommendations to making recommendations on how to provide feedback that may be difficult for clients to hear. Specifically, the chapter brought advice and insight on how to provide feedback that is sensitive, thoughtful, and kind. Before you leave this chapter, come join me in a conversation.

Our Conversation: Between You and Me

Here are two types of situations that you may encounter with regard to making recommendations and providing feedback that is critical of the intervention. Practicing with these common scenarios will help you when you encounter similar kinds of situations in the real world.

1. A group of program implementers has just read the recommendations. However, they are not sure how to move forward. They feel stuck. Oh, dear. An evaluator's role in such a case varies greatly, depending on whether the evaluator is internal or external, or what is included in her (the evaluator's) contract. If I had limited time, I would recommend choosing just one recommendation that seems the most feasible, or maybe even the most challenging, and engaging with the program implementers about that recommendation; it might get them rolling forward. If I had more time, I would recommend holding a workshop with the program implementers to "action" the recommendations (sometimes actionable recommendations still need help being actioned!). *What would you do?*

2. A client has just viciously attacked your evaluation report, incuding its recommendations, and shamed you and your team, in a public meeting. Sadly, this actually happened to my team and me on a large government evaluation. In the moment, all I could think of to say was "I am sorry you feel that way." And we got up and left. *What would you do?*

CHAPTER 17

The Dirty Laundry Chapter

The best-laid plans of mice and men often go awry.
—Adapted from ROBERT BURNS, "To a Mouse"

I have conducted many evaluations in collaboration with, or on behalf of, thoughtful clients who engage with and use evaluation in many ways and for many reasons. These include environmental clients who aim to stop the trafficking of animals, and human rights activists who aim to stop the trafficking of humans; innovative groups that focus on changing children's lives, and nonprofits that aim to change the lives of grownups; governments that want to improve the welfare of their citizens, and foundations that want to change the world. I aim to be a better evaluator for all of these clients.

Even when evaluators are engaging with such thoughtful and committed clients, challenging situations arise. These challenges are often buried in a laundry basket in the back corner of the room, while the clean and pressed laundry items (i.e., journal articles and conference presentations) are hung out for everyone to see. Only in more recent years have evaluators begun publicly sharing evaluation mishaps. This chapter, following the example of these brave souls, presents some common challenges and ways to navigate them.

Thus far in the second part of our journey, we have learned quite a lot about evaluation and being an evaluator. We have learned about the many roles an evaluator can play, yet noted that clarifying an evaluator's role does not capture the essence of being one. We discussed the critical role that values play throughout the entire evaluative process, not just when criteria are needed to judge the intervention's success, and introduced the remaining indispensable and all-influencing "fabulous five plus one"—culture, language, power, politics, and context.

We acknowledged the importance of knowing the evaluation literature, considered some key aspects of evaluation (just enough to get our interest piqued), engaged with the art of providing recommendations, and learned how to provide not-so-nice-to-hear feedback to our clients. These chapters culminate in this final chapter—a chapter that shares some common challenges an evaluator often faces when practicing evaluation.

The process of designing and implementing evaluations is a dynamic, interactive one, influenced by all the factors we have examined in Chapters 1–16. It is a process that almost always involves multiple human beings, all of whom bring their own understandings of evaluation, their expectations of it, and experiences that influence their own emotional response. Thus, in every evaluation, there are multiple human relationships that must be managed in an often complicated situation. There is no textbook or contract provision that can unfailingly tell an evaluator step-by-step how to navigate each of these dynamics. However, this chapter does try to outline some of the more common evaluation challenges that you can expect to face, and provides some strategies to help you navigate these. In short, it aims to help you engage in a real-world evaluation process and think like an evaluator.

The challenges covered in this chapter take place at different stages of an evaluative process: design, implementation, and reporting. The challenges are briefly noted, followed by thoughtful and practical suggestions for engaging with them.

Do not be misled in reading this chapter into thinking that every evaluation process will be a disaster. Some evaluations are "smooth rides" or traverse only small speed bumps. I just have not focused on those experiences because (1) they are not as interesting, and (2) there is no need to provide advice.

Eight Challenges in the Design Phase, and How to Mitigate Them

I have selected eight challenges to share about the evaluation's design phase because they are some of the most common in any kind of evaluative process. Following each challenge, I provide some suggested strategies.

- *Challenge 1.* The evaluation design (or approach) is selected for the evaluator, yet does not appear appropriate to address the client's purpose. There is no perfect evaluation design, but there are decidedly imperfect ones. Every evaluation needs a well-thought-out design that meets a client's needs (e.g., it answers the evaluation questions). It needs to be feasible, ethical, accurate, culturally sensitive, and useful. Challenges can arise when the client proposes a design that appears unlikely to address one or all of these.

 Facilitate or engage in a conversation that aims to identify why the client has requested that design. Ask the client, "What made you select that design? What is it that you like about that design? What do you think that design entails or will provide?" Once you have discerned the reason for the choice, it may become clear that the design is actually appropriate; that the client misunderstood the design; or perhaps it is one that the client has little choice about (e.g., it is required by the funder or their boss).

If it is *not* a required design (just a suggested one) and it is not appropriate, discuss with the client the shortfalls of the chosen design (e.g., why it is not likely to answer the evaluation questions); offer an alternative one (or two or three); and demonstrate to the client (using clear, practical examples) in what ways the designs differ. For a few clients, a theoretical comparison may also be appropriate.

If it *is* a required design, and is clearly not an appropriate choice, find out what can be altered or augmented. On those rare occasions where an inappropriate design needs to be implemented with *no* changes, there are several options. If you are able to meet with the client, articulate the challenges and limitations to him, and document those meetings. If you are unable to meet with the client, document the challenges and limitations of the particular design, and provide this documentation to the client *before* the evaluation commences. The final step is to apply your favorite stress mechanism (e.g., yoga, chocolate, running, music) and march ethically onward, soldier.

• *Challenge 2.* The method of inquiry is selected for the evaluator, yet does not appear appropriate to answer the stated evaluation questions. The difficulty here occurs when a client wants a quantitative approach but is asking questions that warrant a qualitative study, or vice versa. Or sometimes a client requests mixed methods, but only one kind of data is appropriate to answer the evaluation question(s), or the opposite, he requests one kind of data but the questions require a mixed methods design.

As noted for Challenge 1, ask the client why that specific method of inquiry has been requested. Once you learn the reason(s) for the choice, it may become clear that the method of inquiry is one that the client has little choice about (e.g., it is required by the government department or funder) or maybe he just prefers a certain kind of data (i.e., he finds it credible). The first option is to revisit his evaluation questions; perhaps the wording of the questions does not convey the client's needs, and by revising the questions, their method choice becomes appropriate. If the questions do convey their needs, and if there is a choice about the method of inquiry, educate the client, as needed, by explaining why the evaluation questions require a certain method of inquiry. A final option is to do what the client wants, *and* do what is needed, if resources permit. If the client insists on a specific method of inquiry that does not match the question, and the budget does not allow for any augmentation, document the challenges and provide the documentation to the client before the evaluation commences. Then breathe deeply, and either walk away from, or walk further into, the evaluation process.

• *Challenge 3.* The budget is unknown. This is often the case when evaluation opportunities are advertised and an evaluator needs to bid on an evaluation project. The main reason the client is unable to disclose the budget is often related to legal or tendering reasons. However, when a budget is provided (or, at the very least, a budget range), the evaluator is more likely to provide an accurate idea of what *can* be done (vs. what should be done). At the same time, the lack of a specified budget can also happen when working for an organization that, or person who, is inexperienced with evaluation and needs the evaluator to provide budget guidance. A similar example would be when an internal evaluator needs to respond to her boss, who has requested an evaluation design and budget to get "an idea of how much it will cost."

Let's first look at the situation where an evaluator is bidding on an evaluation project with an undisclosed budget (however, a budget does exist). Sometimes there are telltale signs of the budget size. Look for the number of person-days (sometimes called *level of effort* or LOE), the amount of travel, the time frame provided in which to conduct the evaluation (e.g., 30 days or 30 months), and established daily rates for consultants. These clues can *sometimes* be enough to suggest the resources available for the evaluation, and to guide the development of an approach that is likely to meet the client's budget. Now let's bring in the second example, where an evaluator is providing budget guidance, as the next steps apply to both situations.

When there is no guidance with regard to the budget, develop the most practical design that meets your evaluation standards (see Chapter 15 for some ideas on standards) and cost it. Call this Option A. Then remove or cut down on parts that are feasible to change (i.e., it still answers the questions), which will result in a skeleton approach, estimate its costs, and call it Option B. Explain how Option B will provide answers to the questions; then list what it will not do. Next, add components or increase what is being done in Design A (e.g., allow for more inter- views), cost it, and call it Option C. Explain how Option C will enhance the evaluation. Finally, submit (or discuss, as appropriate) all three designs, each with their designated budgets. Note that this process is time-consuming (and for the evaluator who is responding to a tender, note that only one budget may be accepted). A less time-consuming option is to submit budget notes with the budget for Design A, that succinctly suggests various design options (10 interviews in place of 30) and related cost implications.

• *Challenge 4.* The budget is known, and it is known to be too small. It is a challenge when the budget does not support a design necessary to answer evaluation questions. For example, a statistically relevant sample may require administering 2,500 surveys, or reaching data saturation and achieving appropriate triangulation of data may require interviewing 75 people. The problem is that the budget is too small to support that kind of data collection and analysis. Or for the evaluation to be culturally appropriate, the evaluation's Team Lead needs to facilitate intensive meetings with local leadership forums throughout the process, and the budget does not support these kinds of interactions.

There is one general solution to this problem: Negotiate. Negotiate for more funding. Negotiate for addressing fewer questions. Negotiate for a narrower focus. However, do *not* capitulate and conduct an evaluation that does not collect credible data, produce credible findings, and provide a credible evaluation (see Chapter 5 on credibility).

• *Challenge 5.* There is no or little communication at the onset between the evalua- tor and the client (or other evaluation users). Designing an evaluation and not being able to engage, or having limited time, with the potential client during the design phase can be detrimental to the evaluation. With little to no communication between the evaluator and the client at the onset, a situation is created that more than likely leads to challenges in the implementation and reporting phase.

At a minimum, the evaluator and his client need a shared understanding of the evaluation's purpose and the evaluation questions. Ideally, the evaluator is also aware of the client's needs, fears, expectations, and assumptions, which are then used to inform the design of a useful evaluation.

There are a few practical ways of obtaining this information that are dependent on why the communication does not happen. Perhaps there is no budget for meetings to take place during the design phase. If that is the case, look to see if there is a budget to engage at the end of the process, such as through workshops to present findings. If there is such a budget, see if those resources can be shifted to a meeting or workshop at the beginning of the evaluation process; it is better to spend time with a client up front and understand their needs than to meet at the end and find out that you did not. If there is simply a lack of time to meet with the client, ensure that a clearly articulated and extremely detailed design is provided to the client that highlights all key aspects. Key aspects likely include your understanding of the evaluation's purpose and its questions, critical assumptions that inform the design, and potential challenges. (To read more about an evaluation design, see Chapter 15.) Attached to the design should be a detailed report outline (or description of the final product). Ensure that the design, with the attached report outline, is approved by the client. I suggest an actual physical sign-off, or an email clearly stating that the design and report format is approved.

That approval will give you the comfort of knowing that the client is aware, and has a shared understanding, of the purpose, questions, the resulting design, and report structure (what will be provided at the end of the process). Having an approved design and report format (or whatever the evaluation product is) that has been signed can be very helpful when you are engaging with Challenges 5 and 6 in the next section of this chapter ("Ten Challenges to Implementation and Reporting"). Again, engaging with a client and building a relationship at the beginning of a process will often support a smoother implementation of the evaluation and fewer surprises at the end.

- *Challenge 6.* Not enough is known about contextual factors. To develop a feasible and credible evaluation design, an evaluator needs to be aware of how (and whose) values, power, politics, language, culture, and other contextual factors are likely to influence the evaluation. External evaluators often need time to engage with these tangible and intangible factors; even internal evaluators can need time to pause and reflect.

Depending on the time and budget, and also the location of the evaluator in relation to the intervention, there are various options. The most useful solution is to include at least one person on the evaluation team who is familiar with the general (and preferably specific) context of the intervention. If that is not possible (i.e., sometimes evaluators have no say about who is on the evaluation team, or perhaps an evaluator is working solo), consider these options.

If time is short, or the distance is great, conduct some internet research: Explore the organization's, the community's, or other relevant websites. These may provide some tiny clues. If there are adequate time and budget provisions for the design phase, conduct some exploratory interviews that aim to provide contextual insights that can be used to inform the design. If there is no budget provided for the design phase (i.e., time to develop the design), create a two-phase evaluation design that includes time to meet with key people and groups (phase 1), with the intent to gather these kinds of information to inform the final evaluation design (phase 2). Conceptually, these are the same processes. However, practically, in some cases the evaluation design is not a paid part of an evaluator's work, while the "actual" evaluation is (i.e., semantics). And what if an evaluator is just tossed into the thick of things, with no time to engage or prepare for how these factors may influence the evaluation? Just remember to (1) keep breathing, (2) be aware of the fabulous five, plus one (see Chapter 13), (3) seek to identify them as the process moves forward, and (4) be guided by the ethics to which you have committed (see Chapter 12). In sum, do your best.

- *Challenge 7.* The client tells the evaluator that information on the intervention exists. This understanding is then used to develop the evaluation design. However, when the evaluation begins, the evaluator finds out that the information does not exist, or it exists but it is not accessible, not credible, or for other reasons not usable. For example, having an articulated theory of change is core to the evaluation design; however, when the evaluation commences the evaluator finds out that it is of poor quality or is outdated. Or a database exists that has monitoring data, but extensive data cleaning is needed before the data are useable. These and other resulting challenges will negatively influence the evaluation process and have budget and other resource implications.

Whenever possible, build some time into the evaluation design phase to confirm what information exists, its quality, and its accessibility. If doing so is not feasible (e.g., the design phase is short), design the evaluation so that the first step in the evaluation is to explore and investigate anything (e.g., theory of change, database) that the design is dependent upon; then use those findings to inform or refine the design as needed. (Refer to the advice for Challenge 6 with regard to a two-phased approach.)

If neither of these options is feasible, take these steps. First, clarify what program information is understood to be accessible, accurate, and credible. Second, make a detailed list of these items. Third, have the client review, confirm (or make changes as needed), and sign the list. It is a funny thing, having someone sign a document. The formality of the process sends the message of how critical it is to have this information in place and allows for a conversation about the consequences of their not existing (e.g., budget, time). If the list is confirmed, and what was supposed to be there is not usable, you are in a much stronger position to clarify why extra time, funds, or other resources are needed.

- *Challenge 8.* The client requests a specific research design and does not understand how that is different from an evaluation approach. To see an explanation of the differences between the two, see the first question under "Nine Common Questions That Arise during an Evaluative Process," toward the end of this chapter (also see Chapter 2 for a more in-depth explanation).

There are three potential strategies. The first strategy includes taking the educator role and explaining the differences. The second strategy includes taking the facilitator role and encouraging a discussion through asking three questions: (1) How will the intervention be judged in terms of its merit, value, and/or worth, and who decides that? (2) What kind of actionable information is needed that can be used by what decision maker? (3) Who can benefit, and who can be hurt? These three questions will likely open the door to a broader discussion of an evaluation approach, as the answers (and lack thereof) will emphasize key differences between research and evaluation. A third strategy includes taking a negotiator role; select an evaluation approach that you are likely to use, and demonstrate how that approach will guide the evaluation and how it can incorporate the research design (and then negotiate, as needed).

These are some challenges that commonly arise during the design phase of an evaluation. I do not pretend that my advice on ways of responding to these challenges has been exhaustive (nor did I exhaust the list of challenges). But now that we have some strategies for how to mitigate the design phase challenges, let's look at the potential ones that arise in the course of implementing the evaluation and writing the final report. Note that I focus on the final report, as it is the most common product of an evaluation process. As acknowledged in earlier chapters, however, other types of final products exist, such as PowerPoint presentations (also called *decks*), or workshops that use the evaluation's data to create a dialogue and inform decisions.

TEN CHALLENGES TO IMPLEMENTATION AND REPORTING, AND HOW TO MITIGATE THEM

Many things can go wrong once an evaluation has started, no matter how well planned it is. When things go wrong during implementation, they can be detrimental to the evaluation, or they may only be a few blips that barely influence it. Challenges raised about the evaluation report require different kinds of strategies to those for implementation and are addressed separately in this section. I have selected these 10 challenges because they involve not only common problems, but ones that can spell disaster or cause immense frustration (i.e., they fall into the "detrimental to the evaluation" category). I do not always provide a nice textbook strategy for how to address a challenge, simply because I do not have one (despite 20-plus years of trying). However, there is something to be said for simply being aware, and not feeling isolated when (or perhaps I should say if) the challenge happens to you. Let's count down the 10 challenges in reverse order, and explore how to deal with them.

- *Challenge 10.* The evaluation purpose shifts. Sometimes, even after the evaluation purpose has been confirmed several times, that purpose changes during the evaluation's implementation. There could be many reasons for the shift, and many different points in the evaluation when that shift becomes apparent. The suggestions below address some of the different reasons for the shifts that occur at different points in the evaluation process, along with some helpful hints.

If the purpose shifts early in the evaluation process (say, from a focus on understanding how something was done to a focus on how effective the intervention was), explore to see whether and, if so, how that shift can be accommodated. Some considerations for shifting the evaluation approach to meet the new evaluation purpose would include time and budget, while other shifts may require a whole new evaluative skill set (e.g., advanced statistics, facilitation skills).

If findings are presented, and the key evaluation user says, "Oh, that is not what I expected. I thought the evaluation was going to . . ." at the end, there are very few possible strategies. Screaming is one strategy, but is not very professional, so let's dismiss that one. One viable strategy is to review the data and see if the key evaluation user's new needs can be addressed (within time and budget considerations). A second viable option is one to remember for the next evaluation: Provide a detailed evaluation report outline before the evaluation commences, and obtain physical sign-off on that outline. Sometimes, for the client or evaluation user, there is a disconnect between "This is the purpose for the evaluation" and "This is what I expect actually to read at the end." The process of providing a detailed report outline then allows for a discussion (this is what the client wants, and this is what you as the evaluator will aim to provide) and re-clarification of the evaluation's purpose, as needed.

- *Challenge 9.* Data collection goes haywire. Despite well-planned fieldwork, a multitude of unexpected things can happen during data collection that are out of the evaluator's control. Below I have outlined some strategies for dealing with the more common ways that data collection can go awry.

   a. Focus groups and individual interviews are scheduled, but people do not arrive at the designated place.

   Once you realize that people are not arriving for interviews, describe what happened, clearly identify potential solutions, and provide this documentation to the client immediately. The client may want to be involved in identifying or selecting solutions, or he may want the evaluator to "sort it out." One solution is rescheduling the in-person session for a different time. If it is not feasible (e.g., cost, time), consider online options, such as organizing Skype or phone interviews. Another option is to email the questionnaire to the respondents (realize that the data-gathering tool will likely need to be revised for that purpose). While these options may fit within the evaluation's time frame and budget, some options may also negatively influence the evaluation's actual or perceived credibility.

   b. The evaluation plan has budgeted for 35 interviews (1 hour each) with key informants to be recorded and transcribed. However, each key informant speaks for 3 hours and provides useful data. There is now insufficient budget to transcribe or analyze the mountains of data.

If, after several interviews, it becomes clear that there are likely to be more data than anticipated, the client should be notified immediately. Provide the client with three options: have fewer, more in-depth interviews; have a larger number of more superficial interviews; or a provide a budget increase to maintain the current number of planned interviews. These options then provide you (the evaluator) and the client with the opportunity to negotiate and make informed choices. If all the data are collected before the challenge becomes fully apparent (e.g., different team members collected data at the same time, and it is not until all data are submitted that the challenge becomes obvious), other strategies could be deliberated. The first option is to explain the situation to the client and request additional money as needed for the additional analysis time (and perhaps even to cover the lengthier interviews). If additional funding is not an option, consider these possibilities. One is to develop a thoughtful random sampling strategy to select x number of interviews for transcription and analysis, to minimize costs. A second option (unfortunately) is to work for no additional compensation and analyze all data. If selecting the second option (i.e., working for free), consider how much more time is likely needed to complete all the analyses and, once again, communicate that to your client.

c. Respondents provide answers; however, the answers do not adequately inform the evaluation questions.

This is one of the most frustrating challenges you may face when conducting an evaluation. In qualitative processes, perhaps those interviewed tended to focus on other kinds of stories, despite the interviewer's best efforts to redirect them. In a quantitative process, perhaps a majority of the respondents selected "don't know" or "not applicable" for a majority of the evaluation questions. When faced with this situation, you should review the budget and your calendar carefully, and consider whether it would be feasible to revise the interview questions or sampling strategy (as appropriate) and try again. If that is not feasible, consider reviewing secondary data sources to determine whether they can provide useful information. Finally, if all else fails, groan in frustration (this is considered professional when you are immersed in data challenges!). As above, make sure you document your challenges, solutions, and any resulting changes, and provide this documentation to the client as soon as possible.

d. The email list provided to the evaluation team to send surveys to 100 beneficiaries has resulted in 84 bounced-back messages.

First, try to retype the email addresses, which may result in a higher success rate (i.e., perhaps some emails addresses were mistyped). If there is still a high number of bounce-back messages, request another list. If another list is not provided, consider other ways to get the email addresses or to collect the needed data (e.g., obtain phone numbers for the respondents, phone them, and clarify their email, or perhaps conduct an interview by phone). As advised on the previous page, always inform the client as soon as a challenge arises, provide alternative solutions, and note any changes made to the design. For the next evaluation, however, consider these non–mutually exclusive strategies. During the design phase, confirm with the client that they have an updated email list that they use for regular communication. A second strategy is to request more email addresses than needed (if that is an option). In this case, though, having too many data (e.g., with regard to resources for analysis) can become a slight risk. Consider which problem is the lesser of two evils (i.e., the potential of too many data or not enough data) and allow this to influence your choice.

In reviewing Challenges 9 and 10 and the proposed solutions, you will notice five recurring themes. First, the sooner the issues are identified and the client is informed, the better. If problems are hidden, blissfully ignored, not identified in a timely manner, or not engaged with properly during the evaluation process, they will bubble to the surface, most likely when the client is reading the report. Trust me. Second, always provide a description of the problem *and* suggested solutions to the client. Third, clarify any changes to what was planned versus what was done. Fourth, where no obvious solutions exist, offer to meet with the client to discuss a way forward. Fifth? Document, document, document.

Part of implementing an evaluation often includes writing a final report. Let's assume that the report is good quality; if a report is of bad quality, that is a completely different story. Thus the following challenges focus on when a good-quality report (e.g., has met all the criteria set out by the client, empirically answers evaluation questions) is rejected.

• *Challenge 8.* The methodology is rejected. Even when the methodology had been approved at the beginning, evaluation users may question it or reject it at the end. The main challenge is that a methodology cannot be retrofitted; it has already been implemented. (Note, however, that I have had clients request, in a final report, that I change the methodology description to reflect what they want it to say, not what was actually done. To address that kind of issue, read the ethics section in Chapter 12.)

Engage in a discussion with the evaluation user to determine specifically what was not liked, for what reason, and by whom. Conceivably there has been a misunderstanding that can be readily addressed. For example, the way the methodology is described in the final report is unclear to the evaluation user, which has led to some confusion. This is easily fixed through revision (i.e., making it clearer). Or perhaps the rejection is rooted in not understanding the methodology, and the evaluator needs to fill the educator role. Sometimes the problem may not be the methodology at all: Perhaps the client does not like the findings, and attacking the methodology is an approach to discrediting them. People are complicated (as are the circumstance in which they work), and unfortunately this can happen. In situations like these, one option would be to suggest that the report be peer reviewed, with reviewers who are credible to both the evaluator and the client.

• *Challenge 7.* The client or other evaluation user does not like the report structure. For example, the report does not contain, or perhaps look like, what the client or evaluation user expected. Sometimes the client or other evaluation user expects a more focused report, multiple executive summaries, or perhaps a different presentation of the information.

Engage in a discussion with the client to determine exactly what was not liked, who did not like it, and exactly what is needed to change. It may be relatively simple, such as adding a few sentences for clarification, providing more data visualization, or presenting recommendations in a different manner. These are often quick, fixable changes. And then there are the more troublesome reasons, such as the client's expecting an entirely different report structure or product. One option is to rewrite the report in another structure or to provide the different product. The second option is one I am not allowed to print.

A related challenge may also arise when an evaluation question is not answered because there is not enough *credible* evidence to answer it. Although it is common to address data challenges in the methodology (i.e., limitations section) of the report (e.g., to explain the lack of data for a certain question as the reason why the question was not answered), most evaluation users do not automatically look there. They just read the report and do not see their question answered (and criticize the report structure). One strategy is to provide the evaluation question or theme in the body of the report, with a concise explanation of why the question cannot be answered with the existing data. Then direct the reader to the methodology section for further details. While I would like to rule this last one out, hard-earned experience has also shown me that when a client raises these and similar issues, it is sometimes meant to merely discredit the evaluator and/or her findings. Chin up. Tomorrow's another day.

• *Challenge 6.* No conclusive findings. Someone has just spent money on an evaluation, and now the finding is that there are no conclusive findings.

This is a tough one. Although "no conclusive findings" is often an acceptable response in research, it is not so well received in evaluation. No conclusive findings need to be framed as a finding in and of themselves, with suggestions for how to engage with them. See the Listen–Speak–Listen activity (Activity 2.1 in Chapter 2) as a way to engage with these kinds of findings. That suggested process will then hopefully provide insight to inform the evaluation report, or through participating, give clients or other evaluation users better insight as to why the finding is not conclusive.

• *Challenge 5.* "Can you just add a section on . . . ?" Sometimes, after an evaluation report is completed, the client will think of a new question—or remembers one he forgot to ask.

On the one hand, it is inspiring that the evaluation has been so useful that the client wants more answers. On the other hand, to complete an evaluation report that has followed the approved design and outline, answered the agreed-upon evaluation questions with empirical findings, and provided useful recommendations, and then to have the client say, "What about . . ." and add another question that must be answered before the report is approved can be wearying.

Try to understand from where these questions are arising. Has there been a misunderstanding? Then sit down with the client and go through the evaluation design to clarify (and, ideally, address) the misunderstanding. If there has not been a misunderstanding, consider some other options. One option is to "buck up," which is an expression used here to mean "Take a deep breath, and figure out how you can accommodate the client or other evaluation user." Never lose sight of the fact that the client's (or evaluation user's) request likely means that she finds your work useful. Proceed with caution, however, as budget and other resource constraints will influence how much can be accommodated. Another option is to refer to the scope of work (i.e., the contract) to determine whether the request can reasonably be construed as within the existing scope or is completely outside it. Any evaluator who is asked to undertake additional services outside the scope is entitled either to refuse or to ask for an amendment and more time/resources.

- *Challenge 4.* The data and/or data analysis are criticized by the client and/or the evaluation user.

Find out what exactly the client (or evaluation user) is not satisfied with and how they would like it changed or amended. Again, it may be a misunderstanding that only requires a bit of clarification. Or sometimes the client wants additional analysis, or more data presented in the report, and it is feasible to address. However, if the client simply does not find the data credible after the evaluation is completed, your hands are often tied. Here is an example. Several years ago, my evaluation team conducted over 100 qualitative interviews. There was very little diversity in the answers among diverse groups, which was an interesting finding. After reading the report, the client became angry and asked, "Where is all the information from the 100 interviews?" The team explained that even 100 interviews, analyzed and interpreted, do not always equal large quantities of findings. The client was still not happy, even though the data contributed substantially to answering the key evaluation question.

Understand that there are two potential challenges when data are critiqued. One is that the data are critiqued and technically found to be of poor quality. That is not good for you. An evaluator needs to have good data. The other is that the data are critiqued on the basis of someone's perception or misunderstanding of how to assess data. That is not good for you, either; however, there are two possible ways to address it: (a) Educate the client by taking them through some of the analysis, and/or (b) bring in an external peer reviewer whom the client (and you, the evaluator) deems credible to review the data. If neither one addresses the issue at hand, remember, I am with you in spirit. Finally, and as noted previously, sometimes when evaluation users or clients raise these and similar issues, it is meant to merely discredit the evaluator and/or her findings.

- *Challenge 3.* The findings are rejected. There may be various reasons for this. A client or evaluation user may not like a finding because it does not say what he expected or wanted it to say. It may be that something completely and unexpectedly catches the client or evaluation user off guard. Perhaps a finding challenges the current political thinking, or those in power. And so on.

As a first step, if the evaluation report had more than one finding, find out *which findings* are rejected; it might be just one or it could be all of them. Recognize that it is difficult to engage with generic statements such as "The finding is rejected" or "The finding is not liked." Consider requesting a formal statement that clearly identifies which findings are not liked, who did not like them, and the reasons why. As I have noted in other places in the chapter, having a written statement often brings useful formality (and clarity) to the process. Perhaps there was a misunderstanding. For example, the client misconstrued what the evaluator wrote, and the finding simply needs to be written more clearly. Or maybe only one out of 10 evaluation users did not like the finding, which is very different from having all the users reject it. Engage with that one person to identify how to move forward. When there is no discernible reason for the findings to be rejected, explore potential political reasons; doing this may not change the situation, but it may bring useful understanding. If you cannot identify why findings are rejected beyond "I [or other parties] just do not like them," and have tried to engage with the client to resolve the issue without being able to do so, document what you have done and move on to another client. If you are an internal evaluator, there are two unique options. First, explore the possibility of how internal politics (or other contextual issues) influenced the findings being rejected, and use that understanding to inform the next steps and the next evaluation. Second, consider hosting some internal evaluation events to educate the staff on evaluation, which may support having worthwhile evaluation processes in the future.

- *Challenge 2.* The recommendations are rejected.

As a first step, if the evaluation report had more than one recommendation, find out *which recommendations* are rejected; like my response to Challenge 3, it might be just one or it could be all of them. Find out *why* the recommendations are rejected and *who* is rejecting them (so you know with whom to engage). It may be that only slight modifications to the recommendation are needed (e.g., make it clearer). Perhaps it is feasible and ethical to remove the recommendation. Also, consider that the recommendation may be rejected because the finding it is linked to was rejected. In this case, the discussion should move to one that focuses on the finding and away from the one on the recommendation. For a fuller response, see Chapter 16, which is all about the recommendations. Also, since recommendations are often based on a mix of facts, assumptions, and opinions, revisit Chapter 4's discussion on this, which could inform a facilitated conversation with your client or evaluation user.

- *Challenge 1.* Clients or evaluation users want data or findings removed or altered; however, they provide no reason as to why those changes are needed (except "because I said so"). I have saved the dirtiest piece of laundry for last.

Discuss with the client why the data or findings should be removed or changed (e.g., ask them, "What makes you say that?"). Through a discussion you may identify that there is just a misunderstanding that is easily cleared up, or the discussion may unveil acceptable reasons to make the requested changes (e.g., that finding, if published, will do harm to a specific beneficiary group). If, after trying to identify reasons, no valid reasons are identified (as noted, it is just because they said so), your response to the client should be guided by your personal ethics and those professional ethics that you have committed to uphold. In most cases, a report belongs to the client, not to the evaluator; thus the client can make changes without the evaluator's approval (or sometimes, even their knowledge). When I am in this situation, and I do not want to change my data or findings, but the client changes or removes them, I ask that my name be taken off the report and, furthermore, that any changes made be clearly reflected in the report. Of course, I have very little power in these situations to enforce my requests. I still ask. Being told to remove or change data does not happen often; however, being asked to change or remove findings, without providing acceptable reasons for those requests, happens often enough.

Nine Common Questions That Arise during an Evaluative Process

Before we wrap up this chapter, nine additional questions that often arise during an evaluation process need to be addressed.

Chapter 2 was very clear on the differences between research and evaluation, and between researchers and evaluators. However, I am not so clear on the exact differences between a research design (what a researcher does) and an evaluation approach (what an evaluator does). Can you explain these?

There are some fundamental differences, a very nice summary of which has been developed by Wolfgang Meyer (2015). Meyer describes the evaluation process as consisting of 8 steps (recall that different evaluation approaches will actually consist of more or fewer steps, such as UFE's 21 and the CIPP model's 4), and then compares the evaluation process to a research process. I have modified Meyer's summary of differences in Table 17.1.

Note in the table that the key differences occur at the beginning and end of the two processes. The reason the designs are different is that applied research studies a real-world problem to understand it, whereas an evaluator studies an intervention for a problem and renders a judgment about the intervention's effectiveness (see Chapter 2).

Must an implementer plan for an evaluation, or can the implementer just have one when he decides he needs to have one?

This is a tricky question. Sometimes if evaluations are not planned, they are not budgeted for, and when an evaluation is needed, there are no evaluation resources. On the other hand,

TABLE 17.1. The Research and Evaluation Processes: Key Differences and Similarities

Evaluation	Research
Understand the evaluation task. This includes the purpose, key evaluation questions, users, and uses.	Formulate the research problem.
Determine how the intervention is to be valued (assessment criteria).	Clarify what theory is to be tested.
Identify key stakeholders and identify their level and kind of involvement in each part of the evaluative process.	—
Plan and prepare for data collection; this includes developing data collection tools, defining the population, and selecting a sampling approach.	Plan and prepare for data collection; this includes developing data collection tools, defining the population, and selecting a sampling approach.
Collect data.	Collect data.
Analyze data.	Analyze data.
Produce a report or another product (e.g., PowerPoint, poem), often with an executive summary, and share it with users.	Produce a report or publication.
Assist clients in using the evaluation to learn about, improve, change, judge, or otherwise influence a decision or situation. It is actionable.	Engage in scientific discussion.
Note. Shaded rows indicate similarities. Based on Meyer (2015).	

an evaluation can be planned that is not necessary; yet it is done because it *was* planned, not because it is useful. A rule of thumb is to set aside evaluation funding that can be used for an evaluation or other reflective process, as needed. Consider planning routine meetings with program staff and evaluators (if possible) to reflect on monitoring data and informal feedback that encourages evaluative thinking. Do the data indicate that something is going terribly wrong or remarkably right? Does the information cause you to ask, "Why is that happening?" Then plan and implement an evaluation, as needed. See Chapter 1 to read more about evaluative thinking, which plays an important part here.

Why should we do an evaluation? We have monitoring data.

There may be no need to have an evaluation if monitoring data are providing the information the client (or other user) needs to make informed management decisions, meet accountability needs, and there is no requirement to have one. However, consider that an evaluation can provide other types of benefits, such as answers to why something is or is not happening, and can bring the whole element of valuing into the equation. Or consider that having an external team or even an internal person interpreting data from different perspectives, or gathering different kinds of data (or even the same kind of data from different groups), could prove useful. Evaluations also have the potential to identify unintended consequences, both positive and negative. To read more about the differences between monitoring and evaluation, see Chapter 1.

I always work in teams when I conduct an evaluation. I find that sometimes our teams are just rushed out into the field to collect data, and we do not have time to talk about the evaluation approach. Any suggestions?

It is indeed a challenge when an evaluation team is rushed into the field to collect data with little or no preparation time. A multitude of difficulties often emerge when team members do not have a shared understanding of the evaluation's purpose, design, and methods. One potential danger is that the evaluation is implemented differently (or even incorrectly) at different sites. The evaluation Team Lead should be given time to write a descriptive, step-by-step field guide for the teams. She can then use that guide to train her team either in-person or, if there is no budget or time, through a phone or online discussion (e.g., via Zoom, Skype, or GoToMeeting). Worst-case scenario, she can email the guide to everyone. Or in the utmost worst-case scenario, when there is no evaluation guide, ensure that the team members have time to fully review the evaluation design and ask clarifying questions before the data gathering begins.

It seems that if I have a finding that the client is not expecting, it is less likely to be accepted, but if I have a finding the client expects, they question what added value I have brought to the process. How do I deal with this challenge?

It is a conundrum. Whereas some clients can be relieved to have their perceptions or understandings confirmed, evaluation users who have expected to learn something new may wonder about the evaluation's usefulness. While the beginning of an evaluation process may be rushed, it is critical to talk to evaluation users about their expectations. Here is one strategy. Review the evaluation's purpose and questions, and engage in a conversation that assesses the usefulness of their questions *to them*. Drawing from Patton's (2008) UFE process, provide *clearly* made-up data to answer the evaluation questions, and have an evaluation user reflect on how those findings would be used (this could be one-on-one, or done through a more formal workshop with various evaluation users). When the evaluation user says, "Yes, that would be useful to know," keep the question; if he responds, "No, we already know that; it is not helpful," then revise or drop the question. Before you begin the evaluation, remember to have the client sign off on the evaluation design, including its questions *and* a detailed report outline.

Useful evaluations are expensive, aren't they?

Evaluations can be expensive. They can also be inexpensive. A highly participatory evaluation that requires lots of site visits and extensive travel will likely be more expensive than one that requires no travel and gathers secondary data through a desk review. Sending an evaluation team to collect data in rural areas is often more expensive (due to travel costs) than collecting data in a city in which the evaluator resides. However, even on a limited budget, where there is a will, there is a way. I have implemented useful evaluations that have cost less than U.S. $5,000, and have been on evaluation teams where the evaluation cost millions of U.S. dollars and its usefulness is questionable at best. Thus the evaluation's usefulness does not necessarily relate to the cost.

I have a similar question: How much money should be spent on an evaluation?

It depends. There is no hard and fast rule for how much should be spent on an evaluation. Some organizations recommend using 3–5% of the overall intervention's budget for evaluation, while others recommend 7–10% of the overall budget for monitoring *and* evaluation. And some organizations do not provide any guidance. The amount of money spent on an evaluation will depend on the purpose, the evaluation design, the size of the intervention, and the donor, government, and/or implementing organization's appreciation of evaluation, among other factors.

I was just asked to pull together a report of a 3-year evaluation in the final year of the evaluation process, when all data collection was complete. Yet the data are bad: Some data are not credible, while other data are credible but do not answer the evaluation questions. What do I do?

That is a tough situation. Sort through all the data and see what data exist that are credible and do answer the evaluation questions; there may be some. Identify for which questions no corresponding data exist (i.e., the data provided to you do not answer the question). You now have several options, which are not mutually exclusive.

First, clearly describe the challenge in a formal report or in an email to your client. State that there are no data that support answering these (list them) evaluation questions. Then, provide clear, logical reasons why some data are not credible, while other data are credible but not useful. Second, request additional resources to gather primary data. Third, explore whether there are any secondary data (e.g., reports or databases) that can answer the questions. One of the most useful exercises, however, would be to sit down with the evaluation's commissioner and user (who may be the same person) and have a frank discussion on the data challenges. Then facilitate a discussion of what could be done differently in the next evaluation process. This is a form of process use. To read more on process use, go to page 231.

I have the imposter syndrome. I am hired as an evaluation "expert," but I do not feel like an expert. I do not have a degree in evaluation.

Imposter syndrome is the term for a very competent person's fear of being exposed as a fraud, or as someone who does not know as much as others think the person knows. Because there is no clear definition of who is and is not an evaluator, that syndrome seems to run rampant in the evaluation field. (For more on evaluator professionalization and competencies, see Chapter 11.) I have struggled with this syndrome myself, but it has kept me reading, writing, taking short courses, attending conferences, and always trying to learn from my peers. Be confident in what you do know, and aware of what you do not.

WRAPPING UP

The challenges described in this chapter do not even remotely exhaust what you will encounter when designing and implementing an evaluation (if you are keen to learn about some more real-life challenges, read *Evaluation Failures: 22 Tales of Mistakes Made and Lessons Learned* (2018), edited by Kylie Hutchinson). The challenges in designing an evaluation, and implementing one, are discussed for three reasons: first, to provide an inkling of the kinds of challenges that you may face as an evaluator; second, to note that sometimes challenges can be avoided, fully addressed, or mitigated, and sometimes—well, "it is what it is"; and third, to help you think like an evaluator.

The activities of reading the evaluation literature, attending evaluation conferences, taking courses on evaluation, posting on relevant blogs (and reading them), and using other forums where information can be read and exchanged is critical to continuing to grow as an evaluator. It is highly likely that if you have a challenge, someone else has also had the same challenge. Ideally, this person can offer insights, suggestions, and brainstorming; share a laugh; or, at the very least, commiserate with you.

This final chapter does not have a section to have a conversation with me. Rather, I invite you to join me in the Epilogue.

Epilogue

We have come to the end of our journey, and I am glad that you have joined me. Together, we have accomplished many things:

- We have demystified monitoring and evaluation (M&E)—clarifying terms and concepts while learning how to facilitate interactive approaches and activities.

- We have deconstructed the evaluative process while building a scaffold from which to explore and practice monitoring *and* evaluation, and guide others in their exploration.

- We have thought deeply about what it means to be an evaluator and what it means to evaluate, including how values are embedded in every aspect of the evaluative process, and how participants to that process may have different values.

- We have learned about different methods of inquiry, different evaluation approaches, and different evaluation designs.

- We have talked about the multitude of choices an evaluator must make to provide the most accurate, feasible, credible, and useful evaluation to specific evaluation users, at that time, for that intervention, in that context, and with those resources.

- We have learned about evaluation reports and other evaluation products, spent time learning how to provide specific and actionable recommendations, and recognized the importance of providing constructive feedback as critical friends.

- We have learned some evaluation trade secrets, and have even seen some dirty laundry.

In addition to these more technical issues, we have grappled with the very real challenges that stem from the fabulous five, plus one (values, power, politics, language, culture, and context)—factors that subtly guide and influence all decisions throughout the entire evaluative journey. We have recognized that evaluators are responsible for many decisions, processes, and products, and yet have faced the reality that at times, many of these decisions can also be outside an evaluator's control. We have acknowledged that being an evaluator involves more than knowing the evaluation methods, and yet that an evaluator is naught without them. But most of all, we have learned that our clients should expect nothing less than a clear, transparent, thoughtful, ethical, appropriate, and engaging evaluative process from an evaluator who is committed to continual learning, and that we should expect nothing less from ourselves.

While being an evaluator is not a bed of roses, I cannot imagine being anything else. You may not have chosen to be an evaluator; perhaps you are still considering becoming one; maybe you have been one for a long time; or perchance you work with evaluators. Wherever you find yourself in the evaluative journey, each chapter in this book has aimed to inspire you to believe that making a difference through evaluation is possible, practical, and within your grasp. I wish you, and others you bring along with you, an exciting and meaningful evaluative journey.

References

Abma, T. (2005). Responsive evaluation: Its meaning and special contribution to health promotion. *Evaluation and Program Planning, 28,* 279–289.

Alkin, M. C. (2011). *Evaluation essentials from A to Z.* New York: Guilford Press.

Alkin, M. C. (Ed.). (2013). *Evaluation roots: A wider perspective of theorists' views and influences.* Thousand Oaks, CA: SAGE.

Alkin, M. C., & King, J. A. (2017). Definitions of evaluation use and misuse, evaluation influence, and factors affecting use. *American Journal of Evaluation, 38*(3), 434–450.

American Evaluation Association (AEA). (2004). American Evaluation Association guiding principles for evaluators. Retrieved from *www.eval.org/p/cm/ld/fid=51.*

Amo, C., & Cousins, J. B. (2007). Going through the process: An examination of the operationalization of process use in empirical research on evaluation. *New Directions in Evaluation, 2007*(116), 5–26.

Australasian Evaluation Society (AES). (2013, July). *Guidelines for the ethical conduct of evaluations* (rev. ed.). Carlton, Victoria, Australia: Author. Retrieved from *www.aes.asn.au/images/stories/files/membership/AES_Guidelines_web_v2.pdf.*

Babbie, E. (2017). *The basics of social research* (7th ed.). Boston: Cengage Learning.

Babbie, E., & Mouton, J. (2001). *The practice of social research* (South African ed.). Cape Town: Oxford University Press Southern Africa.

Bamberger, M. (2010, November). Reconstructing baseline data for impact evaluation and results measurement (World Bank, PREM Notes, No. 4). Retrieved from *http://siteresources.worldbank.org/INTPOVERTY/Resources/335642-1276521901256/premnoteME4.pdf.*

Bamberger, M., Rugh, J., & Mabry, L. S. (2006). *Real-World evaluation: Working under budget, time, data, and political constraints.* Thousand Oaks, CA: SAGE.

Bateson, G. (1972). *Steps to an ecology of mind.* San Francisco: Chandler.

Bickman, L. (Ed.). (2000). *Validity and social experimentation.* Thousand Oaks, CA: SAGE.

Blaikie, N., & Priest, J. (2017). *Social research: Paradigms in action.* Cambridge, UK: Polity Press.

Bledsoe, K., & Donaldson, S. (2015). Culturally responsive theory driven evaluation. In S. Hood, R. Hopson, & H. Frierson (Eds.), *Continuing the journey to reposition culture and cultural context in evaluation theory and practice* (pp. 3–27). Charlotte, NC: Information Age.

Bowman, N., & Dodge-Francis, C. (2018). Culturally responsive indigenous evaluation and tribal governments: Understanding the relationship. *New Directions in Evaluation, 2018*(159), 17–31.

Brisolara, S., Seigart, D., & SenGupta, S. (Eds.). (2014). *Feminist evaluation and research: Theory and practice.* New York: Guilford Press.

Calhoun, E. A., & Risendal, B. C. (2018). Program evaluation. In E. A. Calhoun & A. Esparza (Eds.), *Patient navigation: Overcoming barriers to care* (pp. 81–98). New York: Springer.

Campbell, D. T. (1969). Reforms as experiments. *American Psychologist, 24*(4), 409–429.

Candel, J. J. (2018). Diagnosing integrated food security strategies. *NJAS—Wageningen Journal of Life Sciences, 104,* 103–113.

Carden, F., & Alkin, M. C. (2012). Evaluation roots: An international perspective. *Journal of Multi-Disciplinary Evaluation, 8*(17), 102–118. Retrieved from *http://journals.sfu.ca/jmde/index.php/jmde_1/article/view/348.*

Chelimsky, E. (1987). What have we learned about the politics of evaluation? *Education and Evaluation Policy Analysis, 9*(3), 199–213.

Chen, H.-T. (1990). *Theory-driven evaluations.* Newbury Park, CA: SAGE.

Chen, H.-T. (1994). Theory-driven evaluations: Need, difficulties and options. *Evaluation Practice, 15*(1), 79–82.

Chouinard, J., & Cousins, J. B. (2009). A review and synthesis of current research on cross-cultural evaluation. *American Journal of Evaluation, 30,* 457–494.

Conley-Tyler, M. (2005, March–April). A fundamental choice: Internal or external evaluation? *Evaluation Journal of Australasia, 4*(1–2), 3–11. Retrieved from *http://journals.sagepub.com/doi/abs/10.1177/1035719X05004001-202.*

Coryn, C. L., Noakes, L. A., Westine, C. D., & Schroter, D. C. (2011). A systematic review of theory-driven evaluation practice from 1990 to 2009. *American Journal of Evaluation, 32*(2), 199–226.

Cousins, J. B. (Ed.). (2007). Process use in theory, research, and practice [Special issue]. *New Directions in Evaluation, 2007*(116).

Cranston, P., Beynon, P., & Rowley, J. (2013). Two sides of the evaluation coin. Retrieved from *www.betterevaluation.org/en/resource/example/two-sides-coin.*

Creswell, J. W., & Creswell, J. D. (2018). *Research designs: Qualitative, quantitative, and mixed methods approaches* (5th ed.). Thousand Oaks, CA: SAGE.

Creswell, J. W., & Plano Clark, V. L. (2018). *Designing and conducting mixed methods research* (3rd ed.). Thousand Oaks, CA: SAGE.

Dahler-Larsen, P., Abma, T., Bustelo, M., Irimia, R., Kosunen, S., Kravchuk, I., et al. (2017). Evaluation, language, and untranslatables. *American Journal of Evaluation, 38*(1), 114–125.

Davidson, E. J. (2005). *Evaluation methodology basics: The nuts and bolts of sound evaluation.* Thousand Oaks, CA: SAGE.

Davidson, E. J. (2010). "Process values" and "deep values" in education. *Journal of MultiDisciplinary Evaluation, 6*(13), 206–208.

Davidson, E. J. (2012). *Actionable evaluation basics: Getting succinct answers to the most important questions.* Auckland, New Zealand: Real Evaluation.

Davidson, E. J. (2014). *Evaluative reasoning* (Methodological Briefs—Impact Evaluation No. 4). Florence, Italy: UNICEF Office of Research—Innocenti.

Davies, R., & Dart, J. (2005, April). The 'most significant change' (MSC) technique: A guide to its use (Version 1.00). Retrieved from *www.researchgate.net/publication/275409002_The_'Most_Significant_Change'_MSC_Technique_A_Guide_to_Its_Use.*

Denzin, N. K., & Lincoln, Y. S. (1998). *The landscape of qualitative research.* Thousand Oaks, CA: SAGE.

Donaldson, S. I. (2007). *Program theory-driven evaluation science: Strategies and applications.* New York: Psychology Press.

Donaldson, S. I. (2009). In search of the blueprint for an evidence-based global society. In S. I. Donaldson, C. A. Christie, & M. A. Mark (Eds.), *What counts as credible evidence in applied research and evaluation practice?* (pp. 2–18). Thousand Oaks, CA: SAGE.

Donaldson, S. I., & Lipsey, M. W. (2006). Roles for theory in contemporary evaluation practice: Developing practical knowledge. In I. F. Shaw, J. C. Greene, & M. M. Mark (Eds.), *The SAGE* handbook of evaluation (pp. 56–75). Thousand Oaks, CA: SAGE.

Drennan, J., & Hyde, A. (2008). Controlling response-shift bias: The use of the retrospective pre-test design in the evaluation of a master's programme. Assessment and Evaluation in Higher Education, 33, 699–709.

Drucker, P. F. (1995). People and performance: The best of Peter Drucker on management. London: Routledge.

Drucker, P. F. (2007). Management challenges for the 21st century. London: Routledge.

Earl, S., Carden, F., & Smutylo, T. (2001). Outcome mapping: Building learning and reflection into development programs. Ottawa, Ontario, Canada: International Development Research Centre.

Fetterman, D., Rodriguez-Campos, L., Zukoski, A. P., & Contributors. (2018). Collaborative, participatory, and empowerment evaluation: Stakeholder involvement approaches. New York: Guilford Press.

Funnell, S. C. (2000). Developing and using a program theory matrix for program evaluation and performance monitoring. New Directions in Evaluation, 2000(87), 91–101.

Funnell, S. C., & Rogers, P. J. (2011). Purposeful program theory: Effective use of theories of change and logic models. San Francisco: Jossey-Bass.

Galdas, P. (2017). Revisiting bias in qualitative research: Reflections on its relationship with funding and impact [Editorial]. International Journal of Qualitative Methods, 16(1), 1–2.

Greene, J. C. (2000). Understanding social programs through evaluation. In N. K. Denzin & Y. S. Lincoln (Eds.), Handbook of qualitative research (2nd ed., pp. 981–999). Thousand Oaks, CA: SAGE.

Greene, J. C. (2007). Mixed methods in social inquiry. San Francisco: Jossey-Bass.

Greene, J. C. (2008). Is mixed methods social inquiry a distinctive methodology? Journal of Mixed Methods Research, 2(1), 7–21.

Greene, J. C. (2009). Evidence as "proof" and evidence as "inkling." In S. I. Donaldson, C. A. Christie, & M. A. Mark (Eds.), What counts as credible evidence in applied research and evaluation practice? (pp. 153–167). Thousand Oaks, CA: SAGE.

Guba, E. G., & Lincoln, Y. S. (1989). Fourth generation evaluation. Newbury Park, CA: SAGE.

Guijt, I. (2014). Participatory approaches (Methodological Briefs—Impact Evaluation No. 5). Florence, Italy: UNICEF Office of Research—Innocenti. Retrieved from http://devinfolive.info/impact_evaluation/img/downloads/Participatory_Approaches_ENG.pdf.

Guin, L. (2002). Triangulation: Establishing the validity of qualitative studies. Gainesville: University of Florida, Extension Institute of Food and Agricultural Sciences.

Haynes, B. (1999). Can it work? Does it work? Is it worth it? British Medical Journal, 319(7211), 652–653.

Hedtke, L., & Winslade, J. (2017). The crafting of grief: Constructing aesthetic responses to loss. New York: Routledge.

Heshmat, S. (2015). What is confirmation bias?: Wishful thinking. Psychology Today. Retrieved from www.psychologytoday.com/blog/science-choice/201504/what-is-confirmation-bias

Hood, S., Hopson, R., & Frierson, H. (Eds.). (2015). Continuing the journey to reposition culture and cultural context in evaluation theory and practice. Charlotte, NC: Information Age.

House, E. R. (2007). Regression to the mean: A novel of evaluation politics. Charlotte, NC: Information Age.

House, E. R. (2015). Evaluating: Values, biases, and practical wisdom. Charlotte, NC: Information Age.

House, E. R., & Howe, K. R. (1999). Values in evaluation and social research. Thousand Oaks, CA: SAGE.

House, E. R., & Howe, K. R. (2000). Deliberative democratic evaluation. New Directions for Evaluation, 2000(85), 3–12.

Hudelson, P. M. (2004). Culture and quality: An anthropological perspective. International Journal for Quality in Health Care, 16(5), 345–346.

Huitt, W., Hummel, J., & Kaeck, D. (2001). Assessment, measurement, evaluation, and research. Educational Psychology Interactive. Valdosta, GA: Valdosta State University. Retrieved from www.edpsycinteractive.org/topics/intro/sciknow.html.

Human Subjects Office/Institutional Review Board, University of Iowa. (n.d.). A summary of the Belmont Report. Retrieved from https://hso.research.uiowa.edu/summary-belmont-report.

Hutchinson, K. (Ed.). (2018). *Evaluation failures: 22 tales of mistakes made and lessons learned.* Thousand Oaks, CA: SAGE.

Jacob, S., & Boisvert, Y. (2010). To be or not to be a profession: Pros, cons, and challenges for evaluation. *Evaluation, 16*(4), 349–369.

Johnson, R. B., & Christensen, L. (2012). *Educational research: Quantitative, qualitative and mixed methods* (4th ed.). Thousand Oaks, CA: SAGE.

Johnson, R. B., & Onwuegbuzie, A. J. (2004). Mixed methods research: A research paradigm whose time has come. *Educational Researcher, 33*(7), 14–26.

Kelly, M. J. (2004). Qualitative evaluation research. In C. Seale, G. Gobo, J. F. Gubrium, & D. Silverman (Eds.), *Qualitative research practice* (pp. 521–535). Thousand Oaks, CA: SAGE.

Kennedy, M. (1983). The role of the in-house evaluator. *Evaluation Review, 7*(4), 519–541.

Killam, L. (2013). *Research terminology simplified: Paradigms, axiology, ontology, epistemology and methodology.* Sudbury, Ontario, Canada: Author.

King, J., & Stevahn, L. (2015). Competencies for programme managers in light of adaptive action: What? So what? What now? *New Directions for Evaluation, 2015*(145), 21–37.

Kniker, T. (2011). Evaluation survivor: How to outwit, outplay, and outlast as an internal government evaluator. *New Directions in Evaluation, 2011*(132), 57–72.

Krueger, R. A., & Casey, M. A. (2009). *Focus groups: A practical guide for applied research* (4th ed.). Thousand Oaks, CA: SAGE.

Kurz, C. F., & Snowden, D. J. (2003). The new dynamics of strategy: Sense-making in a complex and complicated world. *IBM Systems Journal, 42*(3), 462–483.

Kushner, S. (2016). *Evaluative enquiry and democracy: Theory and method.* Charlotte, NC: Information Age.

Lahman, M. (2018). *Ethics in social science research: Becoming culturally responsive.* Thousand Oaks, CA: SAGE.

Levin-Rozalis, M. (2003). Evaluation and research: Differences and similarities. *Canadian Journal of Program Evaluation, 18*(2), 1–31. Retrieved from *https://evaluationcanada.ca/secure/18-2-001.pdf.*

MacDonald, B. (1987). Evaluation and the control of information. In R. Murphy & H. Torrance (Eds.), *Evaluating education: Issues and methods* (pp. 36–48). London: Joanna Cotler Books.

Mark, M. M. (2002). Toward better understanding of alternative evaluative roles. In K. E. Ryan & T. A. Schwandt (Eds.), *Exploring evaluator role and identity* (pp. 17–36). Greenwich, CT: Information Age Press.

Mark, M. M., Henry, G., & Julnes, G. (2000). *Evaluation: An integrated framework for understanding, guiding, and improving policies and programs.* San Francisco: Jossey-Bass.

Marshall, C., & Rossman, G. B. (2016). *Designing qualitative research* (6th ed.). Thousand Oaks, CA: SAGE.

Mathison, S. (Ed.). (2005). *Encyclopedia of evaluation.* Thousand Oaks, CA: SAGE.

Mathison, S. (2008). What is the difference between evaluation and research—and why do we care? In N. L. Smith & P. R. Brandon (Eds.), *Fundamental issues in evaluation* (pp. 183–196). New York: Guilford Press.

Maxwell, J. A. (2013). *Qualitative research design: An interactive approach* (3rd ed.). Thousand Oaks, CA: SAGE.

Mayne. J. (2012). Contribution analysis: Coming of age? *Evaluation, 18*(3), 270–280.

McBride, D. M. (2013). *The process of research in psychology* (2nd ed.). Thousand Oaks, CA: SAGE.

McKegg, K. (2017). *Professionalising evaluation: Propositions, tensions and opportunities.* Paper presented at the Australasian Evaluation Society Conference, Canberra, Australia.

McQuinn, A. (2010). *The sleep sheep.* Frome, UK: Chicken House.

Medical Advocates for Social Justice. (n.d.). The Belmont Report (Summary). Retrieved from *www.medadvocates.org/disciplines/ethics/belmont_report.html.*

Mertens, D. M., & Wilson, A. T. (2012). *Program evaluation theory and practice: A comprehensive guide.* New York: Guilford Press.

Meyer, W. (2015). Introduction to evaluation design: Evaluation design one day course—Part A [PowerPoint presentation]. Retrieved from *www.ceval.de/modx/uploads/pdf/Evaluation%20Design%20*

-%20Block%20%20A%20-%20Introduction%20 (10-07-15).pdf.

Miehls, D. (2011). Neurobiology and clinical social work. In J. Brandell (Ed.), *Theory and practice in clinical social work* (2nd ed., pp. 81–98). Thousand Oaks, CA: SAGE.

Miller, R. L. (2010). Developing standards for empirical examinations of evaluation theory. *American Journal of Evaluation, 31*(3), 390–399.

Miller, R. L., & Campbell, R. (2006). Taking stock of empowerment evaluation: An empirical review. *American Journal of Evaluation, 27*(3), 296–319.

Minnett, A. M. (1999). Internal evaluation in a self-reflective organization: One non-profit agency's model. *Evaluation and Program Planning, 22*(3), 353–362.

Minsky, M. (2006). *The emotion machine: Commonsense thinking, artificial intelligence, and the future of the human mind.* New York: Simon & Schuster.

Morabito, S. M. (2002). Evaluator roles and strategies for expanding evaluation process influence. *American Journal of Evaluation, 23*(3), 321–330.

Morris, M. (Ed.). (2008). *Evaluation ethics for best practice: Cases and commentaries.* New York: Guilford Press.

Newcomer, K. E., Hatry, H. P., & Wholey, J. S. (Eds.). (2015). *Handbook of practical program evaluation* (4th ed.). Hoboken, NJ: Wiley.

Nickerson, R. S. (1998). Confirmation bias: A ubiquitous phenomenon in many guises. *Review of General Psychology, 2*(2), 175–220.

Oxford Living Dictionaries: English. (2018). Retrieved from *https://en.oxforddictionaries.com.*

Palinkas, L. A., Horwitz, S. M., Green, C. A., Wisdom, J. P., Duan, N., & Hoagwood, K. (2015). Purposeful sampling for qualitative data collection and analysis in mixed method implementation research. *Administration and Policy in Mental Health and Mental Health Services Research, 42*(5), 533–544.

Patton, M. Q. (2002). *Qualitative research and evaluation methods* (3rd ed.). Thousand Oaks, CA: SAGE.

Patton, M. Q. (2008). *Utilization-focused evaluation* (4th ed.). Thousand Oaks, CA: SAGE.

Patton, M. Q. (2010). *Developmental evaluation.* New York: Guilford Press.

Patton, M. Q. (2012). *Essentials of utilization-focused evaluation.* Thousand Oaks, CA: SAGE.

Patton, M. Q. (2015). *Qualitative research and evaluation methods* (4th ed.). Thousand Oaks, CA: SAGE.

Patton, M. Q. (2018a). *Facilitating evaluation: Principles in practice.* Thousand Oaks, CA: SAGE.

Patton, M. Q. (2018b). *Principles-focused evaluation: The guide.* New York: Guilford Press.

Pawson, R. (2006). *Evidence-based policy: A realist perspective.* London: SAGE.

Pawson, R., & Tilley, N. (1997). *Realistic evaluation.* London: SAGE.

Picciotto, R. (2011). The logic of evaluation professionalism. *Evaluation, 17*(2), 165–180.

Podems, D. R. (2007). Process use: A case narrative from Southern Africa. *New Directions in Evaluation, 2007*(116), 87–97.

Podems, D. R. (2010). Feminist evaluation and gender approaches: There's a difference? *Journal of Multi-Disciplinary Evaluation, 6*(14), 1–17.

Podems, D. R. (2014a). Feminist evaluation for non-feminists. In S. Brisolara, D. Seigart, & S. Sen-Gupta (Eds.), *Feminist evaluation and research: Theory and practice* (pp. 113–142). New York: Guilford Press.

Podems, D. R. (2014b). [Book review: *Essentials of utilization-focused evaluation*]. *American Journal of Evaluation, 35*(1), 154–157.

Podems, D. R. (Ed.). (2017). *Democratic evaluation and democracy: Exploring the reality.* Charlotte, NC: Information Age.

Podems, D. R., & King, J. A. (Eds.). (2014). Professionalizing evaluation: A global perspective on evaluator competencies [Special issue]. *Canadian Journal of Program Evaluation, 28*(3).

Preskill, H., & Catsambas, T. T. (2006). *Reframing evaluation through appreciative inquiry.* Thousand Oaks, CA: SAGE.

Quesnel, J. S. (2010). The professionalization of evaluation. In *From policies to results: Developing capacities for country monitoring and evaluation systems* (pp. 164–170). New York: UNICEF.

Rogers, P. J. (2007). Theory-based evaluations: Reflections ten years on. *New Directions for Evaluation, 2007*(114), 63–67.

Rogers, P. J. (2016). Understanding and supporting

equaity: Implications of understanding methodological and procedural choices in equity-focused evaluations. In S. Donaldson & R. Picciotto (Eds.), *Evaluation for an equitable society* (pp. 199–213). Charlotte, NC: Information Age.

Rossi, P., Lipsey, M. W., & Freeman, H. E. (2004). *Evaluation: A systematic approach* (7th ed.). Thousand Oaks, CA: SAGE.

Rugh, J., & Segone, M. (Eds.). (2013). *Voluntary organizations for professional evaluation (VOPEs): Learning from Africa, Americas, Asia, Australasia, Europe and Middle East.* New York: UNICEF, IOCE, and EvalPartners. Retrieved from *www.mymande. org/sites/default/files/files/UNICEF%20NY_ECS_Book2_Web(3).pdf*

Ryan, K. (2005). Democratic evaluation approaches for equity and inclusion. *Evaluation Exchange, 11,* 2–3.

Salkind, N. J. (2000). *Statistics for people who (think they) hate statistics.* Thousand Oaks, CA: SAGE.

Schwandt, T. A. (1997). Evaluation as practical hermeneutics. *Evaluation, 3*(1), 69–83.

Schwandt, T. (2009) Toward a practical theory of evidence for evaluation. In Donaldson, S. I., Christie, C. A., & Mark, M. A. (Eds.). (2009). *What counts as credible evidence in applied research and evaluation practice?* (pp. 197–212). Thousand Oaks, CA: Sage.

Schwandt, T. A. (2015). *Evaluation foundations revisited: Cultivating a life of the mind for practice.* Stanford, CA: Stanford University Press.

Scriven, M. (1991). *Evaluation thesaurus* (4th ed.). Newbury Park, CA: Sage.

Scriven, M. (2008). Summative evaluation of RCT methodology: An alternative approach to causal research. *Journal of Multidisciplinary Evaluation, 5*(9), 11–24.

SenGupta, S., Hopson, R., & Thompson-Robinson, M. (2004). Cultural competence: An overview. *New Directions for Evaluation. 2004*(102), 5–19.

Shadish, W. R. (1998). Evaluation theory is who we are: Presidential address. *American Journal of Evaluation, 19*(1), 1–19.

Shadish, W. R., Cook, T. D., & Campbell, D. T. (2001). *Experimental and quasi-experimental designs for generalized causal inference.* Boston: Houghton Mifflin.

Shadish, W. R., Cook, T. D., & Leviton, L. C. (1991). *Foundations of program evaluation: Theories of practice.* Newbury Park, CA: SAGE.

Shaw, J., & Campbell, R. (2014). The "process" of process use: Methods for longitudinal assessment in a multisite evaluation. *American Journal of Evaluation, 35*(2), 250–260.

Sielbeck-Bowen, K., Brisolara, S., Seigart, D., Tischler, C., & Whitmore, E. (2002). Exploring feminist evaluation: The ground from which we rise. *New Directions for Evaluation, 2002*(96), 3–8.

Skolits, G. J., Morrow, J. A., & Burr, E. M. (2009). Reconceptualizing evaluator roles. *American Journal of Evaluation, 30*(3), 275–295.

Snowden, D. J., & Boone, M. E. (2007). A leader's framework for decision making. *Harvard Business Review, 85*(11), 68–76. Retrieved from *https://hbr.org/2007/11/a-leaders-framework-for-decision-making.*

Stake, R. E. (1995). *The art of case study research.* Thousand Oaks, CA: SAGE.

Stake, R. E. (2003). Responsive evaluation. In T. Kellaghan & D. L. Stufflebeam (Eds.), *Kluwer international handbooks of education: Vol. 9. International handbook of educational evaluation* (pp. 63–68). Dordrecht, the Netherlands: Kluwer.

Stake, R. E. (2004). *Standards-based and responsive evaluation.* Thousand Oaks, CA: SAGE.

Stake, R. E. (2010). *Qualitative research: Studying how things work.* New York: Guilford Press.

Stevahn, L., King, J. A., Ghere, G., & Minnema, J. (2005). Establishing essential competencies for program evaluators. *American Journal of Evaluation, 26*(1), 43–59.

Stufflebeam, D. L. (2007). CIPP model checklist. Retrieved from *www.wmich.edu/sites/default/files/attachments/u350/2014/cippchecklist_mar07.pdf.*

Stufflebeam, D. L., & Coryn, C. L. S. (2014). *Evaluation theory, models, and applications* (2nd ed.). San Francisco: Jossey-Bass.

Stufflebeam, D. L., & Zhang, G. (2017). *The CIPP evaluation model: How to evaluate for improvement and accountability.* New York: Guilford Press.

Symonette, H. (2004). Walking pathways to becoming a culturally competent evaluator: Boundaries, borderlands, and border crossings. *New Directions for Evaluation, 2004*(102), 95–109.

Trochim, W. M. (2006, October 20). *The Research Methods Knowledge Base*. Retrieved from *www.socialresearchmethods.net/kb*.

United States Agency for International Development (USAID). (1980). *Logical framework analysis model*. Washington, DC: Author.

United Way of America. (1996). *Focus on program outcomes: Summary guide*. Alexandria, VA: Author.

United Way Valley of the Sun. (2008, July). *Logic model handbook*. Phoenix, AZ: Author.

Vocabulary.com. (n.d.). [Definition of doppelganger]. Retrieved March 30, 2017, from *www.vocabulary.com/dictionary/doppelganger*.

Volkov, B. (2011). Beyond being an evaluator: The multiplicity of roles of the internal evaluator. *New Directions in Evaluation, 2011*(132), 25–42.

Watkins, R., Meiers, M. W., & Visser, Y. L. (2012). *A guide to assessing needs: Essential tools for collecting information, making decisions, and achieving development results*. Washington, DC: World Bank. Retrieved from *https://openknowledge.worldbank.org/handle/10986/2231*.

Weiss, C. H. (1972). *Evaluation research: Methods for assessing program effectiveness*. Englewood Cliffs, NJ: Prentice-Hall.

Weiss, C. H. (1987). Where politics and evaluation research meet. In D. J. Palumbo (Ed.), *The politics of program evaluation* (pp. 47–70). Newbury Park, CA: SAGE.

Weiss, C. H. (1995). Nothing as practical as good theory: Exploring theory-based evaluation for comprehensive community initiatives for children and families. In J. P. Connell (Ed.), *New approaches to evaluating community initiatives: Concepts, methods, and contexts* (pp. 65–92). Queenstown, MD: Aspen Institute.

Weiss, C. H. (1998). Have we learned anything new about the use of evaluation? *American Journal of Evaluation, 19*(1), 21–33.

Weiss, C. H. (2000). Which links in which theories shall we evaluate? *New Directions for Evaluation, 2000*(87), 35–45.

Weiss, C. H. (2003). On theory-based evaluation: Winning friends and influencing people. *The Evaluation Exchange, 9*(4), 1–5.

Weiss, C. H. (2006). The purposes of evaluation in a democratic society. In I. F. Shaw, J. C. Greene, & M. M. Mark (Eds.), *The SAGE handbook of evaluation* (pp. 33–55). Thousand Oaks, CA: SAGE.

Westhorp, G. (2014, September). Realist impact evaluation: An introduction. Retrieved from *www.odi.org/publications/8716-realist-impact-evaluation-introduction*.

White, H., & Raitzer, D. A. (2017). *Impact evaluation of development interventions: A practical guide*. Manila, the Philippines: Asian Development Bank.

White, H., Sabarwal, S., & de Hoop, T. (2014). *Randomized controlled trials (RCTs)* (Methodological Briefs—Impact Evaluation No. 7). Florence, Italy: UNICEF Office of Research—Innocenti.

Wilcox, E., & King, J. (2014). A professional grounding and history of the development and formal use of evaluator competencies. *Canadian Journal of Program Evaluation, 28*(3), 1–28.

Worthen, B. R. (1994). Is evaluation a mature profession that warrants the preparation of evaluation professionals? *New Directions for Program Evaluation, 1994*(62), 3–15.

Yarbrough, D. B., Shulha, L. M., Hopson, R. K., & Caruthers, F. A. (Eds.). (2011). *The program evaluation standards: A guide for evaluators and evaluation users* (3rd ed.). Thousand Oaks, CA: SAGE.

Zhang, G., Zeller, N., Griffith, R., Metcalf, D., Williams, J., Shea, C., et al. (2011). Using the context, input, process, and product evaluation model (CIPP) as a comprehensive framework to guide the planning, implementation, and assessment of service-learning programs. *Journal of Higher Education Outreach and Engagement, 15*(4), 57–83. Retrieved from *http://openjournals.libs.uga.edu/index.php/jheoe/article/view/628*.

Author Index

Subject Index

Note. *f* or *t* following a page number indicates a figure or a table.

About the Author

Donna R. Podems, PhD, is Founder and Director of OtherWISE: Research and Evaluation, an evaluation consultancy in Cape Town, South Africa. She was a Research Fellow at Stellenbosch University for 10 years and is currently a Research Associate at the University of Johannesburg and Assistant Professor at Michigan State University. Dr. Podems has served on the national boards of the South African Monitoring and Evaluation Association and the American Evaluation Association (AEA), and is Chair of the AEA's International Working Group. She edited the book *Democratic Evaluation and Democracy: Exploring the Reality* and has written numerous articles and book chapters on feminist evaluation, process evaluation, principles-focused evaluation, systems evaluation, utilization-focused evaluation, democratic evaluation, and professionalizing of evaluation.